T5-CQD-756

THE GENDER FACTOR: MANAGING PAIN FOR MEN AND WOMEN

William Ackerman, M.D.,
and Hollye Acker

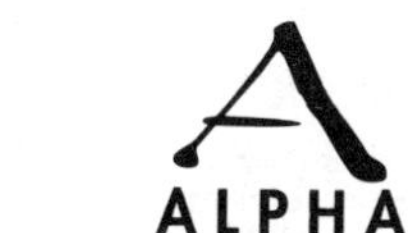

ALPHA
A Member of Penguin Group Inc.

Dr. William Ackerman: This book is dedicated to my wife, Carrie, and to all my patients whose inquisitive questions prompted the need for this book.

Hollye Acker: To my mom and dad—your constant love, guidance, and support have enabled me to achieve my dreams. I love you!

ALPHA BOOKS

Published by the Penguin Group

Penguin Group (USA) Inc., 375 Hudson Street, New York, New York 10014, U.S.A.

Penguin Group (Canada), 10 Alcorn Avenue, Toronto, Ontario, Canada M4V 3B2 (a division of Pearson Penguin Canada Inc.)

Penguin Books Ltd, 80 Strand, London WC2R 0RL, England

Penguin Ireland, 25 St Stephen's Green, Dublin 2, Ireland (a division of Penguin Books Ltd)

Penguin Group (Australia), 250 Camberwell Road, Camberwell, Victoria 3124, Australia (a division of Pearson Australia Group Pty Ltd)

Penguin Books India Pvt Ltd, 11 Community Centre, Panchsheel Park, New Delhi—110 017, India

Penguin Group (NZ), cnr Airborne and Rosedale Roads, Albany, Auckland 1310, New Zealand (a division of Pearson New Zealand Ltd)

Penguin Books (South Africa) (Pty) Ltd, 24 Sturdee Avenue, Rosebank, Johannesburg 2196, South Africa

Penguin Books Ltd, Registered Offices: 80 Strand, London WC2R 0RL, England

International Standard Book Number: 1-59257-360-6

Library of Congress Catalog Card Number: 2004113224

06 05 04 8 7 6 5 4 3 2 1

Interpretation of the printing code: The rightmost number of the first series of numbers is the year of the book's printing; the rightmost number of the second series of numbers is the number of the book's printing. For example, a printing code of 04-1 shows that the first printing occurred in 2004.

Printed in the United States of America

Contents

1. Why You Need to Understand Gender-Specific Medicine ..1
2. Why Genders Respond Differently to Pain 11
3. Understanding the Psychological Aspects of Pain 19
4. Understanding Adjuvant Medicines and Pain 33
5. Assessing Pain with Your Doctor 43
6. Learning About Opioid Drugs and Pain Management ..53
7. Reducing Pain with Nonsteroidal Anti-Inflammatory Drugs 67
8. Learning About Alternative Medicine Practices and Herbs..79
9. Using Topical Analgesics 89
10. Realizing the Effects of Physical Therapy 101
11. Trying Alternative Therapy 115
12. Understanding Neck Pain 129
13. Understanding Back Pain 145
14. Understanding Whiplash 163
15. Understanding Headaches 179
16. Understanding Arthritis..195
17. Understanding Peripheral Neuropathies: Pain in Your Arms, Legs, Hands, and Feet 209
18. Understanding Osteoporosis 225
19. Understanding Irritable Bowel Syndrome and Other Stomach-Related Pains 241
20. Understanding Fibromyalgia 257

21. Understanding Myofascial Pain 273
22. Understanding Facial Pain 289
23. Understanding Angina 305
24. Understanding Complex Regional Pain Syndrome 321
25. Understanding HIV Infections and Pain 337
26. Understanding Raynaud's Disease and Phenomena 353
27. Understanding Shingles 373
28. Understanding Sports-Related Pain 393
29. Understanding Reproductive System Cancer-Related Pain 409
30. New Pain-Management Research and Therapies........429
31. Changing the Perception of Pain Medicine 441

Appendix

Glossary 457

Index 463

Introduction

Everyone has experienced some form of pain in his or her life, whether it be pain from a minor injury or a serious disease or condition. Feelings of pain can be simple or complex and everyone can experience pain differently. It is especially different between men and women.

Our physical and psychological makeup affects how each of us feels and responds to pain. Current research in the field of pain management is uncovering new methods of therapy and medications to relieve our pain. Pain is no longer an entity that is to be feared. With proper self-education and the help of a pain-management doctor, your pain can be controlled effectively. Reading this book is your first step in self-education about your pain.

As you read through this book, you will notice *italicized* words. These words are defined in the glossary at the back of the book.

In Chapters 1 through 5 you will learn why men and women respond differently to pain, why drugs have different effects in men and women, and how to assess pain with your doctor.

Chapters 6 through 11 describe the various treatments that are associated with managing pain. Prescription medications, herbs, acupuncture, reflexology, chiropractic therapy, massage therapy, aromatherapy, and physical therapy are all detailed in terms of the relief they can provide for your pain.

Chapters 12 through 29 are where you will find information about specific types of pain such as back pain, headaches, arthritis, fibromyalgia, angina, shingles, sports-related pain, and cancer-related pain, among many others. These chapters describe the causes and treatment for each type of pain. After carefully reading the chapter that best describes your specific type of pain, you will be better prepared to approach your doctor and explain your pain symptoms. It also will give you some idea of what type of treatment to expect.

Chapters 30 and 31 describe the new pain medications and therapies that are constantly being researched and tested. It is important that you not be afraid of the practice of pain management. Treatment by a properly trained pain-management doctor can help alleviate your symptoms and help you live a healthier, happier life.

After reading this book, you will be more educated about your specific type of pain and how you can control it. Stay optimistic about controlling your pain, whatever it may be. You are on your way to a better feeling of being pain free.

Acknowledgments

Thanks to Ms. Amita Castelberry for her assistance in typing parts of this book when necessary.

Chapter 1

Why You Need to Understand Gender-Specific Medicine

The causes and treatment of pain are different for men and women. The study of the differences between how men and women feel pain and are treated for it is a relatively new branch of medicine. Your age, physical design, hormones, psychological issues, and social issues all play a part in why you feel pain. These things also determine how your doctor will treat your pain. In the future, doctors will be able to design treatments that are specific to men and women. After reading this book, you will know how men and women feel pain, why they feel it differently, and how it can be successfully treated for both men and women.

Sex and Gender: What's the Difference?

Simply stated, your sex (male or female) is determined by your chromosomes (XX for women, XY for men) and your body's particular anatomy. Your gender (man or woman) is determined by your body's anatomical features and social issues.

Concerning social issues, in most cases men have been programmed since they were children to be macho when dealing with pain. When playing in athletic events, boys are often told to "tough it out" when they are hurt. On the other hand, women since childhood have been allowed to express their pain freely. It is socially acceptable for a girl to cry, but it is not so for a boy. These distinct differences are important when your doctor tries to figure out how to treat your pain and other medical problems.

Pain is a very individual and personal experience. Things that cause pain in you may not cause pain in someone else. Without a psychological component to your type of pain, the repeated experience of the same type of pain would not be considered to be as painful as the first episode. This is the reason why a professional football player continues to play in a big game in spite of a broken bone. The psychology of the game distracts the broken-bone pain. Pain perception varies between person to person based on gender and age. When you feel pain, your response is to stay away from everything that would cause you to feel more pain. This is the response that aids your body in tissue healing.

Hormone Differences

Differences between men and women exist with physical characteristics, hormones, and social expectations, just to name a few. One of the reasons men and women feel pain differently has to do with hormones.

Sex differences affect the absorption, metabolism (breakdown of drugs), and excretion (elimination of drugs) of many medications. Women respond more favorably to a class of antidepressant medications called *serotonin-specific reuptake inhibitors,* or SSRIs (for instance, Prozac), than to other antidepressants known as *tricyclics* (for instance, Elavil). Sexual differences between men and women are important with respect to drug action, especially because the menstrual cycle can affect the amount of medication in the blood (blood levels). If a female retains fluid, the excess fluid will dilute the action of the drug. Oral contraceptives (for instance, "the pill") can decrease the blood levels of some anticonvulsant medications such as Dilantin. On the other hand, oral contraceptives can increase the blood level of some medications such as Valium. Hormone replacement in women does enhance the effects of antidepressant medications. Approximately two thirds of antidepressant medications in the United States are used by women.

Women have more side effects with antidepressant-type medications than men. They suffer more fatigue, gastrointestinal affects, and other adverse affects than men. Gonadal hormonal changes in women that occur monthly (before, during, and after the menstrual cycle) alter the metabolism (breakdown of drugs in the liver) of certain drugs and can affect their removal from the body. (C.H. Gleiter and U. Gundert-Remy. "Gender Differences in Pharmacokinetics," *European Journal of Drug Metabol Pharmacokinet* 21 [1996]: 123-8) (M.F. Jensvold, et al. *Psychopharmacology and Women: Sex, Gender, and Hormones.* Washington, D.C.: American Psychiatric Press, 1996)

One of the reasons why men and women differ in the perception of pain results from the effects of the female hormones estrogen and progesterone on the brain and spinal cord (the nervous system). The effects of the menstrual cycle on the nervous system vary before, during, and after menses. In the future, sexual and/or gender differences may allow a doctor to individualize treatments that are specific for each sex. It has also been found that low testosterone in males can also lower the pain threshold.

Central Nervous System Differences

The wiring of the central nervous system is influenced by differences in sex. Male and female brains have approximately the same number of receptors for estrogen and androgen. Estrogen is primarily a female hormone, whereas androgen is primarily a male hormone. A receptor is an area on the outer covering, or membrane, of a cell where hormones or drugs attach and start to take action.

The way receptors respond to drugs and hormones effects the body's response to both drugs and hormones. For example, giving estrogen to a man does not affect his brain like it does a woman. In the same way, giving androgens (male hormones) to a female brain does not cause the same response as in a male. Researchers have therefore concluded that hormone and hormonal receptor differences between men and women also influence the regulation and transmission of the nervous impulses that transmit pain.

Estrogen (the female hormone) affects the central nervous system levels of dopamine and serotonin, which are involved with mood disorders. Women experience more depression than males. Men may have more serotonin receptors, which may be a reason why they suffer from a lower incidence of depression. As a result, a woman's greater sensitivity to pain may be dependent on the fact that she has less serotonin in the brain and spinal cord. Studies show that sex hormones modulate neural function and affect the central nervous system with respect to the perception of pain. Recent studies in rats have shown that hormone receptors for male and female hormones are also present and modulate the function of the peripheral nerves (nerves outside the brain and spinal cord). (C.H. Gleiter and U. Gundert-Remy. "Gender Differences in Pharmacokinetics," *European Journal of Drug Metabol Pharmacokinet* 21 [1996]: 123-8) (M.F. Jensvold, et al. *Psychopharmacology and Women: Sex, Gender, and Hormones*. Washington, D.C.: American Psychiatric Press, 1996)

Why Understanding Pain Is Important

After reading this book, hopefully you will be able to take control of your acute and chronic pain and work with your doctor as a partner in the management of your pain. You are encouraged to stay informed of the new developments in gender-specific pain medicine. This will require some effort on your part. You must keep a pain diary that you can bring with you when you visit your doctor. You will learn how your doctor evaluates your pain and find examples of pain questionnaires in Chapter 5. Find the one that suits you and your doctor the best and be attentive in completing this diary. If you have any concerns or questions about your pain management, discuss it with your doctor. Take control of your pain by becoming better informed as to why you are suffering from pain and the methods available for the treatment of your pain. This can include not only conventional medicine, but also methods that could be offered by complementary and alternative medicine health-care providers.

When you are reading this book, you may be struck by the diversity of factors that affect your pain diagnosis and pain management—whether these factors are hormonal, psychological, physiological, or pharmacological. All these different factors and their various influences on pain may seem overwhelming. Gender is only one of the many factors that affect the extent of different pain syndromes. Pain is a complex and personal experience that is affected by a multitude of factors both inside and outside your body; however, you can control many of the situations outside your body.

Social Issues Affect Pain Perception

Social issues also play a part in how pain will affect you. Pain may begin as damage to your body, but your final experience of pain will be at the brain level with your emotional feelings. Your social and cultural surroundings also can affect the emotions you have about your level of pain.

Studies Show Men and Women Feel Pain Differently

Studies into how and why men and women feel pain differently have begun in the past few years. These studies are important and must cross the life cycle of men and women, because age can also affect hormones and physical characteristics. In the future, your doctor will be able to use such research to design treatments that will work just for you.

Researchers at the University of California at San Francisco have found that men and women respond differently to different kinds of pain-relieving medicines. Depending on the kind of medicine given, both the duration of effect and the degree to which pain was relieved differed in men and women.

Pain perception will vary from person to person. While, men and women report the same number of negative (or adverse) reactions during and following treatment with therapeutic medications, negative effects of medicines are higher and more serious in women than in men. This disparity may be influenced by the fact that women use medications more often than men and in different doses, and also because the different ways the drugs are absorbed, metabolized (broken down), and removed from the body by men and women.

Women often report more migraine headaches and arthritic pain than men. Women also have a greater discomfort for the same type of pain than men and are more likely to develop long-term pain after an injury. Women also use more over-the-counter pain medications and have more doctor visits than men. (Weyland C.M. et al. "The Influence of Sex on the Phenotype of Rheumatoid Arthritis," *Arthritis & Rheumatism* 41 [1998]: 817-822) (Waters and O'Connor. "Epidemology of Headaches and Migraines in Women," *Journal of Neurology, Neurosurgery and Psychiatry* 34 [1071]: 140-153) ("Pain Coping Strategies in Osteoarthritis Patients," *Journal of Consulting and Clinical Psychology* 55 [1987]: 208-212)

Because of these differences, research (called "clinical trials" or "clinical drug research") is being done on why women are more likely to suffer from painful conditions than men and which medications work better for men and women. Media advertising often recommends a certain medication for a specific condition, but none of the advertisements discuss doses with respect to the body size of a man or woman. Body size determines the amount of a medicine needed to treat a painful condition. Take a look at an aspirin bottle label. Does it tell you the dosage for a man or woman? The answer is no.

Reviews of major medical journals show clinical drug studies rarely test to determine how medication will affect men and women differently. Women are excluded from many clinical drug study trials. Because of the potential for pregnancy and the potential harmful effects of a new drug on a developing baby, most researchers have been hesitant to include women in their studies. Early studies mainly consisted of male prisoners.

In 1977 the U.S. Food and Drug Administration (FDA) prohibited women of child-bearing age from being involved in clinical trials. As a result, many drug studies were done only on men until recently. In 1985, a U.S. public health service task force addressed the Department of Health and Human Services and expressed the need to establish a policy that included women in clinical drug studies. In 1990, the Government Accounting Office issued a report and concluded that there was a lack of compliance in including women in clinical drug trials. So in 1993, Congress made it mandatory that women, as well as minorities, be included in clinical drug trials. Also in 1993, the FDA began allowing women of child-bearing age to take part in clinical drug trials. In 1994, the National Institutes of Health issued guidelines to grant applications to confirm that researchers complied with the inclusion of women of child-bearing age in their studies. According to the U.S. Food and Drug Administration's website, www.fda.gov, recent studies in 1997 showed that women exceeded 50 percent of the study participants.

Published clinical trial results today often include data analyzing how the studied drug affected men and women. Data submitted to the FDA for drug approval must include the gender, age, height, and weight of each participant. It also has been recommended that the data include whether any participating women are pre- or postmenopausal, because levels of hormones can affect how much pain is felt.

Anatomic Differences Affect Drug Absorption

The anatomic differences between men and women also influence their reactions to medications. In general, women have lower body weights and organ sizes and a higher percentage of body fat, factors that need to be taken into account when discussing the way the body handles drugs and their use in men and women. For example, the muscle relaxant Valium (diazepam) causes more impairment of voluntary muscle control in women than in men, probably because of lower body weight of women as compared to men.

Differences in drug reactions are caused by differences in the way men and women process drugs. The transport of drugs within the bloodstream and the chemicals that break down drugs differ in men and women. Enzymes in the liver help break down drugs. One of these enzymes is the CYP 3A4 liver enzyme. This enzyme breaks down more than 50 percent of all therapeutic drugs. In women, drugs that have been metabolized in the liver are delivered more slowly to the bloodstream, where they are then sent to the kidneys for excretion from the body. Because more of the pain medications are not taken out of the liver, a higher concentration of these drugs in the liver requires processing. The liver enzymes in women have to process higher concentrations of the drugs than males. Liver enzymes in women may also not metabolize the antidepressants of the selective serotonin-specific reuptake inhibitor class.

Women have a lower stomach acid secretion than men. This can increase the absorption of drugs such as Elavil or Valium, and decrease the absorption of acidic drugs such as Dilantin and barbiturates. Women weigh less than men and have a lower total blood value than men. Body fat is 11 percent higher in women between the ages of 25 and 35. After a drug is absorbed from either the stomach or the small intestine, the drug is distributed throughout the tissues in the body. Drugs that have a high affinity for fat are called fat-soluble drugs. If an individual has a high body fat content, some drugs may rapidly enter the fatty tissue. This action will decrease the level of medication in the blood and make it less effective. However, if repetitive administration of a drug causes a high concentration of that drug in body fat, it will eventually be released back into the bloodstream, which can cause a significantly higher blood level of the drug at that time.

The liver breaks down and eliminates most drugs. Biologic systems, including the liver, may be more efficient in men than in women. Drugs may be eliminated from the body more effectively by the kidneys in men when compared to women. As a result, equal doses of medication could result in a higher blood level of that particular drug in a woman than in a man. This in turn could cause serious side effects in the woman but not in the man.

Sex Hormones Affect Drug Absorption

Men and women differ with respect to their response to medications. Note, therefore, that the dosage for men and women must differ. However, many doctors are unaware of the gender-specific differences between men and women with respect to their responses to medications, as well as the differences between men and women with respect to body weight. An obese woman may require more medication to achieve the same pain relief than a thin woman. Before men and women with painful conditions can be treated properly, many research questions need to be answered with respect to the different effects of drugs on men and women.

As you can see, attention to gender is important not only in the specialty of pain management but also in other medical specialties. Sex hormones influence the effects of analgesics and many other drugs. The menstrual cycle, pregnancy, and menopause affect how drugs react in women's bodies, such that the same drug will have a different effect depending on the stage of the menstrual cycle and whether the woman is pre- or postmenopausal.

When you take a pill, the amount of medication that you are taking may not be appropriate for you depending on the previously mentioned factors. This may be the reason why a drug "just stops working." In some instances, if you mention this to your doctor, the doctor may think you are just seeking more drugs. Many doctors are not aware of the effects of gender on drug activity. As a result, you may be responsible for enlightening and informing your doctor as to the effects of the various drugs with respect to gender specificity. Also remember that gender-specific medicine is a new branch of medicine and that many of the older doctors who practice medicine are not aware of these new developments. The purpose of this book is to make you a better-informed health-care consumer.

The way in which antidepressant medications are absorbed, distributed in the bloodstream, and eliminated by the kidneys differs in men and women. Monthly hormone cycles in women can influence the effects of some antidepressants. Further, oral contraceptives and hormones can alter drug interactions in women. For example, acetaminophen (Tylenol) is made inactive in women taking oral contraceptives when compared to women who are not taking oral contraceptives. High blood levels of estradiol (a female hormone) sensitize a female to thermal (heat) pain. (C.H. Gleiter and U. Gundert-Remy. "Gender Differences in Pharmacokinetics," *European Journal of Drug Metabol Pharmacokinet* 21 [1996]: 123-8) (M.F. Jensvold, et al. *Psychopharmacology and Women: Sex, Gender, and Hormones*. Washington, D.C.: American Psychiatric Press, 1996)

Premenopausal women take longer to empty stomach content such as food and medication. In essence, this means that medications in the stomach are slower to leave the stomach to go into the small intestine. The small intestine has a greater absorptive capacity than the stomach. If a medication is delayed in passage from the stomach to the small intestine, medicine will be absorbed more slowly into the blood. Consequently, the blood level of the drug may be decreased.

The effects of hormones on neurotransmitters in the brain during the premenstrual cycle can affect the sensitivity of neurotransmitters or nervous system receptors. A doctor may have to increase the total dosage of a specific medication throughout the entire menstrual cycle and may have to decrease the medication two to three days after the cycle has been completed.

Oral contraceptives used by some women can decrease the effect of anti-anxiety drugs such as the Valium. Studies are currently investigating whether estrogen can be effective in treating depression in women. The effects of estrogen on certain drugs in postmenopausal women is also currently under study. Men and women respond differently to antidepressant medications. In women, pre- and postmenopausal effects must be taken into account when prescribing an antidepressant medication.

Age Affects Drug Dosing

Age also influences the effects of drugs. Because older people break down drugs more slowly, older individuals typically need a smaller dose of a drug. However, age effects are less prevalent in women than in men. Older men have a decreased ability to excrete drugs than women.

Age can also influence how sensitive you may be to pain. The intensity of pain felt by children lessens as they grow older. As puberty approaches, girls will notice and report more pain than boys do.

Osteoarthritis, which affects 40 percent of middle-age patients and approximately 70 percent of geriatric patients, essentially will have the same degree of input into the central nervous system of men and women. However, patient responses to the degree of pain differs. Women appear to cope better with pain related to osteoarthritis than men. (R.B. Fillingham. *Sex, Gender, and Pain*. n.p.: IASP Press, 2000)

Approaching Your Doctor About Specific Pain

Because men and women respond differently to pain medications, it is important that you develop a "partnership" with your doctor. You should always have input into the treatment methods that your doctor recommends. Your doctor should not be the "boss," and you should not be your doctor's "employee." You and your doctor should establish a partnership when you are first accepted as a patient. Treating and managing painful conditions can be complex. It is important that you feel comfortable with your doctor and be able to tell the doctor anything that will have an effect on your treatment. This will help your doctor determine what kinds of treatment are working for you and which ones should be discontinued or changed.

You should write down the type and intensity of your pain at least twice a day. When you feel pain, write down what type of activity you were doing. This type of daily pain diary will help your doctor chart your treatment progress and possibly determine which things trigger your pain. This may help your doctor determine which types of activities will make your pain better or worse. Write down whether the pain is sharp, dull, burning, or throbbing. Also write down a pain score. Use a range from 0 to 10, with 0 being no pain and 10 being the worst pain ever imaginable. Record all medicines that you are taking, including alternative medications, and discuss these with your doctor. Take your daily pain diary with you each time you visit your doctor so that you can go over it together.

Your doctor also should talk to you about pain relief alternatives that do not include using medications. Yoga, meditation, biofeedback, and hypnosis have all been shown to be effective for pain treatment. Walking, stretching, and simple activities such as chores around the house can result in mental as well as physical improvement.

You also should consider joining a support group. Discussing problems with other people who have similar types of pain problems may help you learn to manage your pain. The Internet is an excellent source through which to find support groups.

The sooner you begin learning about your specific pain condition and what you can do to treat it, the more effective your relationship will be with your doctor. Pain medicine is in its infancy, as is gender-specific medicine. Treatment methods are constantly changing. Do as much research as you can to learn about the different methods available for you to treat your pain. Feel free to discuss them with your doctor and ask any questions that you may have. Understanding your condition will help you to take charge of your own treatment and help make that treatment as successful as possible.

Chapter 2

Why Genders Respond Differently to Pain

Pain costs almost $100 billion a year in the United States. Each year, more than 500 million work days are lost, and 40 million doctor visits are made for the treatment of painful conditions. According to *The Wall Street Journal* in 2001, until the past decade, no new pain treatments had been developed for more than 30 years.

With the beginning of the pain medicine specialty, new methods for the treatment of pain are becoming more available. And as research is developed, new methods that have fewer side effects and are more effective are being developed. You do not need to fear a lifetime of agony as a result of your pain. Research into the processes that cause pain has resulted in the development of more drugs to block nervous system pathways that transmit pain in your body.

Some researchers have implied that gender differences with respect to the treatment and management of your pain are relatively minor. However, other researchers have reported that gender differences significantly influence responses to pain. Which of these opinions is correct? Both may be correct. Be aware that pain research can be influenced by whether the study is in an experimental situation or an acute or chronic pain situation.

During laboratory experiments and clinical trials, gender differences are well documented with respect to pain responses. The problem that exists among doctors who treat pain in their day-to-day practices is that many do not identify these gender differences, which can influence your pain diagnosis and treatment. As discussed in Chapter 1, studies of large numbers of people (epidemiological data) clearly show that women are at greater risk for developing certain pain syndromes than men and that this is a result of hormonal factors and other differences between the sexes.

Hormonal differences between men and women may account for the fact that predominantly those seeking pain management treatment are women. Whether a woman is experiencing her menstrual cycle also significantly influences her response to pain and medication. In other words, a female with a pain syndrome may respond differently from one day to the next depending on where she is in her menstrual cycle. At one time it was thought that the menstrual cycles in animals were obstacles to experimental research. However, with the advancement of gender-specific medicine, it is thought that the menstrual cycles in laboratory animals are opportunities. The problem in doing gender-specific pain medicine studies arises from the emphasis on the equality of the sexes that became dominant in the 1980s. This factor may have delayed the onset of gender-specific medical research.

Many factors determine how well a particular medicine will work on your body. This chapter discusses why men and women respond differently to pain and how each copes with it. (R.B. Fillingham. *Sex, Gender, and Pain*. n.p.: IASP Press, 2000)

Brain and Body Structure Matters

Pain is your body's way of telling you that something is harming your body. For example, chest pain tells you that you may be having a heart attack. Pain will cause your body to become restricted or immobile so that healing can occur. When your pain becomes severe, it tells you to seek medical attention. The problem exists when your body's pain alarm system fails to quit working and the pain continues. When pain becomes uncontrolled, depression, anxiety, and loss of sleep can result, making your perception of the pain worse. The onset of depression or anxiety happens when your pain reduces certain levels of chemicals in your brain and spinal cord.

Pain is an individual experience that is difficult to study. The International Association for the Study of Pain defines pain as an unpleasant emotional and sensory experience that results from tissue injury or the threat of tissue injury. The sensation of pain in different places on your body usually begins with the *peripheral nervous system*. The peripheral nervous system includes all nerves located outside of your spinal cord and brain, such as in your arms and legs. The spinal cord and brain together are called the *central nervous system*. Nerve fibers in the *peripheral nervous system* send painful impulses from nerve endings in your body directly to your spinal cord and brain.

Nerve Fibers That Transmit Pain

There are two main classes of nerve "fibers" that transmit pain in your body. The first class of pain fibers is called Alpha delta fibers. These fibers are able to send sharp pain and transmit pain impulses rapidly. The second class of pain fibers is called C fibers. These are smaller fibers and send burning types of pain more slowly than the Alpha delta fibers. If you were to hit your finger with a hammer, you would experience two components of pain. First, you would feel a fast, sharp pain (Alpha delta fiber), followed by a second slow, throbbing or burning (C fiber) pain. The throbbing or burning pain last longer than sharp pain.

Specific pathways exist that transmit pain information from the damaged part, or "tissue," through your spinal cord to a center of pain perception in your brain. When you are hurt, chemicals called *neurotransmitters* are released by the injured tissue that stimulates your nerve endings to feel pain. As a result, the pain you feel comes from the place of your tissue injury. The effects of several of these *neurotransmitters* have been studied well. Some of these chemical substances make your nerve endings more sensitive to pain. This process is called *transduction.*

If a type of *neurotransmitter* called prostaglandin is in the hurt area of tissue, the size of your blood vessels will grow and increase your blood circulation to that area. This will cause you to have swelling, redness, and warmth in the injured area. The pain impulse travels along the length of your nerve to a junction where the nerve enters the spinal cord. This junction between the nerve and the spinal cord is the command center for many pain syndromes. *Transmission* occurs when the pain impulse from the injured tissue flows to the junction at your spinal cord. From this area, the sensation of pain is transmitted to the back of your spinal cord. When the pain impulse reaches your spinal cord, it can lessen your sensation of pain. This process is called *modulation.*

Nerves "talk" with each another when *neurotransmitter* chemicals are released, causing other nerves around the injured area to transmit painful impulses. Another chemical released from injured tissue is *bradykinin.* Bradykinin causes C fibers to transmit pain, and also causes another type of *neurotransmitter* called prostaglandins to be produced. Prostaglandins decrease the level of pain tolerance that C fibers can withstand, which causes an increased sensitivity to feelings of pain. There are some medications available that can block these prostaglandins from casing pain. A common prostaglandin blocker is Ibuprofen.

When the pain fibers enter the spinal cord, they terminate in different parts of the spinal cord. Nerve cells in the spinal cord receive and respond to pain impulses from both the large and small fibers. Activation of receptors by the continual bombardment by pain impulses can result in a significant increase in your pain. The spinal cord is "upregulated" to magnify pain impulses and result in excruciating disabling pain.

Nonpain Transmitting Fibers

Another type of pain fiber exists that transmits impulses from the peripheral nervous system to the spinal cord. The third fiber that is important in understanding the transmission of pain are large nerve fibers called A beta fibers. These fibers respond to nonpain-producing stimuli such as touch, pressure, or movement of joints. These fibers also end at the spinal cord. They are important because these nerves can either activate or inhibit pain impulses.

Pain and Nonpain Fibers Working Together

The convergence of different types of nerves including pain-producing nerves as well as touch and pressure producing nerves can be a source of an unusual experience referred to as referred pain. Referred pain occurs when an individual feels pain, for example, in the shoulder when the actual pain producing tissue is the heart as is noted when an individual suffers a heart attack. This referred pain from the heart travels to the shoulder because some of the receptors in the spinal cord also receive nervous impulses from both the *peripheral nervous system* and arms and legs as well as within the organs within the body. In this case, the brain misinterprets the location of the injured tissue stimulus.

When a hammer strikes a finger, rubbing the injured finger can result in considerable pain relief. This phenomenon was explained in 1965 by two pain researchers who published the gate-control theory of pain. Their studies revealed that only a limited amount of sensory information can be processed by the brain and spinal cord at any given moment. When pain fibers from the periphery such as the arms or legs, activate pain transmission cells in the spinal cord, signals from the nonpain-producing large fibers can inhibit or increase activation of these the pain impulses from these pain transmitting nerves. As a result, pain impulses appear to be dependent on a balance of activity in both the large and small fibers. This is the basis of the gate-control theory of pain. When the balance of nerve activity is directed toward the pain transmission fibers, the gate is open which allows transmission of painful signals to go from the spinal cord to the brain. On the other hand, when the large nonpain fibers predominate electrical impulses, the gate is closed and the pain signals are decreased. In some instances they may be completely blocked.

Once the pain impulses have reached the spinal cord, the pathways for pain are crossed. Pain originating from peripheral nerves on the left side of the body is transmitted to the spinal cord on the right side of the body. Pain transmission then reaches the brain by two main pathways, called tracts.

Chronic pain can make pain nerve endings more sensitive which results in more pain that continues to worsen over time. After a while the pain from the pain transmitting fibers can "cross wires" with the large nerves that transmit touch and movement sensation so that even a slight change in movement or light touch can cause severe agony to a patient.

Gender differences in body structure and brain function develop when a fetus is still in the mother's womb. These differences show themselves in childhood. These factors combine with family lifestyles and school and sociocultural sex roles to act uniquely on the individual. All of these events factor into gender-specific patterns of pain perception. During adolescence, gender differences in pain syndromes emerge, such as dysmenorrhea in women and cluster headaches in men. Smoking and other dangerous activities can influence the onset of these chronic pain syndromes in both men and women.

Serotonin and Depression

When acute pain becomes chronic, a self-perpetuating cycle of maladies can occur, resulting in changes in your body as well as behavior that makes your pain worse. For example, after an injury, changes can occur in the regrowth of damaged nerve endings and where pain nerves connect with other nerves. This can result in muscle tension, making muscles extra sensitive because they are tense rather than relaxed. The increased stress from chronic pain can increase the release of a naturally occurring chemical in the brain called norepinepherine, eventually leading to its depletion and resulting in depression and exhaustion. The depression can magnify the physical pain, which in turn depletes serotonin in both the spinal cord and brain.

Persistent pain can decrease an individual's sleep. This depletes the body's supply of endorphins, chemicals that decrease pain. With the depletion of endorphins, pain can become worse. As a result of the increase in pain, people often place themselves into guarded positions to avoid pain. However, these unnatural positions can strain other muscles, which in turn spread more pain to other parts of the body. Other, unused muscles shrink, or atrophy, with a resulting loss of strength causing more discomfort. The goal and purpose of pain medicine is to interrupt this vicious cycle.

Different Hormones Affect Pain Perception

Some pain syndromes are affected by changes in sex hormones. For example, migraine headaches resolve during pregnancy as a result of elevated blood levels of progesterone. Experimental animal pain responses are reduced during lactation as a result of increased progesterone. When estrogen decreases (following menopause, for instance), joint pains increase in females.

In men, a decrease in testosterone will increase the frequency of angina. With an increase in testosterone, cluster headaches are more prevalent in men. With an increase in progesterone, testosterone, and estrogen, both men and women experience an increase in temporomandibular jaw (TMJ) pain.

Positron Emission Tomography (PET) scanning has shown areas in the brain where sex steroid hormones can affect gender differences in pain control. A PET scan is a nuclear medicine device which enables a physician to assess functional activity of tissue. PET scan imaging has determined that pain can vary from person to person. Furthermore, studies have shown that pain within each person is based on life experiences.

Endorphins, mentioned previously, can shut the gate to pain. Endorphins are natural morphinelike drugs (chemically related to opium) that switch off the pain alarm. Several types have been identified that modulate pain at the spinal cord and the brain. Because pain can affect breathing, blood flow, heart rate, and digestion, the body naturally releases endorphins to deal with pain. Moreover, pain can affect the limbic system, which is a complex area of nerve pathways in the brain that controls emotions such as mood, self preservation, rage, fear, and pleasure. Certain areas of the spinal cord contain high concentrations of endorphin receptors. The body also produces enkephalins and dynorphins, two neurochemicals also involved in pain modulation. Another important neurochemical is gamma aminobutyric acid (GABA), an inhibitory pain mediator. GABA inhibits pain transmission in the spinal cord.

Genetics also produce gender-related pain differences. Gender-linked genetic disorders affect both males and females. Chromosome differences in two strains of mice have revealed different perception to opioid therapy in male mice. Stress can influence an animal's response to pain. There is a difference in stress-induced analgesia between male and female rodents, with the females having a greater pain response to stress. The reason for this observation is unknown and is believed not to be a result of the effect of hormones. On the other hand, estrogen, a female hormone, regulates the formation of the pain transmitter chemical substance P as well as some of the other chemicals in the nervous system that do cause pain.

Women go through a 5- to 10-year period of menopause. During this time, changes occur in hormones, most notably a decrease in the hormones in the female bloodstream. In men hormone changes occur over approximately 20 years. Body structure changes occur in both males and females. Lifestyle changes also occur during this time. Increases in the incidence of disease occur during this time in both men and women. There also is an alteration of drug metabolism in both men and women.

During adulthood, social roles and lifestyles become entrenched. Be aware that health-care providers also have ideas that have become entrenched with respect to gender specificity in pain management. Not only does lifestyle affect one's perception of pain, this in combination with nutrition and hormone status combine to affect one's perception of pain.

Nicotine can have a gender-specific effect on pain. Doctors usually ask their patients about recent nicotine use. When conducting research, however, many researchers fail to ask their subjects about nicotine consumption. It has been shown that nicotine increases the amount of stimulus needed to cause pain in men but not in women. (R.B. Fillingham. *Sex, Gender, and Pain*. n.p.: IASP Press, 2000)

Tailor Your Treatment

It is obvious that men and women differ with respect to pain. This is also true with regard to the treatment of pain. Doctors are beginning to realize that men and women respond differently to different pain therapies.

The best overall pain-management treatment is one that is tailored to the male and female patients as individuals. A flexible combination of pharmacological agents and physical therapy and/or manipulative therapy needs to be individually designed for each patient. Communicate to your doctor that you do not want to have random physical and manipulative therapy applied for your pain. You must be active in helping your doctor determine which therapies are best for you.

Chapter 3
Understanding the Psychological Aspects of Pain

Men and women perceive and respond to painful experiences in different ways. Hormonal influences on pain perception were discussed in Chapter 1. Debate that has spanned many generations continues over who can stand more pain, men or women.

In this chapter, you will learn how your own psychology affects how you perceive your pain and how pain is perceived differently by men and women. Anxiety, pain thresholds, and pain tolerance will be discussed. You will learn about psychological methods of treatment for your pain, including biofeedback, relaxation, and hypnosis. Behavioral medicine specialists such as psychiatrists and psychologists may be able to help with your emotional disorders associated with your pain. It is important for you to keep the psychology of your pain in mind as you begin to take control of your total pain treatment.

The Psychology of Pain Perception

The International Association for the Study of Pain (IASP) defines pain as an unpleasant sensory and emotion experience associated with tissue injury as a result of trauma (for instance, bone fracture) or disease (for instance, cancer or shingles).

Pain is psychological in that it is a mental processing of sensation impulses that reach the pain center in the brain, whereas pain "intensity" depends on how an individual reacts to pain. Injury or illness experienced when young may influence the way an individual relates to pain. When pain becomes chronic, it becomes a personal problem. However, pain can also become a social problem, perhaps disrupting the family and resulting in loss of self-esteem.

The following findings relate to how an individual's psychological state influences his or her perception of and response to pain:

- Patients who have strongly negative emotions about a situation experience more pain.
- Women have more negative emotions about situations in general than men and, therefore, have a higher incidence of pain. However, women cope better with pain than men.
- Family members' and friends' pain may influence an individual's own pain. For example, women whose immediate family members were experiencing significant pain experienced more clinical pain and complained of more severe pain themselves. In general, men do not demonstrate this effect.
- In general, women have a lower tolerance to pain than men. A higher level of anxiety in women may be somewhat responsible for their increased pain sensitivity. In 1998, a *Washington Post* article reported that although women are more sensitive to pain than men, they appear better able to handle it.
- In 1998 *The Wall Street Journal* reported that women and men report different responses to pain. An article in the *Journal of the American Medical Association* in 1998 reported that girls and boys have different responses to pain and that these pain responses begin early in their lives.

As already stated, pain is an unpleasant sensory as well as an emotional response to tissue trauma. "Nociception" is the avoidance of a painful stimulus. For example, if a match is placed against your skin, you will quickly move away from the heat of the match. This is a nociceptive response to prevent tissue damage. Following the initial tissue response, the psychological aspects of suffering then become manifest. You can be classified as a "wimp" or as "tough" following an injury. However, we do observe this in children following a fall. Some children cry loudly and seek attention, whereas others pick themselves up and continue what they were doing without a whimper. Even though the tissue trauma can be the same for multiple individuals, the response to pain is individualized based on education, psychological makeup, gender, and cultural influences.

Gender Differences

"Pain medicine" as a specialty has evolved in a short time to realize that pain is a multidimensional entity influenced by psychological, neurological, social, ethnic, and cultural factors. Before the advent of this specialty, many doctors looked only at tissue injury and not at the patient as a whole.

Pain cannot be observed or objectively measured. Instead, a pain "diagnosis" is based on verbal and nonverbal communication from the individual suffering pain. People communicate their pain through their behavior. These behaviors, such as limping or grimacing, can be seen by others and result in attention being given to the suffering individual. Doctors should diagnose pain based on both physical and psychological data. Physical data may include a physical examination and interpretation of x-rays, CT scans, and multiresonance imaging (MRI) images. Doctors use this information to tailor therapies (successful, one hopes) to the individual patient.

For reasons not entirely understood, women suffer from more disability than men in general. Further research is needed to unlock the mystery of human behavior and its relationship to disabling painful states so that chronic pain will cease to become a major cause of both physical and psychological disability. (R.B. Fillingham. *Sex, Gender, and Pain*. n.p.: IASP Press, 2000)

Anxiety Issues

Because emotional factors can affect pain perception and intensity, a pain specialist's complete assessment of pain should include not only a physical examination but also analysis of the psychological, emotional, and behavioral aspects of pain. Such analysis may prove challenging because many patients are reluctant to discuss painful psychological issues with their pain-management doctor (and it is more socially acceptable to seek medical rather than psychiatric care).

The purpose of "behavioral medicine" is to relieve anxiety and depression and to decrease pain intensity. Techniques used include biofeedback, relaxation training, and hypnosis. Because anxiety and depression can make people less able to cope with persistent pain, consultation with a behavioral medicine specialist can prove extremely beneficial. Sadness, hopelessness, insomnia, and feelings of worthlessness are all associated with depression. Anxiety is characterized by apprehension and fear or a sense of doom. Doctors need to recognize the stressors that are causing anxiety and address them with their patients. Signs and symptoms of anxiety include loss of appetite, diarrhea, fainting, increased heart rate, and sexual dysfunction.

Personality greatly influences an individual's response to pain and his or her chosen coping strategies. In general, people who have underlying anxiety are more likely to seek higher doses of pain medications. Understanding how people cope with stress is helpful; this is a task aided by discussion with the patient's family. A psychological history should include questions about depression, sleep disruption, preoccupation with body pain, reduced "everyday activities," fatigue, and loss of sexual interest. People with "psychogenic" pain make illness and hospitalization a primary goal. Psychological stresses such as anxiety and depression make pain more intense and less tolerable.

Psychologists have analyzed pre-injury personalities to identify types of people who may be more likely to develop pain syndromes. These studies conclude that there does not appear to be an unstable personality that predisposes to reflex sympathetic dystrophy or other chronic pain syndromes. *Reflex sympathetic dystrophy*, an extremely painful nervous system condition, was once thought to be caused by psychological disorders. Reflex sympathetic dystrophy is further discussed in Chapter 24.

According to psychological studies made after reflex sympathetic dystrophy and similar types of neuropathic (nerve injury) pain syndromes have resolved, a predisposing psychological factor is rarely associated with the pain syndrome. In some instances, however, a person's psychological makeup may control his or her sympathetic nervous system. In 1964, the behavioral aspects of seven patients' chronic reflex sympathetic dystrophy involving an extremity were reported. In each of these seven cases, financial compensation was the main motivating factor, for which these seven individuals maintained signs and symptoms of reflex sympathetic dystrophy, including each individual's chronic disability. Anxiety over potential long-term disability can actually lead to a disability in some patients. As you can see, psychological factors can affect the length of time one experiences a painful syndrome.

Pain is a subjective complaint and is affected by a patient's emotions. Unfortunately, persistent pain can change a patient's behavior. Persistent pain can increase patient anxiety and depression. As a result, it is difficult for a doctor to ascertain whether the pain came first or the psychological dysfunction. Most pain patients can benefit from behavioral treatments designed to improve their ability to cope with pain.

Psychotherapy may help patients realize what is actually causing pain to be chronic. In some instances, a psychiatrist or a neuropsychologist can significantly decrease a patient's pain. If your pain-management doctor wants you to consult a psychologist or a psychiatrist, don't think that your doctor thinks that you have a significant psychological problem. The opposite is true. Psychologists and psychiatrists often operate multidisciplinary pain centers. Multidisciplinary, in this case, means that a panel of different health-care providers evaluates your pain; as a team, these professionals attempt to diagnose and successfully treat (alleviate) your pain. Psychologists not only diagnose and treat behavioral disorders, they may also suggest pain-treatment alternatives. To treat your pain, however, a behavioral medicine specialist must identify any underlying precursors that could make you resistant to pain treatment.

Thresholds and Pain Tolerances

"Pain" is difficult to define because it relates to people's subjective complaints and behaviors. As previously stated, pain varies in duration and intensity. Most people with pain, whether acute or chronic, are able to adapt in a normal manner. Other people have an extreme disruption of their lives and develop chronic pain syndromes in which the pain itself becomes a disease, serving no useful biological purpose. At the time of injury, pain serves a useful purpose: warning the body to cease activity and allow healing. When pain persists after the tissue has healed, it serves no known biological purpose.

Ultimately, pain affects society because of the loss of contributing, productive individuals disabled by pain. In 1976 Fordyce suggested that pain behavior is a learned response that can be modified. If a patient receives extra attention from a spouse or family members, the pain behavior is "reinforced." This is an example of pain causing a benefit or a "positive reinforcement." On the other hand, if an individual loses work and income because of pain, pain intensity usually decreases, allowing the individual to return to work. This is an example of "negative reinforcement."

Both the patient and the doctor need to identify situations that reinforce pain behavior. Patients can use a pain diary to help identify what behavior signals pain, and a family conference may help to identify the positive reinforcements (rewards) of pain, such as a doting spouse, being excused from household chores, and so on. Some people appreciate extra attention given to them by family members, attention that perhaps was not available before the painful condition. Others use pain to avoid psychologically painful situations, such as workplace problems with co-workers or a supervisor, and use it to avoid going to work and dealing with colleagues. People may also use pain to avoid social or family gatherings.

Behavioral Medicine Specialists

When doctors fail to relieve pain, patients may find that a consultation with a behavioral medicine specialist such as a psychologist or psychiatrist may prove helpful. If pain provides a way to escape difficult psychological situations, this should be addressed. Most people with pain respond to routine treatments, such as oral medication and nerve injections of anti-inflammatory drugs (corticosteroids, for instance) as well as physical or manipulative therapy. When an individual fails to respond to these methods, psychological intervention is necessary.

Pain patient behaviors that should be closely watched include frequently talking about pain, moaning, and frequently going to doctors and refusing to work. Doctors should observe and note blatant pain manifestations. Pain behavior is influenced by environmental consequences. Suffering is the conceptual component of pain that denotes a persistent negative affect. Suffering is composed of depression, fear, and isolation.

The concept of pain is complex. Philosophers have argued for years whether pain is an emotion or a sensation. Some theologians in the Middle Ages thought that pain was a penalty. It has been described as a punishment for sin. Pain is essentially a behavioral subjective phenomenon.

Dr. Gerald Aronoff, a noted psychiatrist with a specialty in pain medicine, has reported that patients with chronic pain share many of the following characteristics: preoccupation with pain, strong dependency needs, feelings of isolation, an inability to attend to self needs, and an inability to appropriately deal with repressed anger and hostility.

Many patients with chronic pain exhibit masochistic behavior patterns. Pain can gratify an individual's need to suffer and receive constant attention from a family member or health-care professional. Pain and disability can cause dependency upon others to assist in activities of daily living, such a cooking, cleaning, laundry, and so on. Many chronic pain patients have suffered emotionally traumatic childhoods; a history of this trauma should be sought by the doctors caring for these patients.

Pain may significantly increase when there is low self-esteem. When an individual attempts to suppress emotions, muscle tension may occur. Muscle tension can contribute to both body pain and tension-type headaches. (R.B. Fillingham. *Sex, Gender, and Pain.* n.p.: IASP Press, 2000)

Emotional Disorders and Psychology

Emotional disorders can also be associated with chronic pain, including somataform disorders, somatization disorder, conversion disorder, psychogenic pain disorder, and hypochondriasis. These emotional disorders will affect a patient's response to a chronic pain syndrome.

In a *somataform disorder*, physical symptoms are compatible with a physical disorder, but there is no evidence of any clear psychiatric or physical problem. These patients overanalyze their bodies and have a tendency to look for abnormal symptoms.

A *somatization disorder* is a chronic disorder that usually begins before age 30 and primarily affects women. With it, an individual complains of many symptoms but has few physical findings to confirm their complaints. These individuals consult many doctors to validate their symptoms and may even consent to multiple injections by a pain-management doctor or even a surgical procedure for the treatment of pain.

A *conversion disorder* results from an emotional conflict unrelated to bodily disease but resulting in loss of function of a part of the body. An example is losing the use of a hand without an obvious physical problem or injury. These individuals exaggerate the magnitude of their complaints.

Psychogenic pain disorders are complaints of pain without adequate physical findings. These individuals exhibit neurotic behavior. Neurotic behavior is a behavior that you realize is abnormal such as anxiety. Individuals seeking financial compensation may exhibit psychogenic pain disorders.

Hypochondriasis is a disturbance that involves an unrealistic interpretation of physical disease. These individuals have a preoccupation with the belief that they have a serious disease and are preoccupied with their physical symptoms.

Malingering is uncommon but implies a conscious fabrication of an illness for personal gain. These individuals are often seeking financial compensation or may be seeking narcotic analgesic drugs such as morphine or Dilaudid.

However, before diagnosing an individual of faking an illness, a doctor must thoroughly investigate a patient's complaint and exclude any possible real illness.

The pain-prone patient is often an individual who had a traumatic childhood, perhaps with a history of physical and/or emotional abuse or a history of chronic pain or disability. Individuals who feel unloved are prone to use pain to meet ungratified needs. These individuals frequently try to manipulate others and have a tendency to burden their families.

Various psychological tests are available to evaluate pain patients. A common test is the Minnesota Multiphase Personality Inventory Test (MMPI), which evaluates multiple dimensions of a pain patient. The Beck Depression Scale can be used to assess depression. The MMPI, consisting of 566 questions, is widely used by psychologists working with pain patients, but cannot consistently distinguish between psychogenic and tissue damage pain. However, people with high hypochondriasis and hysteria scores and lower depression scores may have a physical basis for their pain, rather than a conversion reaction. The MMPI test also proves useful in assessing emotional disorders that occur secondary to a pain experience and personality factors that could affect an individual's response to pain treatment.

A problem with labeling pain as psychogenic is the assumption that the actual cause of the affected patient's pain is unknown. This assumption may be false, because the physical reason for many pain syndromes may be unclear or unknown. This is a problem in workman's compensation or bodily injury cases. If, following an examination, a doctor paid by an insurance company cannot find a reason for a claimant's pain, the patient is often labeled as a malingerer, which unfortunately ruins the patient's credibility with a judge or jury. Remember, however, that the diagnosis of psychogenic pain is a diagnosis only of exclusion. That is, a diagnosis made by excluding the diseases to which only some of your symptoms may belong, leaving one disease as the most likely diagnosis, although no conclusive tests or findings establish that diagnosis for certain.

Most chronic pain patients are *not* malingers. Acute and chronic pain is disabling. Most patients do not want to suffer. A desire to avoid pain is a strong desire.

Most pain doctors want to minimize the use of drugs and medicines. No medicine is without potential dangerous side effects. This is why most pain-management doctors use injection therapy and prescribe physical and/or occupational therapy and make referrals to chiropractors or other nonconventional health-care providers. In the past, the failure of injections or drugs to relieve pain resulted in referral to a psychologist or a psychiatrist for treatment of psychiatric or behavioral problems. Today these specialists are essential to pain management. In fact, a psychiatrist is a medical doctor, and a psychologist has a Ph.D. Not only can psychiatrists prescribe medications for pain, they also attend to mental and emotional conditions that may be contributing to pain. (A psychologist cannot prescribe medication.)

Psychological assessments and treatment are now part of the total approach to managing those experiencing chronic pain. Psychologists can teach relaxation techniques and biofeedback and use hypnosis to decrease pain, complementing physical therapy, pharmacological therapy, and injections. Therefore, you should not feel offended if your pain-management doctor wants to send you to a psychologist. Instead, welcome this method and be aware that the psychologist will help you take control of your own pain. Remember that pain medicine is not a "cookbook" approach to diagnosing and treating pain. A multidisciplinary approach, one that treats the whole patient, is the proper way to manage your pain.

Psychology and Treatment Methods

Placebo medicine studies help us to further understand the role of psychology in chronic pain. Pain may be considered a result of a tissue injury signaling the brain to experience pain. However, placebo medications, defined as inactive drugs such as sugar pills, can significantly decrease pain.

When doing any type of study evaluating the analgesic effects of a particular new medicine, a placebo group must be included. For example, chronic migraine headache sufferers asked to participate in a study evaluating a new headache medication will be divided into two groups. One group will be prescribed the active, or "study," drug, whereas the other will be given either an inactive drug or no drug. If a participant experiences significant pain relief from the inactive drug or the sugar pill, he or she has experienced a placebo effect: essentially, pain relief from no medication.

The placebo effect demonstrates that a psychological component affects the perception of painful stimuli. People with high expectations that the drug they are receiving are powerful pain relievers will likely experience a decrease in pain after taking placebo drugs. The expectation of significant pain relief psychologically causes relief.

People's expectations when seeing a pain doctor or receiving medications, nerve injections, and psychological therapy will also affect their pain response. Those who do not expect relief, on the other hand, will probably not experience pain relief. For this reason, each individual has control of his or her painful situation.

Consider New Methods

Monitor new methods of pain relief with your doctor. New methods become available on a month-to-month basis as a result of ongoing research. Some of these methods can prove extremely useful, whereas others may not. Be aware also that some of the new methods that become available may not have included a placebo group. You can check the Internet, especially the National Library of Medicine website, to find out whether placebo-controlled studies were done on the method that interests you. If this method was not compared to a placebo, stay away.

Unfortunately, many pain-relieving methods touted on television and in reputable magazines are not "placebo controlled." (That is, a placebo group was not a part of the study looking at the method's effectiveness). To properly assess a drug or a treatment method, read the medical literature. Again, the National Library of Medicine has an excellent website. If you do not have a computer, access the Internet at a public library, or ask your doctor for copies of research. Don't allow yourself to become a guinea pig! If a placebo can provide you with pain relief, why expose yourself to a drug?

Take Control of Your Pain

You can observe the pain patterns of animals to realize that in humans there must be a strong psychological component to a chronic pain syndrome. For example, a dog or cat can be struck by an automobile and sustain significant trauma. In most instances, however, the animal is back functioning within a short time. An animal has no secondary gain issues and does not anticipate having significant monetary compensation for an injury caused by a careless driver. However, humans can have prolonged pain following an accident only to have the pain relieved following a large jury settlement. This observation is referred to as the "green police" treatment.

If you truly believe that you will get better and that you will conquer your pain syndrome, you will. The effect of prayer also has been documented as a powerful analgesic. An orthopedic surgery textbook tells of an individual with two lumbar disk ruptures. This individual had weakness in a leg. The orthopedic surgeon used MRI images and clinical evaluation of the patient to determine surgery was necessary. The patient also had significant pain. However, when the patient's church congregation prayed for his relief, his pain dissipated in a day. A repeat MRI revealed no disk rupture. The numbness in the extremity also disappeared. This is one of many documented cases of the power of prayer.

If you truly believe that a method will work, in most instances it will. Would you be angry at your doctor if you were given a placebo pill for the treatment of pain? If you got relief from the placebo pill, would you feel that you have a mental problem? The answer to this question should be absolutely "no!" That you received relief from a placebo pill means that you can control your pain. Congratulate yourself and your doctor! Moreover, you should be *happy* with your doctor. That you are able to control your pain means that you are less dependent on drugs, nerve blocks, and other methods for pain relief. The goal of any pain-management practitioner is to have you control your pain symptoms. Try to take control of your pain and do not let your pain control you.

Another study looked at postsurgery cancer patients who were given saltwater (saline) injections and had a significant decrease in postsurgery pain. Individuals may even have side effects associated with placebos. If you are a participant in a study, the side effects of the actual drug studied are noted and written down for you. A placebo response can be as high as 35 percent with side effects experienced in as many as 19 percent of cases. For instance, individuals responded to flavored water with demonstrated signs of drunkenness when they were compared to a group that had flavored alcohol drinks.

Some researchers report that the placebo effect is related to your body's release of *endorphins,* naturally occurring chemicals that we have in our bodies to control pain. A placebo, furthermore, may reduce anxiety. Anxiety can increase the perception of pain. People with positive expectations prior to taking medications generally have more positive results. This finding may be related to endorphin release from the brain and spinal cord. Expectation is a learned trait. This is one reason why a placebo response is not evident in children. Expectation depended on an individual's life experience and personality. Hostility with a treating doctor will decrease expectation. On the other hand, respect for a doctor's abilities will increase positive expectations for successful pain relief.

Biofeedback and Relaxation Treatment

Other methods used by psychologists for the management of pain include relaxation and biofeedback training. These methods are used to treat both acute and chronic pain syndromes. Relaxation is also frequently used to control pain associated with labor contractions. Used properly, relaxation can also decrease the body's metabolic activity and preserve energy. Learning to manage pain through relaxation methods enables people to consciously control pain and become proactive in their own pain management.

Biofeedback is another method frequently used by psychologists to manage pain. An electromyogram, which measures muscle contractions in different parts of the body, can be used for biofeedback training and pain evaluations. Other measurements include skin temperature and brainwave forms. When muscles are tense, skin temperature is less than in surrounding tissues because of a decrease in blood flow. Biofeedback techniques can increase blood flow to muscles and skin and increase your temperature. This can be used in combination with relaxation training to manage pain; both techniques are more commonly used by women than by men. Biofeedback has been used to treat many chronic pain syndromes, including muscle-tension headaches. People with migraine headaches, phantom limb pain, and reflex sympathetic dystrophy can also respond to biofeedback training.

Success of biofeedback for the treatment of muscle-tension type headaches ranges from 50 to 60 percent. Individuals who have attempted self-relaxation for the treatment of muscle-tension headaches do not improve as much as individuals who have had formal biofeedback training by a psychologist. Relaxation training has also been shown to decrease muscle-tension types of headaches. The advantage of relaxation training is that it is easier to learn and more cost-effective. Biofeedback training can be much more expensive. Your psychologist may give you relaxation tapes to take home to help you decrease muscle tension.

Migraine headaches have been successfully treated with biofeedback. On average, females have a higher incidence of migraine headaches than males. Biofeedback training can result in a 50 percent reduction in severe migraine headache pain. Some studies advocate combining biofeedback and relaxation training for the treatment of migraine headaches. Which would you prefer, medications or psychological treatment for the treatment of your migraine headaches? Both can be equally effective. The decision is yours. Some individuals would rather not take medications, whereas others prefer to skip the time that it takes to learn biofeedback or relaxation techniques.

Relaxation treatment has also been shown to be effective for the management of lower back pain. Most back pain is caused by sustained muscle tension. Relaxation training relaxes muscles and increases blood flow and oxygen delivery while removing excessive buildup in muscles of lactic acid. Be aware, however, that muscle relaxation is not effective in all people. Further, no method described in this book is 100 percent effective for pain control. If you suffer from arthritis of the spine, muscle relaxation will not completely relieve your arthritic pain. Biofeedback has also been shown to be helpful in the management of back pain, especially if related to increased muscle tension. If you suffer from TMJ (temporomandibular joint pain), relaxation techniques and/or biofeedback may also provide you with significant pain relief.

You may know someone who has torticollis of the neck muscles. This is a twisting of the head to one side as a result of contractions of the neck muscles. Biofeedback has been shown to be effective in the management of some of the pain associated with these chronic spasms of the neck muscles. Biofeedback and relaxation methods have been shown to decrease menstrual pain as well as some arthritic pain in addition to phantom limb pain. It is exciting to note that you can have long-term pain relief for some of the chronic pain syndromes if you are properly trained in relaxation and/or biofeedback and practice these methods at the onset of pain. Biofeedback can train you to have some control over your bodily processes.

Biofeedback and relaxation techniques continue to be studied for the relief of various pain syndromes. If your doctor does not offer you a choice of either of these methods, let your doctor know that you are interested in either or both of these useful analgesics.

Hypnosis Treatment

Hypnosis is another tool used by psychologists to relieve pain. Hypnosis has a long history of use in various pain syndromes. Hypnosis reduces awareness of painful stimuli by providing suggestions or images that divert attention away from painful stimuli. Hypnosis is a state of consciousness that differs from the normal waking state and is characterized by a significant response to suggestions, although not everyone responds to hypnotic therapy.

Hypnosis can decrease or inhibit pain impulses to the brain's pain center as well as pain impulses in the spinal cord. Hypnosis can create the expectation of pain reduction. As mentioned previously, the expectation that a method will provide pain relief often means the method will succeed. Hypnosis has been used for the management of cancer pain and postoperative pain. Some anesthesiologists have used hypnosis during surgery. People with headaches can also find relief with hypnosis. A study published in 2000 demonstrated that hypnosis can decrease the need for narcotic medications after surgery. Hypnosis has also been shown to be effective in the management of labor pain.

Imagery is an important component of hypnosis. Hypnosis causes a deeply relaxed state, diverting attention from pain. When you have pain, if you visualize the pain as a bright red color, you can use imagery to lighten the red to a pink color, which is analogous to a reduction in your pain. If you have burning pain over your skin from shingles, you may imagine cool water and ice being placed over your burning skin. These suggestions and images may prove useful to reduce pain. Although hypnosis is used to reduce pain, it is difficult to completely eliminate it. However, it can decrease pain to a tolerable state. You are probably now aware that hypnosis uses positive suggestions. You are advised that you will feel calm, warm, and relaxed. Negative suggestions, such as "Your pain will be completely eliminated," are not frequently used. Negative suggestions do not give you adequate imaging. A study published in 2000 demonstrated that 75 percent of individuals typically receive significant pain relief from hypnosis.

Working with a Psychologist

A psychologist can also help you manage pain through "cognitive-behavioral management" of pain. Cognitive processes are those means by which we become aware of situations. These processes include reasoning and decision making. Behavior is your response to a stimulus. In doing this type of psychological pain relief, your psychologist will analyze your thoughts and feelings as well as your beliefs and what behavior response you use on a painful stimulus.

Chapter 4

Understanding Adjuvant Medicines and Pain

Adjuvant drugs are medications used to facilitate the effects of other pain medications such as opioids and nonsteroidal anti-inflammatory drugs. Antidepressant medications and anticonvulsant medications may be used as adjuncts to opioid pain medications such as morphine, Oxycontin, and Dilaudid and so-called nonsteroidal anti-inflammatory drugs (or NSAIDs) such as Motrin and Naprosyn for the control of pain. Anticonvulsant medications not only treat mood disorders but also many pain symptoms. A combination of these drugs is also useful for the management of pain associated with nerve hyperirritability.

In this chapter, you will learn how adjuvant drugs have an affect on your feelings of pain. It will cover tricyclic antidepressants, monoamine oxidase inhibitors, selective serotonin reuptake inhibitors, antidepressants, anticonvulsants, and muscle relaxers. These types of adjuvant medications can help relieve some of your pain so that you will not just be relying on pain reliving medications.

Tricyclic Antidepressant Medications

Antidepressant drugs can decrease pain intensity from unbearable to more bearable, although they will not completely resolve pain. Side effects such as dizziness and sedation caused by higher doses of tricyclic antidepressants cause doctors to increase doses of antidepressants only very gradually over several weeks. Initially only low doses of antidepressants such as a tricyclic are needed. However, the dose needed to control pain will usually need to increase over time.

A tricyclic antidepressant used commonly for pain is amitriptyline (Elavil). This agent can cause constipation and dry mouth, and some patients complain of dizziness when they stand quickly. Sedation and tremors may also be seen, and weight gain and sexual dysfunction have been reported. Some people even complain of craving chocolate. An overdose of tricyclic antidepressants or related drugs may cause a dangerous and even fatal abnormality of heart rhythm.

Tricyclic antidepressants in combination with opioids can cause more constipation than either of the drugs used alone. No antidepressant should be stopped without the advice of a doctor. When stopped suddenly, anxiety, vivid dreams, nausea, vomiting, and dizziness may result. Because of the frequent side effects associated with tricyclic antidepressants, a newer class of antidepressant drugs called selective serotonin reuptake inhibitors (SSRIs) with fewer side effects are starting to take their place. Some of the tricyclic antidepressant drugs may have an effect on acid production in the stomach. Some of these drugs can actually decrease acid production and be of some benefit in patients who suffer from ulcers, reflux, or gastritis.

Monoamine Oxidase Inhibitor Medications

Another class of antidepressants is monoamine oxidase inhibitors (MAOIs). This class is used for significant depression and is not usually used for pain management. These drugs have a high incidence of side effects; overdoses can be lethal. These drugs increase the appetite of some patients. This class of drug increases the concentration of epinephrine, norepinephrine, and dopamine in the central nervous system, and when combined with foods such as cheese and wine high in tyramine may cause severe hypertension. For this reason, MAOIs should not be used by people with preexisting hypertension.

Side effects of MAOIs include constipation, nausea, vomiting, dry mouth, drowsiness, and dizziness. Sexual dysfunction may occur. If an MAOI is taken with meperidine (Demerol), a significant and potentially lethal elevation in body temperature can occur. MAOIs can also be associated with liver damage. Blood tests of liver function, therefore, should be monitored for anyone taking this medication. Examples of MAOIs include Marplan and Parnate. The only time that a pain-management doctor sees a patient taking these drugs is when a patient is referred by another doctor who was treating the patient for severe depression.

Selective Serotonin Reuptake Inhibitor Medications

A more recently developed class of antidepressant drugs is the selective serotonin reuptake inhibitors (SSRIs). The first of this class was fluoxetine (Prozac), introduced in 1987. Overall, this class of drugs causes fewer side effects than the tricyclic antidepressants or the MAOIs. The SSRIs exert their pain modulating and antidepressant effect by increasing serotonin levels in the central nervous system. This neurochemical is extremely valuable in reducing pain. Other SSRIs include piroxitine (Paxil), sertraline (Zoloft), and fluvoxamine (Luvox).

A more recent SSRI, venlafaxine (Effexor), has been studied for its pain-modulating effects in chronic pain. This particular selective serotonin reuptake inhibitor has been shown to be effective in the control of pain in many painful disorders. The selective serotonin reuptake inhibitor class of drugs can cause nausea and diarrhea. Jitteriness and lack of sleep have also been reported as side effects in a small number of patients. Other individuals complain of sedation. If sedation is a problem, the medication should be taken only in the evening. The drug can be used as a nonaddicting sleep aid. A decreased libido is occasionally associated with this class of drugs. Some news media outlets have even reported that Prozac may lead a depressed patient to commit suicide. The drug itself does not cause suicide tendencies in the patient. These types of people have strong suicidal ideations and probably should have been hospitalized while antidepressant medications were started. An individual who is sincere about committing suicide should be placed immediately under the care of a psychiatrist.

Be aware that SSRIs can decrease the efficacy of the opioid analgesics hydrocodone or oxycodone if taken in combinations with these agents. Both opioids are broken down in the liver to morphine, a chemical reaction that can be slowed by the SSRIs. As a result, less morphine is produced for pain relief.

A new selective serotonin reuptake inhibitor, escitalopram oxlate (Lexapro), is now available to patients. This medication does not interfere with the transformation of oxycodone and hydrocodone to morphine. Consequently, its use with these drugs will not decrease the efficacy of the opioid prescribed. Patients must be told that the selective serotonin reuptake inhibitors can cause generalized muscle pain in a small number of patients. Muscle pain is not associated with tricyclic antidepressant use.

"Atypical" Antidepressant Medications

Trazodone (Desyrel) is essentially in its own antidepressant class and is known as an atypical antidepressant. Like other classes of antidepressants, this drug exerts its effect by increasing serotonin in the brain and spinal cord. It is not as potent as the tricyclic antidepressants but it does cause drowsiness and may be used to enhance sleep. Side effects include dizziness and dry mouth. Priapism, a painful, persistent erection, is one of the most serious side effects and may precipitate a visit to an emergency room for treatment. The incidence of priapism in males is 1 in 10,000. The drug should be stopped immediately if there is any change in erectile function.

Studies have demonstrated that antidepressants can lessen the pain of the following syndromes in many patients: phantom pain, acute herpes zoster, postherpetic neuralgia, cancer pain, cluster headaches, migraine headaches, reflex sympathetic dystrophy, and tension-type headaches. Is one class of antidepressant more effective than another? The drug of choice depends on the incidence of side effects.

Anticonvulsant Drugs

Anticonvulsant medications, which are used to treat seizures, may also be effective in the management of pain. They are most effective in treating pain related to direct injury of either a peripheral nerve or the brain and spinal cord. Anticonvulsant medications may also be useful for the treatment of some types of cancer pain, headaches, reflex sympathetic dystrophy, phantom pain, postherpetic neuralgia, and trigeminal neuralgia. Common anticonvulsant drugs used for the treatment of pain include gabapentin (Neurontin), carbamazepine (Tegretol), valproic acid (Depakote), clonazepam (Klonopin), phenytoin (Dilantin), and lamotrigine (Lamictal).

Neurontin is the most frequently prescribed anticonvulsant medication because it has the least side effects. It is also the most studied anticonvulsant for the management of pain. Neurontin and other anticonvulsants relieve severe, lancinating pain. All anticonvulsant medications can cause lethargy and drowsiness, but gabapentin has the lowest incidence of these side effects.

Anticonvulsant medications exert their effects on the chemicals that transmit impulses in the central and peripheral nervous systems. By increasing "neurotransmitting" chemicals, such as GABA, pain impulses are less readily transmitted from the peripheral nerves to the brain. As a result, less pain is experienced. Several anticonvulsant drugs affect the movement of sodium into and out of the nerve cell. By inhibiting sodium from going into the neuron, a hyperexcited nerve can be made less irritable, decreasing the transmission of pain impulses down the nerve.

All the anticonvulsant medications can have side effects such as lethargy, fatigue, confusion, or sedation, and may have interactions with other medications. For this reason, when someone has been prescribed an anticonvulsant, he or she must tell his or her pain-medicine doctor. The potential for drug interactions is important with any drug. Tegretol (carbamazipine) can cause anemia as well as decrease platelets in a patient's bloodstream. For this reason, any patient taking Tegretol should have periodic laboratory tests done.

Topamax (topiramate) is an anticonvulsant medication that has found recent use for weight loss. Some doctors also prescribe this medication for the management of pain associated with reflex sympathetic dystrophy. Patients may experience trouble with concentration or memory with this agent, a side effect that occurs equally in men and women.

With respect to gender specificity, there appears to be no significant gender differences when men and women take gabapentin. In many instances, a patient's ability to excrete drugs is decreased due to a patient's age. Gabapentin dosage should be decreased for elderly patients (both men and women) because of their decreased ability to excrete the drug in the urine.

Gender differences in antidepressant treatments, including responses and side effects, have been studied. Because of the breakdown in the liver and the absorption of the drugs from the gastrointestinal tract into the blood, women have higher blood concentrations of tricyclic antidepressants such as amitriptyline than men. As a result, gender-specific recommendations for the prescribing of tricyclic antidepressants should be considered. Men are more responsive to selective serotonin reuptake inhibitors (SSRIs). Men have lower blood levels than women, but a greater affect is noted in men than in women.

Some studies note that women may better respond to selective serotonin reuptake inhibitors than tricyclic antidepressants. In another, men responded more to a tricyclic than to a selective serotonin reuptake inhibitor. Women taking selective serotonin reuptake inhibitors are more likely to report side effects of nausea and dizziness, whereas men reported increased urinary frequency and sexual dysfunction.

With respect to tricyclic antidepressants, women complain more of nausea, whereas men report increased urinary frequency and sexual dysfunction. Men appear to respond quicker to a tricyclic antidepressant than women. The exact mechanism responsible for differences in males and females is unknown. One hypothesis suggests selective serotonin reuptake inhibitors are important for female biophysiology but are not as important for males. Preliminary studies report that estrogen, a female hormone, enhances serotonin activity. This has led to the finding that hormone replacement therapy in postmenopausal women enhances selective serotonin reuptake inhibitor efficacy. The consensus among doctors knowledgeable in gender-specific medicine is that the gender and menopausal status of women should be taken into consideration when prescribing antidepressant medications.

Sex hormones such as estrogen, progesterone, testosterone, and dehydroepiandrosterone (DHE, a male hormone) have a significant effect on brain functioning through interactions with neurochemical transmitters. Alteration of these hormones will interfere with mood, behavior, and pain responses in the brain. A current study is looking at the possible antidepressant effects of hormones. The effects of hormone therapy on pain perception will also be studied.

Muscle Relaxants

Muscle relaxants are used to treat increased contraction of muscles. When a muscle is contracted, blood flow and oxygen delivery are decreased. Reduced oxygen causes a buildup of lactic acid with sustained contraction, which can lead to burning pain. All of these events collectively result in muscle pain. Two classes of muscle relaxant medications can be taken to relieve muscle pain. One, an antispasmodic drug, is used to treat severe chronic muscle spasms; the other, a "centrally acting" muscle relaxant, works at the level of the brain and spinal cord and is useful in treating more mild muscle contractions. People with cerebral palsy, who suffer from sustained painful muscle contractions, require an antispasmodic muscle relaxant. People with episodic muscle pain are best treated with centrally acting muscle relaxants.

A muscle "spasm" is an increase in muscle tone not under the control of the affected individual that increases during movement of the muscle. It is mostly seen with stretching of the muscle. Muscle spasms result from decreased transmission of nerve impulses to the muscle. People with spinal cord injuries can have muscle spasms even though the nerves to the muscles are damaged. Antispasmodic drugs can act within the central nervous system, especially the spinal cord, to decrease muscle contractivity and even exert a depressant effect on the muscle itself. Examples of centrally acting antispasmodics include benzodiazepines (for instance, Valium), baclofen (Lioresal), and tizanidine (Zanaflex).

Because of the potential side effects associated with muscle relaxants in general, people suffering from pain generally attempt other modalities first. These modalities should include stretching exercises, range of motion exercises, and heat/cold packs. Water aerobics may help reduce the pain associated with muscle spasms. The heat of the water can be soothing and can directly relax tense muscles. Only when these modalities have failed should one consider the use of muscle relaxant drugs.

Drugs Used for Muscle Relaxants

Valium, a benzodiazepine, exerts its effect on the central nervous system by decreasing the excitability of nerves going to the muscle. Valium is an especially effective drug for people with spinal cord injuries and resulting muscle spasms. It is also used for people with spasms from cerebral palsy and those that follow a stroke. Valium can also be used for muscle pain following an injury. Unfortunately, Valium and other benzodiazepines can cause drowsiness, dizziness, decreased muscle strength, and can be addictive. Valium is also used for the treatment of anxiety, although anxiety and depression can also be side effects of the drug. If Valium is stopped immediately, seizures may occur. Because Valium is highly addictive, it is rarely used by pain-medicine specialists.

Baclofen (Lioresal) is another antispasmodic drug. Like Valium, Baclofen decreases conduction in the nerves that go to muscles and is used in the treatment of painful muscle spasms associated with spinal cord injuries and other conditions. Baclofen causes less sedation than Valium; however, sedation can occur if the dose is too high. With smaller doses, side effects are few to none; the dose can then be slowly increased to allow the body to adjust to its effects. Addiction potential with baclofen is much less than with Valium. Baclofen's effects are not as long lasting as Valium's; more frequent dosing may be necessary.

Dantrolene (Dantrium) is another antispasmodic drug. Unlike the antispasmodics so far discussed, Dantrolene exerts its effects on muscle tissue, directly reducing muscle tone. Dantrolene can cause dizziness and confusion. Dantrolene is also used to decrease spasms associated with spinal cord injury and stroke. Because it results in significant muscle weakness, it is not used in patients who have to walk, including most people being treated for pain, and is mostly used in those who are bedridden. Dantrolene can cause liver injury. For this reason, patients must have periodic blood tests to measure liver function.

Tizanidine (Zanaflex) is a drug frequently prescribed by pain-management doctors. This medication works at the spinal cord level and lasts about four hours, reducing muscle spasms and also decreasing sharp and burning pain. It can boost the effects of opioid drugs. Like most muscle relaxants, Zanaflex has side effects, including dry mouth, fatigue, and occasionally dizziness. It can also decrease blood pressure. If the medication is abruptly stopped, an elevation in blood pressure may occur, which can be pronounced in people who already have high blood pressure. Unlike Valium and baclofen, Zanaflex can decrease muscle spasms without causing muscle weakness.

Zanaflex decreases transmission of impulses in the nerve fibers that transmit pain from the arms and legs to the spinal cord and ultimately the brain, making it effective not only by decreasing muscle spasm but also by inhibiting firing of the nerves that transmit pain impulses. The drug does not interfere with day-to-day life because it causes little sedation and dizziness. The absence of muscle weakness makes it safe to use in people who need to get about for work and so on. This medication may cause headaches, dry mouth, and, rarely, hallucinations. Patients may want to suck on ice cubes or chew sugarless chewing gum to counter the drying effects. Because this medication can decrease blood pressure, people taking it should have their blood pressure carefully monitored, especially if they are taking antihypertensive drugs. Devices to measure one's blood pressure are readily available at most drugstores.

As previously stated, the centrally acting muscle relaxants are used for more mild muscle pain or spasms. These agents include carisoprodol (Soma), chlorzoxazone (Paraflex), cyclobenzaprine (Flexeril), methocarbamol (Robaxin), and metaxalone (Skelaxin). All drugs decrease pain by decreasing muscle spasms. Use of these drugs should include physical therapy for individuals with acute muscle injuries if the pain persists for more than two weeks. Heat and cold packs should also be used in combination with these medications. These centrally acting muscle relaxant drugs are useful in situations where there has been a muscle strain in addition to pain and swelling in the muscle tissues. Studies demonstrating the effects of skeletal muscle relaxants have shown improvement in muscle problems when compared with placebo pills. All of these mild muscle relaxants have been shown to be effective, but Flexeril is most effective for chronic use. Soma may cause sedation. It has abuse potential and has a street value among substance abusers.

Flexeril, which is chemically related to the tricyclic antidepressants, has antidepressant activities in addition to its effects on decreasing muscle spasms, and is an excellent medication to induce sleep. It does not decrease muscle strength and is not effective for spasticity associated with strokes or spinal cord injuries. Flexeril reduces the number of pain impulses that reach the pain center in the brain. Flexeril is recommended for short-term use. Long-term use studies remain to be completed. Side effects include drowsiness and dry mouth. Flexeril and other muscle relaxants should not be used with alcohol. Alcohol should not be consumed when any medication is used.

Soma will relax muscles somewhat through its effects on the central nervous system, causing sedation, which relaxes muscles. It is not useful for treating spasms associated with spinal cord injury or strokes. This drug can cause mental irritability and difficulties with sleep (despite causing drowsiness and dizziness). People should not drive or operate machinery when taking *any* muscle relaxant medications because it can decrease their overall response time.

Skelaxin is a muscle relaxant that is prescribed by many pain-medicine doctors. It has the fewest side effects of all the mild centrally acting muscle relaxing medications. It can be used safely in geriatric patients (because these patients can become easily sedated). This drug causes minimal sedation or dizziness. Dizziness is to be avoided, especially in elderly patients because a fall can cause a hip fracture or other bone fracture because their bones are brittle. In some patients, it may cause gastrointestinal upset, including nausea and vomiting.

Muscle Relaxants for Muscle-Overuse Injuries

Muscle relaxants can be beneficial in muscle-overuse injuries. Another study has demonstrated the beneficial effects of a muscle relaxant on overuse injuries especially in females. An overuse injury is a result of chronic overuse rather than from a single traumatic event. With overuse, there is an accumulation of muscle damage that is a result of insufficient recovery time from minor muscle injury.

Chronic use can result in microscopic injury to the muscle tissue. The repair of the muscle tissue or ligament tissue may be incomplete before further use occurs. The effect of increased mechanical stimulation can stimulate pain receptors in muscle tissue. Females suffer more frequent ligament injuries or muscle injuries than males, especially during certain times of the menstrual cycle. It is known that ligaments in pregnant patients are lax during pregnancy. Female hormone levels contribute to the laxity of the ligaments. An increase in hormones during pregnancy has been shown to decrease the pain associated with rheumatoid arthritis. Women may be more prone to overuse injuries because of the differences between males and females with respect to hormonal factors and connective tissue stress tolerances. Flexeril appears to be the muscle relaxant that is most studied for the treatment of these injuries.

Studies on Muscle Relaxants

With respect to gender specificity, studies have demonstrated that women may have a more profound response to benzodiazapines than males. Valium can enhance the chemicals in the brain and spinal cord that can inhibit pain impulses. Valium in high enough doses may also suppress seizures. With respect to the control of seizures, there are no gender differences between males and females. On the other hand, it is the effects on pain that are more pronounced in the female patients. The exact cause is not known but may be hormonal related. Studies with Zanaflex reveal that gender has no effects on the breakdown of the drug in the liver, the effects of the drug on receptors, or on the excretion of the drug by the kidneys.

Studies comparing Skelaxin and Flexeril report that Skelaxin appears to have better muscle relaxing results than Flexeril but lacks the sedative effects that Flexeril possesses. The tolerability as well as the effectiveness of Skelaxin was superior to Flexeril in some studies. Gender specificity was not addressed in these investigations, and no gender-specific results were reported.

Studies from a military center have demonstrated that the short-acting muscle relaxant may be most effective for the first four days following a muscle injury. The efficacy of the drug may decrease after that. On study, comprised of a majority of male subjects, suggested that the short-acting muscle relaxant should be used primarily after an acute injury to a muscle group.

Gender specificity with respect to muscle relaxants has not been studied in depth. The reason is probably related to the fact that most muscle relaxants available today are a result of original studies of the male population. These studies were done before the advent of gender-specificity interest with respect to pharmaceutical agents. As new muscle relaxants are developed, it is anticipated that the pharmaceutical companies will include gender-specific studies in their clinical trials as recommended by the FDA.

Chapter 5
Assessing Pain with Your Doctor

Several different techniques are available for your doctor to use in determining your level of pain. Commonly used techniques include verbal, visual, and psychological tests. Both you and your doctor are responsible for documenting and recording trends in the intensity and frequency of your pain. This information tells each of you whether your pain has really improved or whether it has worsened. Charting your pain levels will help your doctor see your long-range pain trends, which are ultimately more important than your day-to-day pain trends.

You may wonder why you need to measure your pain. A pain-experience measurement is extremely valuable to both you and your doctor. It provides a baseline for your doctor to assess any therapy or medications you are currently taking, and it also helps your doctor to prescribe future therapy methods. Your doctor also needs to be able to determine how much disability you have in order to prescribe the appropriate types of therapy for you.

Many of the test instruments mentioned in this chapter enable doctors to diagnose a specific pain condition. They also help doctors determine whether the patient is truly in pain or just making it up. You should be able to easily understand the test you are being given so that it is as accurate as possible at measuring your level of pain.

After reading this chapter you will be able to see that you and your doctor can use several different pain-assessment forms to monitor your pain-medicine therapy. Which form is best for you? There is no definite answer to this question. The assessment form that you feel most comfortable with and one that you will use is the best pain assessment for both you and your doctor. These assessment scales help you and your doctor plan an individualized pain-management program. Look over your pain-assessment evaluations carefully. If you are not decreasing your pain, or if your pain is becoming worse, you and your physician must evaluate other treatments for your pain. You and your doctor must develop a partnership in the control of your pain.

Determining What Type of Assessment to Use

Your doctor will depend on you for accurate and reliable answers to questions about the pain you feel. Because pain involves many aspects such as sensory, emotional, and behavioral factors, it is difficult to measure the amount of pain you feel based on one thing. Your doctor will carefully instruct you as to how to report your pain when going through a pain-assessment test.

The choice of a pain-assessment test depends on the needs of both you and your doctor. A functional evaluation, such as reports of your daily activities, must be included in your assessment. If your doctor does not ask about your daily activities, voluntarily tell him or her your further limitations with respect to work, recreation, dressing, fixing meals, and any other daily activities.

Use a daily pain diary and tell your doctor whether your pain is becoming worse or is getting better. This will enable your doctor to assess your medication and therapy needs. Positive effects of therapy are best assessed when your doctor keeps a database of your pain progression. This type of data is easily stored on a computer. This type of database is even more valuable because your doctor can graph important data from each of your visits.

The assessment and measurement of pain has received considerable attention in the past two decades. Progress continues to be made in developing pain-assessment tools. You or your doctor should not oversimplify your pain assessment. The objective reports you are able to give, as well the observations your doctor is able to make about your behavior, are important to accurate pain management decisions.

Health-Care Provider Assessment

Because pain is subjective and can be observed only by you, it is important that the reports of your pain levels come from you. This will give your doctor a more accurate measurement of the type of pain you are experiencing. For example, if you just complain of a toothache, your doctor will have almost no way of knowing how severe your pain is.

On occasion, your doctor will need to rate your level of pain if you are not able for some reason to identify your level of pain. In general, you should be able to accurately describe your level of pain. If you are not able to rate your pain yourself, it should be done only by your doctor or other type of health-care provider.

Each doctor's approach to managing pain may differ. Therefore, it is important that you and your doctor have a healthy doctor–patient relationship and that your doctor understands your situation. The situations and causes of each person's pain differ, and therefore, your doctor may suggest different combinations of methods to help relieve your pain.

Using Pain Assessment Forms

The current methods doctors have available to measure your pain are imperfect. The perception of pain is based on many things that affect you, and can range from memories of a previous painful event to psychological influences. Pain is not necessarily just a sensory experience, but it is also a result of processes that occur at a higher level in the brain, making pain a psychological experience.

There is no general consensus among pain medicine doctors as to the best test for the measurement of pain. An ideal test for the assessment of pain must bring together experimental as well as clinical knowledge. Right now, there are no adequate tests that can differentiate gender with respect to the assessment of pain. In order to provide adequate pain management, a doctor must combine all of the data given by you concerning your pain complaints. Hopefully a universally accepted pain assessment test will become available in the near future. In the meantime, you and your doctor must talk not only about pain complaints, but also about your feelings of depression and anxiety during each office visit. You and your doctor must develop a healthy relationship so that the appropriate pain modalities can be rationally prescribed specifically for you.

Taking a Verbal Assessment

Pain is subjective and does not allow itself to be measured accurately. In other words, it is impossible to visualize "pain." When your doctor interviews you about your pain complaints, he or she will begin by asking the following questions: the time of the onset of your pain, the location of the pain on your body, how long it lasts, and how often it occurs during the day. Your doctor will also ask you whether your pain is sharp, dull, or cramping. You should tell your doctor whether your pain is mild, moderate, or severe. Women in general are more able to express their pain experiences than men. You must provide your doctor with enough information so that he or she can come up with a reasonable and accurate diagnosis for you.

What follows is an initial pain-assessment form. This assessment addresses your pain and psychosocial issues and leaves room for your doctor's evaluation of your condition. Your doctor will give you a copy of this assessment form. You will be asked questions such as when the pain began, how long it lasts, what makes it worse, what makes it better, what medications you are taking, what effects medications are having on your pain, and what your emotional status is during episodes of pain.

One way of assessing your pain is to use a numeric scale. This is the simplest method for attempting to measure your pain. During this test, you are asked to rate your pain on a scale of 0 to 5 or to use words such as "none," "slight," "moderate," or "severe." This assessment is also a quick, simple, and reliable way to evaluate the effectiveness of any medications you are taking to manage your pain.

On the numeric scale, 0 equals no pain, 1 equals mild pain, 2 equals moderate pain, 3 equals distressing pain, 4 equals horrible pain, and 5 equals excruciating pain confining you to bed rest. This method is easily understood and may be helpful in guiding the treatment plans your doctor creates for you.

Another type of verbal scale asks you to rate your pain on a scale of 1 to 10, with 1 being equivalent to pain that is barely noticeable, and 10 relating to excruciating pain. A verbal numeric scale is easily understood. All you have to do is choose a number to represent your level of pain.

The following numeric pain-intensity scale is the most popular test used by pain-medicine specialists. You circle a number on the scale that corresponds to how much pain you feel. It only uses numbers from 0 through 10 along the length of the horizontal scale. A score of 0 indicates no pain, whereas a score of 10 means that you feel the worst pain ever imagined.

Today's Date:

Name: Age:

Address: Birthdate:

I. Pain History

1.) When did the pain start?

2.) Where does it hurt?

3.) How often does the pain occur?

4.) What makes the pain worse?

5.) What makes the pain better?

6.) Describe the pain:

7.) Is the pain better now than in the past?

8.) When was your pain the worst?

9.) Do you notice any other problems associated with your pain?

II. Pain Goals

1.) Realistically, how soon can we correct your pain?

2.) What is your pain scale goal?

III. Doctor's Examination

IV. Imaging/Tests

V. Treatment Plan

An initial pain-assessment form.

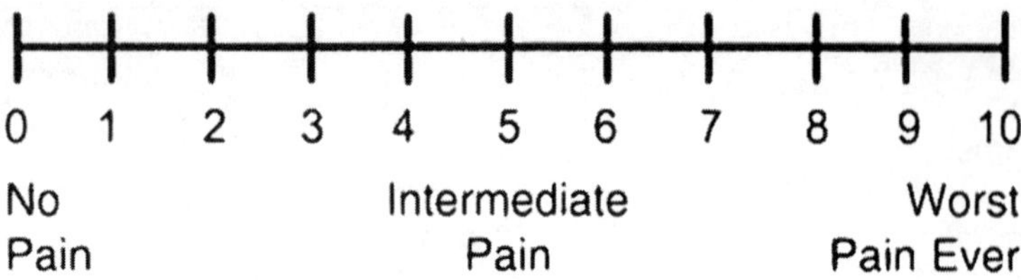

A numeric pain-intensity assessment.

Another method used by some doctors is a pain diary. This is a descriptive report you keep to assess your pain. The pain diary shows a written account of your day-to-day experiences. It can be used to help diagnose the cause of your pain. The value of the pain diary is that you and your doctor can monitor your day-to-day variation of painful states and your response to therapy. You need to keep a diary of your pain patterns when you are sitting, standing, and lying down. Also record sleep patterns and sexual activity. You also must note the amount of pain medication you are taking and whether it lessens your pain. Because pain can interfere with eating patterns, keep a diary of the amount of food you eat and at what time you ate. Be sure to include any types of recreational activities and whether your pain felt better or worse afterward.

The following is a sample of a pain diary that you may find useful. You have to be diligent in your record keeping. This form enables you to record an entire month of pain-intensity scores, your activities, the location of your pain, and a medication log. Your physician will find this diary extremely helpful in working with you to plan your pain therapy.

Date	Duration	Location	Severity	Treatment	Response	Comments

A pain diary form.

Giving a Visual Assessment

Pain drawings offer a visual way to evaluate your pain. You will be asked to shade in areas on a human figure outline that correspond to the areas of your pain. The drawing will help your doctor determine where your pain is coming from and how widespread it is on your body. Over time, your pain drawings can be compared to show the changes of your pain and how you are responding to therapy.

The following is a sample pain-assessment tool that includes diagrams for you to shade to tell your doctor whether your pain is confined to one area of your body or whether your pain is widespread throughout your body. This form allows you to shade the areas of your body where you are feeling your pain.

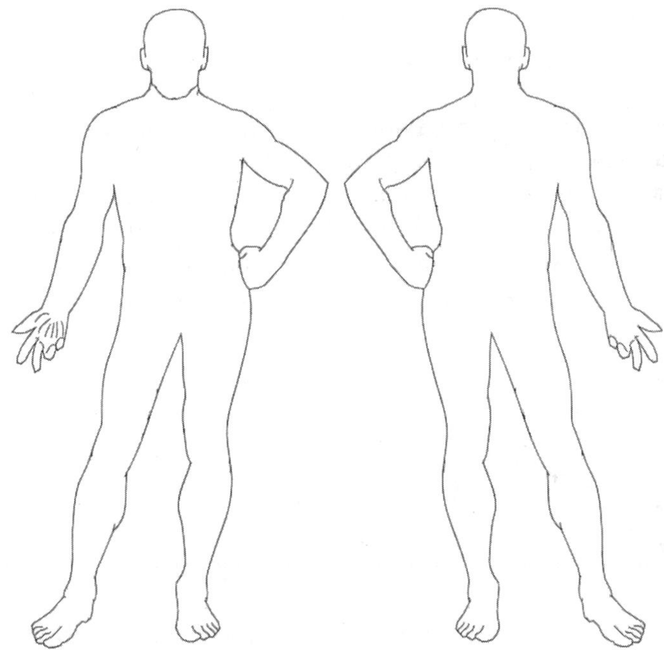

Shading Pain Assessment Form.

A common method of determining the behavioral component of your pain is for you to be directly observed by your doctor. You must be observed while sitting, walking to and from the office, and getting in and out of vehicles. Your doctor will focus his or her attention on the area of your major pain complaint.

Behavioral influences affecting your perception of pain include the amount of medications you use and the number of doctor visits required. Limping and facial grimacing also are appropriate behavioral evaluations of pain. Depression and anxiety are emotional factors that can be measured by tests.

Because the experience of pain is impossible to measure directly, your doctor must observe your displays of appropriate or inappropriate physical behavior. After observing your behavior, your doctor may classify you using the following four-class system: Class 1 consists of patients with low physical injury but high levels of abnormal behavior patterns related to their pain. Class 2 consists of patients with lower physical injury and low behavior pattern abnormalities. Class 3 consists of patients with significant tissue injury in addition to high behavioral pattern abnormalities. Class 4 consists of patients with a high tissue injury and a normal behavioral patterns.

A visual analog scale is another method of assessment that attempts to measure your level of pain. Instead of choosing a number, you are asked to mark a point on a horizontal line that is labeled with "no pain" at one end and "the worst possible pain" at the opposite end. The line is divided into 10 equal spaces, and you choose a number from 1 to 10 based on your level of pain. It is slightly more difficult to administer than the numeric method, but some doctors and researchers think that the visual analog scale is more accurate than the numeric scale for pain measurements.

On the following form you will circle a point on the line that indicates how much pain you feel. Descriptive words are placed along the horizontal scale, which enables you to describe the severity of your pain.

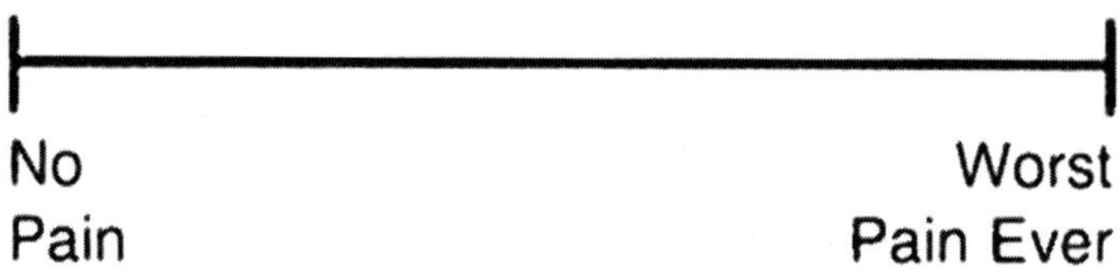

A visual analog scale assessment form.

Another visual scale that is easy to use, especially for children, is the face scale. It shows pictures of happy to grimacing faces and patients are asked to circle the face that shows what kind of pain they feel.

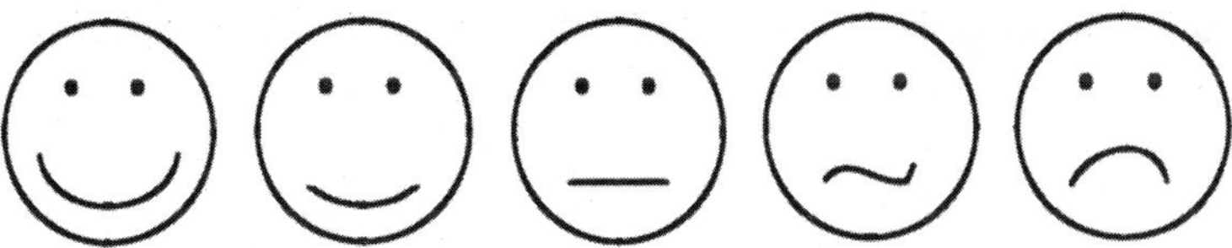

Graphic Rating Scale Assessment Form.

Gathering a Psychological Assessment

Using descriptive words is one method of describing your pain. Self-reports have been used by doctors since 1939. A pain-rating index consists of groups of words associated with pain. This index has been incorporated into the McGill pain questionnaire, a type of verbal assessment that uses word descriptors that are valuable in discriminating between different pain syndromes.

For the following pain assessment form you will circle the words that best describe your pain. Since they are in no particular order, there is no obvious progression of pain shown.

Moderate
Severe
Mild
No Pain
Barely Noticeable
Excruciating

A descriptive pain-intensity scale assessment form.

A McGill pain questionnaire is a method for assessing pain psychologically. A McGill pain questionnaire gives a multidimensional pain score. You are given 20 word sets that describe a different dimension of your pain. You are asked to select words relevant to your pain from each of these 20 sets. For example, one set includes the words "jumping," "flashing," and "shooting." Another set includes the words "tingling," "itching," "smarting," and "stinging." You circle the word that relates closest to the pain you feel throughout the 20 word sets.

This questionnaire is difficult to administer as well as to interpret. However, it has characteristic response patterns for different pain syndromes such as back pain, arthritis, and cancer. The validity of this questionnaire continues to be studied.

The McGill pain questionnaire consists of four different parts. The first part consists of a human figure drawing on which you are instructed to mark the location of your pain. The second part is the pain-rating index that contains 78 words divided into 20 groups. Each set contains up to six words. Five of these groups describe tension or fear. Each word is assigned a value according to its position within a subclass. The third part of this test asks additional questions about prior pain experiences, as well as the location of the pain and current usage of pain medications. The fourth part consists of a present pain intensity index. This aspect of the test requests a pain score from 0 to 5 with word descriptors such as no pain, mild pain, discomforting pain, distressing pain, or horrible and excruciating pain. These words also are assigned different values. All the values are added to obtain a total score. All the scores are then evaluated to attempt to assess your total pain experience.

The problem with this test is that there is no specific mechanism within the test itself to determine which component truly reflects your pain experience. The value of this test, however, is that it treats pain as a multidimensional experience. There also is a short form of the McGill pain questionnaire that has been developed. This questionnaire contains fewer words and categories than the long form. This test is sensitive to evaluations of reduction in pain experiences. This test is also more useful for rapid evaluation of data following procedures or surgery.

Chapter 6

Learning About Opioid Drugs and Pain Management

Opioids are a type of medication used to relieve pain. Opioids are a class of drugs which depress the central nervous system to relieve pain. An opioid is a drug that acts similarly to morphine. Some opioids are found naturally in the environment, whereas others are made in a lab. A *narcotic* is a similar type of medication. However, it applies to drugs similar to morphine as well as to any type of substance that could cause you to become dependent on it.

Morphine is the drug that has been studied the most with respect to the treatment of pain. Morphine was named after Morpheus, the Greek god of dreams. It is prepared from the liquid of the opium poppy plant. Morphine was the first opioid ever used for pain relief. Naturally occurring types of opioid drugs include morphine and codeine. Man-made types of opioids include fentanyl, meperidine (Demerol), and methadone. Altering naturally occurring opioids will produce a semi-synthetic drug, such as heroin.

It is not uncommon for a doctor to prescribe opioids for treating severe pain. However, doctors are sometimes afraid of prescribing these drugs because of the potential for abuse. If prescribed properly, however, opioid drugs are safe and effective for treating both cancer and noncancer types of pain. It is important that you understand how opioids work and how you should use them properly if they are prescribed to you for the treatment of your pain.

In this chapter, you will learn how opioids work, as well as the difference between narcotics and opioids. You will also learn how to take care of yourself if you are using opioids for treatment of your pain. Addictions and their effects will be discussed, along with drug abuse, alcohol abuse, smoking, and illicit drug use. If you will be using opioids to treat your pain, it is important that you educate yourself on how they work and how they can interact with other chemicals in your body.

How Opioids Work

Opioids bind themselves to receptors on nerves in your body that are located in your *central nervous system* and in the *peripheral nerves* in your arms and legs. When the opioid attaches to one of your receptors, it turns it on. When the receptor is turned on like this, the number of pain sensations that reach your brain are lessened.

Opioid drugs can either be classified as weak or strong, depending on how they interact with the opioid receptors in your body. Codeine and propoxyphene (Darvon) are considered weak opioids. All others are considered strong opioids.

All opioid drugs provide pain relief by decreasing the amount of chemicals that transmit pain. With this decrease in the chemicals that transmit pain, your overall pain impulses are dampened or may not even reach the brain at all. Some opioid medications can alter your mood or occasionally cause you to experience euphoria or excitement. Changes in the chemicals that exist in your brain cause these types of mood changes. When you take opioids over a large time span of weeks or months, you can build up a tolerance to the effect of the opioids. When you become tolerant to the opioid, its ability to relieve your pain is lessened, and more of the drug is needed to relieve it.

Agonists and Antagonists

Opioid drugs can be further classified into three categories: *agonist, antagonist,* and *mixed agonist/antagonist. Agonist* drugs such as morphine attach to two of the three opioid receptors in your brain and spinal cord to provide pain relief by switching the receptors on. *Antagonist* drugs bind to all three types of receptors throughout your body. When they bind to the receptor, they do not switch the receptor on. The *mixed agonist/antagonist* drugs stimulate activities at the opioid receptors, but do not allow them to be switched on.

Morphine is classified as a naturally occurring agonist drug. It has been made into a slow-release formula. The slow-release morphine (MS Contin) needs to be taken only every 12 hours. It allows a gradual release of morphine as the pill passes through your stomach and intestine.

Codeine is considered a weak agonist *drug* and is not commonly used for severe pain management. It is often used for mild pain, whereas morphine is used for more severe types of pain. Codeine also is less likely to cause addiction than other opioids. When codeine enters your body, it is converted into morphine, which produces its pain-relieving effects.

Receptor Effects

An example of a synthetic opioid is methadone. Methadone lasts a long time in the body. This drug offers an advantage to patients because less-frequent dosing is required. Methadone is an excellent medication for use in patients who have some component of their pain that is related to nerve inflammation such as shingles (discussed in Chapter 27) or reflex sympathetic dystrophy (discussed in Chapter 24). Propoxyphene (Darvon) is a drug that is related in its chemical structure with methadone. Its pain-relieving effects have been claimed to be less than that of aspirin. The advantage of this drug is that it has novacainelike activity. It has been shown in animals to be a potent local anesthetic. This drug may be effective in patients suffering from mild cases of shingles or mild cases of nerve inflammation as seen in the later stages of reflex sympathetic dystrophy where the patient is getting progressively better. Meperidine (Demerol) can cause seizures if it is administered for a long time in patients. The medication fentanyl was originally used for anesthesia during surgery. However, fentanyl can now be administered by a patch or by a lozenge. It is also available in a sucker form for administering to children. Fentanyl is one of the most powerful drugs that have been mentioned.

The fentanyl (Duragesic) patch was introduced in the late 1980s. It became popular for the treatment of chronic cancer pain. In patients who are unable to swallow or have persistent diarrhea, the patch will provide continuous pain relief. The effects of fentanyl are 70 times more powerful than morphine. It is readily absorbed through the skin. The patch holds the fentanyl in a small amount of alcohol in a gel. The gel is deposited in a drug reservoir within the patch. Between the reservoir and the skin is a membrane that is regulated by various-size holes. An adhesive layer keeps the patch attached to the skin. When the patch is applied to the skin, the drug spreads through the holes in the membrane to the skin. The fentanyl is then concentrated in the outermost layer of the skin. As the drug is deposited in the skin, it is gradually taken from the skin into the bloodstream. It takes at least 60 minutes before any fentanyl actually is detected in a patient's blood. It takes approximately six hours before pain relief is felt. After the initial patch, placement of subsequent patches does not have a delay in the onset of pain relief. It should be noted that an increase in temperature will increase the absorption of the drug from the patch. This can cause side effects or even an overdose of the fentanyl. The patients using the fentanyl patch should not use a heating blanket, sun lamp, or a warm bathing tub. In cancer patients, patient acceptance is high. Occasionally patients using the patch will have an episode of temporary pain called breakthrough pain. This pain is seen if a patient becomes overly active. A fentanyl lozenge (Actuic) has been introduced which has a relatively fast onset. The fentanyl lozenge can be used to enhance the effects of the fentanyl patch.

Tramadol (Ultram) is a synthetic chemical similar to codeine. It also increases serotonin and norepinephrine in your brain and spinal cord. These are two chemicals within the central nervous system that decrease feelings of depression. Serotonin and norepinepherine also decrease the number of pain impulses that ultimately reach your brain. Tramadol also can be combined with acetaminophen (Ultracet) to provide mild pain-relieving effects.

Butorphanol (Stadol nasal spray) and nalbuphine (Nubain) are agonist/antagonist drugs. Butorphanol is available as a nasal spray and is now in a generic form. Nalbuphine is another agonist/antagonist drug that is available only intravenously.

Effects of Morphine on Men and Women

Side effects of opioids can include drowsiness, alteration in mood, and mental clouding. If the dosage is too high, your ability to concentrate can be affected. Opioid drugs can decrease your breathing rate. If the dosage of the opioid is high enough, it is possible for you to completely quit breathing. Nausea and vomiting are common with all the opioids. The opioid drugs can decrease pupil size. This is a result of stimulation of part of a nerve of the eye that controls the opening and closing of the pupil. The morphinelike drugs decrease the cough reflex and can be useful in this matter. If the dose of the opioids is too high, it can decrease your blood pressure. Opioids can cause constipation. They cause constipation by decreasing the ability of the stomach and bowel to push food through to the rectum. Some of the agonist drugs also can cause hives.

Animal studies have demonstrated the differences between males and females with respect to responses to opioids. Male rats have demonstrated greater pain relief with morphine than female rats following painful stimuli. In another laboratory study, there were no sex differences reported with fentanyl and buphrenorphine. The same types of effects have been found in people.

It is imperative that your pain be controlled and that you must be treated with both dignity as well as compassion by the treating doctor even if you have a history of substance abuse. The problem exists in that many drug-seeking individuals will seek out a pain-medicine doctor to receive opioid drugs. This type of behavior ultimately leads to state regulations that ultimately make it more difficult for legitimate patients to get prescriptions for their medications.

The following are ten behaviors that are compatible with addiction:

1. Selling prescription drugs
2. Prescription forgery
3. Theft of drugs from other individuals
4. Diluting and injecting oral pills
5. Obtaining prescription drugs from nonmedical personnel
6. Concurrent use of alcohol with an opioid drug or a tranquilizer and repeated drug escalations despite warnings from the individual's health-care provider
7. Repeated visits to other doctors or emergency rooms to obtain drugs
8. Men who drink more than four drinks per day
9. Women who exceed three drinks per day
10. An individual under the age of 40 who admits to marijuana and also smokes cigarettes

These are some criteria for those who are at risk for addiction. Other risk factors for addiction are people who feel inadequate or have poor stress-management skills. People who have multiple life stressors are prone to addiction. Increased substance abuse was noted in New York after the 9/11 terrorist attack. Those with a previous history of physical, emotional, or sexual abuse may be prone to substance abuse. A family history of severe depression can make a person more prone to drug addiction. A family history of substance abuse is an additional risk factor. Regular contact with drug-using individuals is also an additional risk factor for the development of drug addiction. For the majority of patients, there is a low risk of an addiction being caused by their doctor's prescribed treatment plan. As a result, the treating doctor should focus on the goal of reducing their patient's pain.

Most pain-medicine doctors require that a patient sign a contract when the patient is admitted into the doctor's practice. The contract states that the patient will obtain pain-relieving medications from only one doctor and will use only one pharmacy. These contracts are usually mandated by state medical boards.

A doctor treating a patient with significant pain must provide comfort to the patient. Each year, more than a million patients are prescribed opioid analgesics but do not develop addiction. A study published in 1996 reported that there was no significant difference in the rate of substance abuse among patients with severe chronic back pain versus a controlled group with no back pain. An important conclusion was derived. These investigators concluded that severe pain is not associated with an increased risk for substance abuse. If you are taking medications for pain relief, your chances of becoming addicted are extremely low.

The cost of alcoholism and drug dependency places a huge burden on society. Drug and alcohol addiction taxes the health-care system, harms family life, and threatens the public safety. Drug addiction crosses all social boundaries. It affects both genders as well as every ethnic group and people in every tax bracket. Drug addiction and alcoholism are diseases that may be caused by genetic susceptibility as well as personal misbehavior. Substance abuse contributes to more deaths and disabilities each year than any other cause.

Approximately 18 million individuals in the United States have alcohol problems, and approximately 6 million individual have a drug problem. Approximately 50 percent of all adults have a family history of alcoholism. Approximately 9 million children live with a parent who is dependent on either alcohol or drugs. Twenty-five percent of all emergency room visits and 33 percent of all suicides as well as more than 50 percent of all homicides are alcohol or drug related. Fifty percent of all traffic fatalities are alcohol related. Approximately 50 percent of people who die in fires have elevated blood alcohol levels. Alcoholism and drug addiction cost the American economy approximately $276 billion per year in lost productivity, health-care costs, crime, and motor vehicle accidents. Problems that occur in the workplace include absenteeism, tardiness, problematic interactions with supervisors, mistakes in work, as well as incomplete work. Both alcoholism and drug addiction are diseases that affect both physical and behavioral health. Substance abuse has become America's primary health problem.

Problems also exist when substance abuse occurs in the cancer setting because cancer patients usually require large doses of morphine or morphinelike drugs. This is a complex problem. Misuse of opioids in cancer patients is extremely rare among patients who have no history of drug addictions. However, misuse is higher in patients who have a history of a previous drug addiction. Studies have revealed that approximately 5 percent of cancer patients have a history of substance abuse. A history of drug addiction in cancer care management can undermine patient treatment compliance. Doctors must be trained to recognize drug abuse behavior so that proper treatment can be implemented.

It is important in the management of any severe chronic pain condition that you and your family overcome the fear that you will become an addict. You and other patients must have the opportunity to use proper opioid medications to control severe pain. It is imperative that you and other patients do not endure unnecessary pain and suffering. Both you and your doctor must understand the terms "tolerance," "physical dependency," "substance abuse," and "pseudo-addiction."

Psuedo-addiction occurs when a patient seems to crave a drug when indeed their pain is undertreated by their doctor. Unfortunately, some physicians incorrectly interpret this behavior as addiction. Pseudo-addiction can be seen in patients suffering from cancer or severe noncancer pain. These patients appear to be obsessed with obtaining opioid medications or escalate their medications to achieve pain control. This behavior is seen when patients have severe pain but their pain is not adequately managed by the amount of medication that they have been prescribed. These four entities must be distinguished from true addiction, which is a craving and a compulsive desire to obtain a drug.

Alcohol Abuse: The Differences Between Men and Women

Alcoholism is not a new addiction. At one time, drug addiction and alcoholism were considered "moral" problems that resulted from weakness and lack of will power. In the 1960s there were more than 70 million users of alcohol in the United States. This number has greatly increased since then. Six percent of the adult population today, more than 17 million, can be classified as alcoholics.

Alcoholics are individuals whose alcohol consumption seriously impairs their ability to function in activities of daily living. The incidence of alcoholism is increasing. The incidents of alcoholism tend to be higher in the middle and upper socioeconomic classes.

The average age for an alcoholic is 45 years of age. The life span of an alcoholic is 12 years shorter than the nonalcoholic individual's life span. In general, males account for a higher number of alcoholics than females. In Scandinavia, the ratio of male to female alcoholics is 23:1. In Britain the ratio is 2:1, and in the United States the ratio is approximately 5:1.

Alcohol is a depressant that affects the higher brain centers. Alcohol decreases the inhibition control centers of the brain. As a result, behavioral restraints decline. As alcohol consumption increases, coordination decrease occurs and the perception of cold and pain is dulled. The alcoholic experiences a sense of warmth and well-being. As a result, the alcoholic's self-esteem and adequacy increase. When in a drunken state, an individual's worries are temporarily left behind. During a drinking binge, an individual can be stimulated emotionally, but intellectual functions are impaired. Intoxication occurs when the alcohol content in the bloodstream reaches 0.1 percent. Speech and vision are impaired. When the blood level reaches 0.5 percent an individual will become unconscious. At 0.55 percent, the alcohol potentially lethal.

The prevalence of lifetime alcohol abuse is higher in patients with a bipolar disorder. More men than women meet the criteria for lifetime alcoholism. However, the risk of alcoholism is higher in women than men. There are gender differences in the prevalence, risk, and clinical correlates of alcoholism in individuals with bipolar disease. Individuals with bipolar disease can be more prone to chronic pain. Individuals injecting alcohol who also are prescribed pain medications that contain acetaminophen (Tylenol) can have potentially lethal liver problems. When a doctor is assessing a pain patient, the history should include whether the individual has a history of alcohol abuse. Neuron loss is essentially equal in men and women with comparable alcohol-abuse histories. Note that female alcoholics are more susceptible to brain gray matter injury than males. Women achieve higher blood alcohol levels than men with the same intake of alcohol.

With consideration to the gender specificity, women are more vulnerable than men to the adverse consequence of alcohol use. As stated previously, women achieve higher concentrations of alcohol in the bloodstream and will become more impaired than men after drinking equivalent amounts of alcohol. Women are more susceptible than men to alcohol-related organ damage and to trauma from motor vehicle accidents as well as interpersonal violence. Men are more likely than women to become alcohol dependent. Women's drinking problems are more common between the ages of 26 and 34 and among women who are divorced or separated. Alcoholism in women is more prevalent among Caucasians. (Martin and Bryant. "Gender Differences in the Association of Alcohol and Illicit Drug Abuse Among Persons Arrested for Violent and Property Offenses," *Journal of Substance Abuse* 13 [2001]: 563-81)

Women absorb alcohol differently than men. Women have less total body water than men with the same body weight. As a result, women achieve higher concentrations of alcohol in the blood after drinking equivalent amounts of alcohol. As an analogy for body water and alcohol concentrations, one should think of a shot glass and an ice-tea glass. If one puts the teaspoon of sugar into the shot glass, which has considerably less water than the ice-tea glass, one would expect the shot glass liquid to be sweeter than the ice-tea glass liquid. The ice-tea glass sugar has been diluted. This is the same principle that applies with total body water and alcohol effects. Women eliminate alcohol from their bloodstreams faster than men. Apparently the female liver metabolizes the alcohol faster than the male. This demonstrates enzyme differences between men and women.

Women are more vulnerable than men to alcohol-related organ damage. Women develop alcohol-induced liver disease over a shorter period of time after consuming less alcohol than men. Women are more likely to develop hepatitis and cirrhosis than men. A woman's increased risk for liver damage may be related to the female hormone estrogen.

Magnetic resonance imaging studies (MRI) suggest that women are more vulnerable than men to alcohol-induced brain damage. Men and women who consume one or two alcoholic drinks per day have a lower death rate from coronary artery disease than do heavy drinkers or abstainers. Moderate to heavy alcohol consumption can increase the risk for breast cancer in females.

Women who drink alcohol experience more sexual victimization than women who do not drink alcohol. Women who have been sexually abused in childhood are more likely than other women to experience alcohol-related problems. Furthermore, physical abuse during adulthood has been associated with women and alcohol abuse-related problems. The fact that alcohol induces higher incidence of organ damage in women than men is due to gender differences in the breakdown of alcohol in the liver. Damage that occurs to the brain associated with alcohol is higher in women than in men and is probably due to differences in brain chemistry between males and females.

Women and men respond differently to pharmaceuticals as well as alcohol. Of the 10 prescriptions drugs that were withdrawn from the U.S. market since January 1997, 8 caused greater health risks for women. The higher risk for women is linked to the physiological differences between men and women. The number of adverse effects related to pain management with opioids is more serious in women than men. The differences are related to the way in which drugs are taken up from your stomach and your small intestine into your bloodstream, the effect of the breakdown of the liver, and the elimination of the drugs through the kidneys.

With these facts in mind, you would expect that the amount of drug and the frequency of dosing should differ between men and women.

Smoking and Illicit Drug Use: The Differences Between Men and Women

Smoking can be a risk factor for possible addiction. Nicotine may affect men and women differently. Nicotine can enhance aggressive moods in men but have calming effects on mood changes in females. When nicotine is combined with alcohol, the nicotine enhances the effects of alcohol in women. On the other hand, in men nicotine dilutes the sedating effects of alcohol.

Women are less successful than men in quitting smoking. Women experience more severe withdrawal symptoms than men during smoking cessation. Women who do quit smoking relapse more often than men, which is probably due to the more negative emotions experienced by women.

Women who smoke a pack of cigarettes per day have a six fold increased risk of heart attack compared to women who have never smoked. In male smokers, there is a threefold increased risk. Smoking increases the risk of coronary artery disease in younger women as a result of inhibiting valuable estrogen hormones in the female's body. Smoking also increases the level of the LDL cholesterol (bad cholesterol) in women significantly more than in men. This again is probably due to a hormonal affect. Women who smoke are more prone to develop chronic pulmonary disease than males. Smoking can increase the risk of diabetes more in females than in males. The incidence of illness from secondhand smoke is higher in women than in men.

With respect to illicit drugs, the electric activities within a man's brain when measured by the electroencephalogram (EEG) are changed by cocaine abuse while there are no changes when a woman abuses cocaine. Women are less likely than men to experience symptoms of paranoia when smoking cocaine as compared to men. Women who take amphetamines perceive the effects of the drug differently than men.

Self-Education on Addictions

As you learned in this chapter, men and women differ with respect to the effects of prescription opioids, alcohol, nicotine, and illicit drugs. It is unknown how many patients who are receiving pain medications are taking the other substances that are mentioned. As previously stated, alcohol and acetaminophen can have potentially lethal interactions. The effect of nicotine on mood in female patients can ultimately have an effect on pain perception and could potentially decrease the efficacy of opioid medications. Patients who are taking any opioid medication should not use alcohol or illicit drugs. It is furthermore recommended that tobacco substances not be used.

Research continues with respect to substance abuse and addiction. The American Society of Addiction Medicine continues to promote research in the field of addiction medicine. Doctors need to change their attitudes, knowledge, and practices about how pain is treated differently in men and women. Many doctors who have no training in pain medicine often underestimate the power of the pain-relieving effects of opioids and overestimate how long they can have an effect on your feelings of pain. The only way to properly administer opioid medications for pain control is for your doctor to carefully assess and reassess your level of pain each time you come in for a visit.

Doctors have been criticized for either not prescribing, prescribing too much, or prescribing too little opioid medications for pain management. The stories of abuse of opioids as pain relievers can make it appear that opioids are dangerous and addictive. Oxycontin has even been called "hilly-billy heroin" in some articles. Some medical communities have even recommended banning this drug. The problem only exists with the few people who choose to actually abuse Oxycontin. In reality, it is an extremely effective drug for the management of many chronic pain syndromes.

Public, patient, and self-education is the key to eliminating fears associated with opioid addiction. As long as you do not have a substance-abuse disorder, the likelihood that you will become addicted to opioids is extremely rare. The American Pain Society is requesting that legislatures avoid making policies that establish barriers to keep opioid drugs from the people who need them. The fact that some people abuse opioids should not be a barrier to keeping opioids from people who actually need them. Everyone needs to be educated about the important role of opioid drugs in pain management. (Chen and Kandei. "Relation-ship Between Extent of Cocaine Use and Dependence Among Adoles-cents and Adults in the United States," *Drugs and Alcohol Dependence* 68 [2002]: 65-85) (C.H. Gleiter and U. Gundert-Remy. "Gender Differences in Pharmacokinetics," *European Journal of Drug Metabol Pharmacokinet* 21 [1996]: 123-8) (Compton, et al. "The Specificity of Family History of Alcohol and Drug Abuse in Cocaine Abusers," *American Journal on Addictions* 121 [2002]: 85-94) (Martin and Bryant. "Gender Differences in the Association of Alcohol and Illicit Drug Abuse Among Persons Arrested for Violent and Property Offenses," *Journal of Substance Abuse* 13 [2001]: 563-81)

Chapter 7

Reducing Pain with Nonsteroidal Anti-Inflammatory Drugs

You may benefit from a drug that you see advertised as well as the many other drugs available at your pharmacy. For example, nonsteroidal anti-inflammatory drugs (NSAIDs) can decrease your pain if you suffer from the following: rheumatoid or osteoarthritis, headaches, menstrual pain, or generalized acute and chronic pain. Some of the NSAIDs are used for pain and for inflammation.

Like opioids, NSAIDs are a class of drugs that have similar chemical structures and properties and are effective for many forms of pain. Unlike opiods, NSAIDs do not cause addiction. But, be aware! NSAIDs can have serious side effects, including bleeding from the stomach and intestines, and are responsible for as many as 10,000 deaths per year when used in prescribed doses.

This chapter will teach you about the different types of NSAIDs and how they work to relieve your pain. You will also learn about the benefits and risks associated with using NSAIDs, as well as why they work differently in men and women. Be sure to read the section on risks associated with using NSAIDs, as it will tell you if you should avoid using them if you have certain conditions.

How NSAIDs Work

The NSAIDs, including aspirin, are widely used worldwide. They may be the most widely used drug in the United States. These drugs are used not only for menstrual cramps but also for arthritis, headaches, and minor muscle strains and ligament and tendon sprains. The newer NSAIDs are used for postsurgical pain and are noted to be effective for the control of pain in general. NSAIDs were not traditionally given for postoperative pain because NSAIDs can inhibit clotting mechanisms and cause you to bleed from your surgical incision. The newer NSAIDs (Celebrex, Vioxx, and Bextra) can be given to you after surgery for pain control and you will not have any bleeding problems associated with one of these drugs. Vioxx, one of the newer NSAIDs, is reported to be as effective or in some studies more effective than some opioids such as Oxycodone for the management of your pain. The NSAIDs in general are classified as weak acids. This means that they are absorbed from your stomach or small intestine at different rates into your bloodstream at a rate that is dependent on the pH of your stomach or small intestine. That is why aspirin is buffered.

NSAIDs can exert their effects in your extremities. Following your hammer injury, NSAIDs will decrease pain and swelling in your finger. However, NSAIDs have also been found to be effective in relieving pain related to some spinal pain disorders. You may have strained your back before. A NSAID is an excellent medication for pain control following a back sprain.

Acetaminophen (Tylenol) does have some weak anti-inflammatory properties. Acetaminophen is a nonacid drug. Acetaminophen exerts its effects in the brain and spinal cord as well as in your arms and legs.

It is beneficial for you to know how NSAIDs work. Then you will know whether this class of drug is appropriate for the management of your pain. As you probably know, many NSAIDs are available over the counter at your pharmacy. To understand NSAIDs' function in general, as well as the new classification of NSAIDs that you see in the media, you should understand the pathway of the formation of prostaglandins. This will enable you to make a rational choice with your physician for the choice of the best NSAID for you, whether it is one of the older NSAIDs or one of the newer NSAIDs or just an aspirin.

The nonsteroidal anti-inflammatory medications are usually combined with other analgesics to decrease the overall experience of your pain and suffering. These drugs are used to decrease the overall pain experience without resorting to the need for the increased use of morphinelike medications. Opioid drugs act primarily in your brain and spinal cord. The nonsteroidal anti-inflammatory drugs exert their pain-relieving effects in your peripheral nervous system as well as in your brain and spinal cord. By combining these two different mechanisms, your physician can have better control of your pain that originates from the peripheral nervous system.

Prostaglandin Inhibitors

As stated previously, prostaglandins desensitize nerves that propagate painful stimuli. When you injure your finger hammering a nail, prostaglandins are formed at the area of the tissue injury. Prostaglandins are important in many normal physiological states as well as pathological states. Prostaglandins are ultimately synthesized as a result of trauma or normal secretion from the outer aspects of various cells. The outer cover of your cells in your body is called the cell membrane. Within this cell membrane are fatty substances that contain arachidonic acid. Arachidonic acid is present in all of your cell membranes.

In response to a cell stimulus such as a hit with a hammer, the arachidonic acid in your cell membrane is released and is quickly converted to different types of prostaglandins. A chemical in your body called cyclooxygenase (COX) ultimately converts the arachidonic acid to the various prostaglandins.

Your arachidonic acid formation from your cell membranes can be broken down in your body and mixed with other chemicals to form leukotrienes. These leukotrienes are formed and released from the white blood cells. These chemicals are important in the formation of inflammation (redness, swelling, warmth) in areas of your body as well as allergic reactions. Histamine production in your body released from your body's Mast cells is also involved in allergic reactions.

There are two types of cyclooxygenase chemicals in your body called cyclooxygenase I (COX I) and cyclooxygenase II (COX II). Prostaglandins causing pain can be formed in your body as a result of tissue trauma and COX 2 activity, but your body needs "good prostaglandin" to maintain normal physiologic functions. When prostaglandins are formed, they sensitize the peripheral nerve endings to other pain-causing substances in your body, which causes enhanced pain. The prostaglandins do not cause pain themselves but make the nerve endings more sensitive to other pain-producing chemicals such as bradykinins in your body. Occasionally the pain can become more pronounced than one would expect with a normal painful stimulus such as the hammer hitting your finger. The prostaglandin can make your skin much more sensitive than the pain usually associated with a hammer blow.

Prostaglandin inhibition in the brain and spinal cord produces pain relief. In the past decade, the two structures of cyclooxygenase were discovered. The two cyclooxygenase chemicals are called COX-1 and COX-2 enzymes. Enzymes in your body speed up biological reactions. COX-1 is present in most tissues under normal conditions. COX-2 is formed following tissue trauma. The older NSAIDs decrease the effects of both COX-1 and COX-2 activity. Side effects exhibited by NSAIDs are the result of inhibition of the COX-1 chemicals. Recently, NSAIDs have been developed that are specific for the COX-2 chemicals. These new drugs do not inhibit the COX-1 chemicals. This is significant because you need a normal level of COX-1 enzymes in your body.

Prostaglandins in females can be associated with primary dysmenorrhea. There are two types of prostaglandins that can cause strong contractions of the muscle of the uterus. Prostaglandins can furthermore decrease the calibers of arterial blood vessels in tissue, which causes a decreased blood flow as well as decreased oxygen to tissue. A decrease in oxygen to tissue will result in pain. Dysmenorrhea seen in female patients is a result of increased pain in the pain-containing nerves in the uterus as well as increased muscle contractions and decreased blood flow to the tissue.

Different Classes of NSAIDs

NSAIDs are divided into different classes of NSAID, depending on the drug's chemical structure. There are three classes of NSAIDs. The first are the carboxylic acid and enolic acid groups. This general class includes ibuprofen, naproxen, indomethacin, and ketolorac. The second are the benzenesulfonic acid derivatives such as Celebrex, Vioxx, and Bextra. The third group is the thenol group, which includes acetaminophen. In spite of having different chemical structures, all these medicines do provide anti-inflammatory effects. You should be aware that acetaminophen has only mild anti-inflammatory properties.

Great optimism abounds since the release of the cyclooxygenase-2 inhibitors. The advent of these drugs is important because NSAIDs are the most commonly used analgesics worldwide. Prostaglandins can be formed within minutes following tissue injury. The problem with the COX-2 enzyme inhibitors is that some moderate pain requires inhibition of both COX-1 and COX-2 enzymes. In these instances, your physician may prescribe a mild analgesic such as Darvon (propoxephene). A new NSAID is being developed with both COX-1 and COX-2 inhibition that has equal pain-relieving properties against each of the two COX enzymes but has minimal side effects.

Recent studies report that the COX-2 enzyme may be involved in some forms of cancer. COX-1 and COX-2 may also be involved in the formation of atherosclerotic plaque. COX inhibition may provide you with relief or even prevention of plaques and cancer. COX-2 inhibitors have been approved by the FDA for the treatment of individuals with osteoarthritis as well as rheumatoid arthritis. Vioxx and Celebrex have been approved by the FDA for the treatment of patients suffering from acute muscle and bone pain. If you suffer from arthritis, both COX-1 and COX-2 enzymes may be present in your inflamed joints.

COX-2-inhibiting NSAIDs are now used for postsurgical pain management. If you are to have surgery, your surgeon may give you a COX-2 inhibitor before your procedure to decrease your pain postoperatively. These COX-2 drugs are useful because they do not result in postsurgical bleeding. On the other hand, if you are taking traditional NSAIDs, you must notify your surgeon and anesthesiologist if you are to have surgery. The traditional NSAIDs can increase bleeding during or after your surgical procedure. Some recent studies have advocated the presurgical use of the new COX-2-inhibiting NSAIDs to prevent postsurgical pain associated with RSD following hand or foot surgery. The rationale for using NSAIDs postoperatively is to decrease your need for opioid medications.

If you are to have a dental procedure, you should be aware of the fact that there are recent published studies that postdental pain patients respond better or equal to Vioxx than to Oxycodone (an opioid drug). Postsurgically, the adverse effects of NSAIDs are similar to the adverse effects of NSAIDs in the general population. Gastrointestinal hemorrhage has been reported even with the new COX-2-inhibiting drugs. Delayed healing of fractures can be seen with the traditional NSAIDs. In rabbits, COX-2 inhibitors decrease healing of bone fractures. However, in humans, there is no evidence to date that indicates that a COX-2-inhibiting drug will delay fracture healing. Ask your physician if you may safely take a COX-2 NSAID for pain control if you have a healing fracture.

Other Uses for NSAIDs

The new COX-2 inhibitors can be used for mild to moderate pain of essentially any etiology, including some gynecological disorders. COX-2 inhibitors are useful in the treatment of dysmenorrhea, which can be disabling in female patients. The NSAIDs and especially the COX-2-inhibiting NSAIDs are extremely useful for the management of your joint pain. Arthritic entities that can be successfully treated include osteoarthritis as well as rheumatoid arthritis and ankylosing spondylitis. If you have arthritis, your pain will be present for your lifetime. NSAIDs have been shown to drastically improve the quality of your life if you have arthritis. If you consider the risks and benefits associated with NSAID use, you may agree that you may risk the chance of gastrointestinal discomfort if you can manage your pain. On the other hand, you probably do not want to risk bleeding to get pain relief. Talk to your physician about the risks and benefits of taking a NSAID. Opioid medications are indicated for your pain management if your pain becomes intolerable.

In addition to joint pain, the COX-2-inhibiting NSAIDs can be used for your muscle pain, including fibromyalgia. Fibromyalgia is not an inflammatory entity. However, a drug such as Vioxx is FDA approved for the onset of acute muscle pain. This drug is recommended over an opioid drug for pain management if you have fibromyalgia. Remember that opioids can cause addiction. They can also cause you to become depressed by decreasing your pituitary function. If you are already depressed, you should minimize opioid use.

Other uses for NSAIDs that you might find useful include the treatment of migraine headaches as well as tension headaches. NSAIDs can be used for pain management in cancer patients who have mild to moderate pain. If the pain progresses, opioid medications can be added. NSAIDs are especially useful in bone pain. Some tumors can invade your bone. This pain can be agonizing. New COX-2-inhibiting drugs are currently being tested and will be in pharmacies in the near future and these could provide you with better pain relief than the current COX-2 inhibitors.

In addition to the treatment of arthritic conditions such as osteoarthritis and rheumatoid arthritis, it is possible that the COX-2 inhibitors may provide protection against some forms of cancer as well as Alzheimer's disease.

NSAIDs have proven to be effective agents in decreasing the progression of preterm labor in human studies. By decreasing uterine contractions, a significant decrease in the patient's premature labor pain should be expected. The COX-2 enzyme has been demonstrated to cause breast tumors in mice. A prostaglandin produced by COX-2 in breast tumors can stimulate estrogen synthesis in the tumor and the surrounding tissue around the breast tumor. COX-2 inhibitors are being studied as well as NSAIDs in general to see whether breast tumors can be retarded.

A concern has been addressed in the academic community regarding an increased incidence of heart attack in individuals in a study who were taking COX-2 inhibitors. The older NSAIDs are known to decrease the clotting of your blood and can decrease your risk of a heart attack. Because the COX-2 drugs do not affect clotting, it was suspected that their use could be associated with a higher incidence of a myocardial infarction risk. The general consensus now is that if you are prone to have a heart attack (obesity, hypertension, angina) you should take an aspirin with the COX-2 inhibitor. It is recommended that you take the aspirin initially in the morning, and toward the afternoon you should take the COX-2 inhibitor. A baby aspirin in addition to the COX-2 inhibitor may be given instead of a whole aspirin.

Using NSAIDs to Provide Menstrual Pain Relief

Women can experience painful menstrual periods. The pain can be sharp, intermittent, or dull and aching. The pain is usually in the pelvic area or lower abdomen. Painful menstruation affects about 40 percent of menstruating women. Ten percent of these women are incapacitated for one to three days. Painful menstruation is the leading cause of lost time from school and work among women of childbearing age. Pain associated with menstruation may precede the actual menstruation by several days. The pain usually subsides as the menstruation subsides.

Mild pain during menstruation is normal, but excessive pain is not. Severe menstrual pain that disrupts normal activities is called dysmenorrhea. There are two types of dysmenorrhea. Primary dysmenorrhea is menstrual pain that occurs in normal healthy women. Secondary dysmenorrhea is menstrual pain that is associated with an underlying disease such as endometriosis, fibroids, and so forth.

Prostaglandins are causative chemicals associated with primary dysmenorrhea. Prostaglandin levels are much higher in women with severe menstrual pain than women who have only mild pain. Use of nonsteroidal anti-inflammatory drugs has a success rate of 80 percent. NSAIDs have been shown to be useful in the management of the pain associated with dysmenorrhea. Because the NSAIDs are used only for a short period of time, an older NSAID or a newer COX-2 inhibitor can be used for this painful condition.

Female hormones are believed to be responsible for the increased production of prostaglandins in women who suffer from dysmenorrhea. Patients with dysmenorrhea sometimes require opioids, however, the initial analgesic chosen should be a NSAID. Oral contraceptives are also sometimes indicated for the management of the severe pain. (*Bonica's Management of Pain*. n.p.: Lippincott Williams and Wilkins, 2001) (Carl Germano and William Cabot. *Nature's Pain Killers*. n.p.: Kensington Books, 1999)

Risks Associated with NSAIDs

As stated previously in this chapter, some prostaglandins can have beneficial effects on your body. Some prostaglandins inhibit acid production in the stomach. These "good" prostaglandins can stimulate mucus production in the upper gastrointestinal tract. This effect can decrease the incidence of ulcers. Therefore, the goal of your physician is to not cause a decrease in your body's good prostaglandins. The older NSAIDs would decrease these "good" prostaglandins in your body and could cause ulcers. These older NSAIDs could also cause you to have gastritis, which in turn would cause stomach pain, nausea, vomiting, and diarrhea. A small number of patients would develop gastrointestinal bleeding and would die. If you have a history of ulcers, you should not use the traditional NSAIDs.

In addition to causing ulcers, the older NSAIDs could cause you to bleed from your stomach or elsewhere. These older NSAIDs inhibit proper platelet function. Platelets are needed by the body to form blood clots. NSAIDs that decrease the COX-1 enzymes in your body could cause bleeding. You must inform your physician if you develop rectal bleeding or develop dark "tarry" stools. Aspirin decreases your chance of having a heart attack by decreasing your body's ability to form blood clots readily. You should not take NSAIDs if you are taking blood thinners. You should not take aspirin for 10 to 14 days prior to any surgery or major dental work. You must not use garlic, gingko, or vitamin E when taking NSAID medications. These herbal remedies can cause you to bleed if you are taking NSAIDs. Increased bleeding following the use of NSAIDs has been reported in patients having abdominal surgery, hysterectomies, or tonsillectomies. Patients who use NSAIDs are more prone to postoperative bleeding than individuals who do not regularly use NSAIDs. If you have any concerns about drug interactions, ask your physician.

You should not use NSAIDs if you have a history of any of the following:

- A history of a gastrointestinal bleed
- A history of a peptic ulcer or gastrointestinal intolerance to these medications
- A bleeding history or a history of bruising easily
- If you are taking blood thinners
- A history of kidney disease
- If you are a geriatric patient

"Good" prostaglandins regulate blood flow to your kidneys. These good prostaglandins contribute to normal excretion of water from your kidneys. On the other hand, other prostaglandins can cause a decrease in the blood flow to your kidneys and disrupt renal function. In kidney failure, sodium and water retention occur, causing you to appear swollen. Potassium can be elevated in your bloodstream as well. If your potassium becomes too high, your heart rhythm can be adversely affected. Overall hypertension may occur, which can cause you to have severe headaches. Ultimately, chronic use of nonsteroidal anti-inflammatory drugs can cause significant damage to your kidneys. You should ensure that your physician assesses kidney function every six months. The development of more recent NSAIDs does not spare the effects of NSAIDs on your kidney function. The effect of NSAIDs on your kidneys can occur within a few days from the time that you begin to take the drug. Again, have your kidney functions tested periodically.

Liver damage can occur following chronic nonsteroidal anti-inflammatory use, and you must be aware of this side effect. Liver damage occurs in approximately 3 percent of patients receiving NSAIDs. Therefore, liver function tests must be performed periodically if you are taking NSAIDs long term. If the whites of your eyes become yellow, notify your physician immediately. Nonsteroidal anti-inflammatory drugs increase the activity of your "bad" prostaglandin. This particular prostaglandin sensitizes your tissues to the pain effects of other chemicals from the nerve endings. Nonsteroidal anti-inflammatory drugs have "ceiling effects." Ceiling effect means that if your pain is decreased with a certain dose of NSAID, for example, any higher dose will not give you greater pain relief. If you have severe pain, your doctor can increase the dose until you experience pain relief. Drugs such as morphine have no ceiling effect. They can be administered in increasing doses, which will decrease pain responses. However, be aware that an excessive dose can stop you from breathing.

Even though nonsteroidal anti-inflammatory drugs are used for inflammatory pain such as arthritis, the Food and Drug Administration (FDA) has approved some of the NSAIDs for mild to moderate pain. Ketorolac can be used in the recovery room after surgery and can be administered in your muscle or in your vein. There is also an oral form of the drug that can be used by you for pain management. You should not use this medication for more than three to five days because of the possible serious side effects to your liver.

Motrin, Advil, and Nuprin are trade names for ibuprofen. These drugs are approved for the use in pain management. Nalfon can also be used strictly for pain management in situations where noninflammatory pain is present. If you suffer from fibromyalgia, for example, which is not an inflammatory disease, some of the NSAIDs are approved for pain control.

If you do not want a narcoticlike drug, one of the NSAIDs can be used. Dolobid and Naproxen are two brand name drugs that you can use for pain control. Diflunisal (Dolobid) has a longer duration of action than aspirin and longer than many of the other NSAIDs. It is effective for pain management and has a longer duration of action than the ibuprofen drugs or the fenoprofen drugs. Naproxen has also been successfully used for generalized pain.

You should be reminded that these drugs can cause you gastrointestinal upset and should not be used long term. They are excellent medications for you to use for three to four weeks. Do not risk your overall well-being. When taking over-the-counter NSAIDs, be sure to inform your doctor.

Prostaglandins can cause you to have a fever. NSAIDs can be effective in decreasing your fever. NSAIDs do affect the smooth muscle of the uterus as well. Prostaglandins can also relax the muscle in the lungs. Some prostaglandins inhibit gastric acid secretion in the stomach and make mucus secretion, which is another protective mechanism for the stomach. Other prostaglandins can increase gastrointestinal motility. The "good" prostaglandins can regulate the blood flow to the kidneys as well as sodium/potassium exchange. If the sodium/potassium exchange is compromised, you may retain sodium as well as fluid, which can increase your blood pressure. The "bad" prostaglandins can sensitize nerve endings to pain. As you can see, the many types of prostaglandins have many different functions. This is why you and your physician need to select the right drug for your pain.

You have read in this chapter that NSAIDs are not without potential serious problems. These drugs can also cause less serious effects such as peptic ulcer disease as well as gastritis and belching. NSAIDs can also cause you to experience diarrhea. Rarely have NSAIDs been implicated in kidney failure. NSAIDs decrease your blood's ability to form a blood clot. However, this may not be an entirely adverse event, because the use of an NSAID could protect your heart from a heart attack. NSAIDs have been reported to adversely affect the liver. You could develop jaundice from chronic use of NSAIDs. NSAIDs should not be used if you have a fractured bone. The use of NSAIDs may delay healing of your fracture. NSAIDs may affect cartilage repair in your joints if you suffer from osteoarthritis. If you have pain associated with osteoarthritis, it is recommended that the newer COX-2 enzyme inhibitors be prescribed.

The older NSAID drugs such as ibuprofen (Advil) inhibit both the COX-1 and COX-2 enzymes. The new class of NSAIDs are called COX-2-specific inhibitors. These drugs include Celebrex, Vioxx, and Bextra. They are collectively called COX-2 inhibitors because they exert their pharmacological effects by suppressing the COX-2 enzyme. Because the COX-1 enzyme is necessary for normal functioning of the body, it is essentially preserved by using a COX-2 inhibitor. The development of the COX-2 enzyme inhibitor is a significant development from the older nonsteroidal anti-inflammatory drugs, which inhibit COX-1 and COX-2 enzymes. You should remember that inhibition of COX-1 is related to the adverse effects caused by NSAIDs. Ask your physician about the side effects of the NSAID prescribed to you.

Why Men and Women Respond Differently to NSAIDs

With respect to gender specificity, previous studies directed at the more traditional NSAIDs reveal that male patients respond better to the effects of the traditional NSAIDs than females. The problem with earlier studies is that most of the original studies were done on male patients. In female patients, production of estrogen, the female hormone, may increase the number of prostaglandins present at any one time. This increase in any number of prostaglandins may attenuate the efficacy of NSAIDs. On the other hand, studies with the COX-2 inhibitors suggest that there is no greater analgesic effect in men versus women.

There are no further studies as the field is new and the studies on the effects of these drugs are also new.

Chapter 8

Learning About Alternative Medicine Practices and Herbs

"Conventional medicine" is considered to be practiced by individuals who have a medical doctor degree (M.D.) or a doctor of osteopathy degree (D.O.). Conventional medicine also includes methods practiced by allied health-care professionals such as physical therapists, occupational therapists, psychologists, and registered nurses. Other terms for conventional medicine include *allopathy, mainstream medicine,* and *orthodox medicine.* In contrast, *complementary* and *alternative medicine* are referred to as *unconventional* or *nonconventional medicine* as well as *unproven health care.*

Practitioners of alternative medicine hold to the theory that germs can cause illness only if there is an imbalance in various body systems allowing the germs to thrive. They believe that the body's internal environment is healthy and must be kept healthy, and that everyday exposure to germs does not result in illness. (B. Goldberg. *Alternative Medicine, The Definitive Guide.* Berkeley: Celestial Arts, 2001)

The following is a definition for alternative medicine specialties by the National Center for Complementary and Alternative Medicine. "Complementary and alternative medicines are practices and products that are not currently considered to be part of conventional medicine."

Complementary and alternative medicine practices change and update continually. Those therapies that have been thoroughly investigated and that are proven to be safe and effective eventually do become adopted into the conventional health-care system.

Complementary and alternative medicines, unlike many conventional medicine therapies, are designed to help you develop control over your overall health. If you are going to use any of these methods, you are encouraged to learn the side effects of some of these medications as well as learn about drug interactions with medications that you currently may be taking. Inasmuch, do not be afraid to tell your physician what complementary medicines you are taking.

The purpose of this chapter is not to condemn or advocate the utilization of *nonconventional medicine* practices and substances but to educate you so you can be aware and therefore have some control over what method of pain management works best for you.

Alternatives Gaining Acceptance

Medical professionals are beginning to recognize the benefits of alternative medicine. As an example, the National Institute of Health Office of Alternative Medicine was established in 1992. In addition, there has been a significant increase in professional interest in the area of alternative medicine. Right now, about 30 medical schools are currently offering at least one elective course on alternative medical therapies. The attitudes of medical school faculty toward the use of complementary medicine practices are important to alternatives gaining acceptance.

Here are some other ways that alternative medicine is gaining acceptance:

- Some health plans have announced their intention to incorporate payment for some *alternative medicine* practices into their insurance coverage.
- Some managed care corporations have revealed their intentions to include *alternative medicine* practices for payment.
- Some state governments are considering legislation pertaining to the practice of *alternative medicine* by health-care professionals.

If you are going to use a natural substance or therapy, you are responsible for your own care. You must not self-diagnose. You must discuss your symptoms of pain with your physician before taking any nutritional supplement. Remember, medicine is a drug used to treat disease and is manufactured for this purpose. A supplement is not manufactured as a treatment for disease. A vitamin is a supplement and is not used to treat a disease per se.

There are risks and benefits that you should be aware of when using alternative medications and therapies to manage your pain. In addition, the alternative medications you take could react with the prescription medications your doctor has given you and cause you even more problems. If in doubt, consult the *Physician's Drug Reference* for herbal medicines. This will advise you about safe doses and any precautions and drug interactions that you may need to be aware of.

Complementary and Alternative Support

There was a study published in the *New England Journal of Medicine* in 1993 that was a survey of individuals. More than 30 percent of those surveyed chose alternative medicine over conventional medicine methods to prevent and treat disease.

In 1994, Congress passed the Dietary Supplement Health and Education Act. In passing this act, Congress recognized that many individuals believed that dietary supplements offered health benefits. The bill gave dietary supplement manufacturers freedom to produce more products and to provide information about their products' health benefits.

The Food and Drug Administration (FDA), on the other hand, is responsible for overseeing any claims by the dietary supplement manufacturers to the truthfulness of these claims. The Federal Trade Commission regulates the advertising of all of the dietary supplements. You should be aware that the quality control standards for natural substances are a problem within this industry. Some of the manufacturers of these products will not have the amount of substance in the natural medication as stated on the container label.

You must do your own research to determine whether the natural substance that you are taking has an accurate dosage as stated on the container label for the product. Remember the drug can be actually less than what the label states. A good rule of thumb for you to consider is that if one product is much cheaper than an identical product, you may want to consider purchasing the more expensive product. The reason for this is that companies that follow appropriate standards usually have their own quality-control systems in effect. As a result, they will have a higher overhead and will have to charge more for the natural medication.

In an Atlanta medical school, 200 full- and part-time medical school faculty were given a survey concerning alternative medicine practices. The 24-item survey was given to each medical school faculty member. Three of the 24 items requested participants to respond to a list of 30 specific alternative medical therapies, which included the following:

- Whether they saw alternative medicine as a legitimate medical practice.
- Whether they have had personal experience with alternative medicines and felt that they were effective.
- Whether they have had training in alternative medicine science.

Eighty-five of the responders said they have had training in at least one alternative medical therapy. Fifty-seven percent of the responders said they had training in five or more alternative medicine therapies. More than 80 percent had a personal experience with at least one alternative medical therapy and close to 50 percent of the responders reported personal experience with five or more different alternative medical therapies. Almost 90 percent of these alternative medicine experiences were rated effective. Only 3 percent were rated not effective. Less than 1 percent of the medical school faculty felt that these therapies were potentially harmful.

The results of this Atlanta medical school study demonstrated that the medical school faculty had a positive exposure to alternative medical therapies. This study is important because medical school faculty members have the responsibility for the education and training of future physicians.

Clinical Trials

The NIH does award grants for the study of research in complementary as well as alternative medicines. Clinical trials are being done throughout the United States with respect to complementary and alternative medicines. You may want to participate in one of these trials. Trials with respect to herbal medicines are an important part of the medical research process. The results from clinical trials can define better ways to treat your painful conditions.

A clinical trial is a research study in which a therapy is tested on individuals like yourself to ensure that what is being tested is safe and effective. Always remember that clinical trials have risks. Before participating in a clinical trial, discuss this trial with your primary care physician.

To find out about ongoing clinical trials—for example, studies on arthritis and neurological disorders—go to www.nccam.nih.gov. You also may want to access the National Library of Medicine online (www.pubmed.com). PubMed contains a database from which you can search for "complementary medicine" to find citations to recently published scientific articles on this subject.

Homeopathic Medicine

Homeopathic specialists prescribe dilutions of natural substances from plants, minerals, and animals. Homeopathy has been around for more than 200 years. About 500 million people around the world receive homeopathic treatment each year. (B. Goldberg. *Alternative Medicine, The Definitive Guide*. Berkeley: Celestial Arts, 2001) The World Health Organization has recommended that homeopathy is a system of traditional medicine that should be integrated with conventional medicine, which is considered the traditional approach to medicine. It is important to know that the U.S. Food and Drug Administration recognizes homeopathic remedies as official drugs and regulates their manufacture. This is unlike the herbs used for medicinal use. Homeopathy qualities of medicine are used frequently by conventional physicians in Europe. In Britain, homeopathy is a part of the national health system.

The basic principles of homeopathy are that a disease can be destroyed and removed by a type of medicine that is able to produce the disease in humans. (B. Goldberg. *Alternative Medicine, The Definitive Guide*. Berkeley: Celestial Arts, 2001) In other words, a substance that in large doses would produce symptoms of a disease can be used in very small doses to cure it. In conventional medicine, this is called the theory of antibiotics. Homeopathic practitioners adhere to the fact that the more a substance is diluted, the more potent it is. In conventional medicine, it is believed that a higher dose of the medicine will lead to a greater effect.

The purpose of diluting out substances in homeopathic medicine is to avoid side effects. Homeopathic practitioners adhere to the fact that illness is different for every person. Homeopathic treatments are unique for each patient. Homeopathic medicine emphasizes that patients are individuals and have individual signs and symptoms of an illness and should be treated only on an individual basis. The entire individual is treated, which includes the physical, psychological, and spiritual portions of each person.

Naturopathic Medicine

Naturopathic medicine treats disease by using your body's natural ability to heal itself. Naturopathic practitioners invoke healing processes by using a variety of treatment options based on your particular needs. In naturopathic medicine, disease symptoms are a sign of your body's attempt to heal itself naturally.

Naturopathic medicine gets its data from Chinese, Native American, and ancient Greek cultures. Naturopaths recommend healing of the person and not the disease. Naturopathic medicinal treatments will include doses of natural substances that are much higher than those used by practitioners of homeopathic medicine. (B. Goldberg. *Alternative Medicine, The Definitive Guide*. Berkeley: Celestial Arts, 2001)

Herbal Medicine

Even though your primary care physician may not "believe" in complementary and alternative medications, you should not be afraid to approach your doctor with the fact that you are taking herbal medications. This is important not only because of possible drug interactions, but because some substances such as garlic and gingko can decrease your blood's ability to form a blood clot normally. This could result in excessive bleeding. It is extremely important if you are about to have a surgical procedure that you let your surgeon know you are taking an herb that can thin your blood. You surgery may need to be delayed until your blood's ability to form a normal clot has been restored.

Which Alternative Medications Work?

To best choose a natural product to decrease your pain, you should know which chemicals in the body produce pain. With this knowledge, you can pick the analgesic best suited to relieve your pain. If you have joint pain, for instance, you will want to use an *alternative medicine* that has anti-inflammatory properties. If you are injured or have inflammation, your body makes a variety of chemicals that transmit pain impulses to a pain-processing center in your brain. These chemicals include the *prostaglandins, cytokines, substance P, glutamic acid,* and *nitric oxide.* Nitric oxide is a gas that is a pain chemical transmitter in your *nervous system.* This should not be confused with *nitrous oxide,* which is used for pain control in dental procedures.

The following remedies are anti-inflammatory substances that you may want to use as a *prostaglandin inhibitor* to relieve your pain:

Tumeric has anti-inflammatory and *antioxidant* effects and has been shown to inhibit *prostaglandin* formation. This drug should not be used if you have gallbladder disease. No significant health risks or side effects with use of this drug have been reported to date. The average dose is 3 grams of tumeric per day. This dose can be divided up into 1-gram doses and be taken 3 times per day with meals. For example, you may take 1 milligram with each meal for a total dose of 3 grams.

Ginseng has anti-inflammatory effects and is used in *homeopathic* medicine for the treatment of rheumatoid arthritis. You should not use this medicine if you have hypertension. Do not use ginseng with caffeine. Exercise caution if you use ginseng along with any antidiabetic medicine or insulin. You should not use ginseng with MAOI inhibitors, which are used to decrease your blood pressure. Do not use ginseng in combination with diuretics. Side effects include sleep deprivation, nosebleeds, headaches, nervousness, and vomiting. The average daily dose of this root is 1 to 2 grams. Do not take more than 2 grams per day. The 2 grams can be divided up and taken 3 times a day.

Resveratrol is an *antioxidant* and a *COX-2 inhibitor* that some believe prevents heart disease and cancer. It is largely found in the skin of red grapes. Therefore, many people obtain resveratol by drinking red wine. This substance can prevent clot formation, whereas the conventional *COX-2 inhibitors* do not prevent clot formation. The usual dose is no more than 600 mg per day. There are no known side effects or drug interactions for resveratrol itself.

Fish oils contain the omega-3 fatty acids and can decrease *prostaglandins.* Fish oils are used for the treatment of rheumatoid arthritis. You may also use fish oils for the control of joint pain. The most common side effect that you may experience with fish oil supplementation is mild stomach upset. The fish oils can decrease your blood's ability to clot. If you are taking blood-thinning drugs, you should not take fish oils, because it will give you an increased risk of bleeding. You may safely take up to 10 grams of fish oil per day.

N-acetylcysteine is an amino acid produced by your body that will decrease *prostaglandin* formation. It can help prevent some diseases and boost your immune system. You should not take this drug if you are taking carbamazepine (Tegretol). Side effects include headaches, nausea, vomiting, and stomach upset. The recommended dose is 200 milligrams 3 times a day.

Cayenne is an anti-inflammatory medication that is helpful for the treatment of muscle pain and arthritis. This drug may be helpful for inhibiting the release of *substance P* as well. Cayenne side effects include diarrhea and intestinal colic. It can decrease your body's ability to form a normal blood clot. It also can reduce the effects of aspirin, so you should be aware of this fact if you are taking aspirin as a blood thinner. High doses of cayenne over a prolonged time can cause kidney and liver damage. You should not use this drug for more than two days in a row. After two weeks you may use it again for two days. The daily dose of cayenne should not exceed 10 grams.

Glucosamine, an over-the-counter dietary supplement, has been reported to be effective as a nonsteroidal anti-inflammatory medication for the control of pain associated with osteoarthritis, but without the normal side effects associated with NSAIDS (Muller-Fassbender H, et al. Glucosamine sulfate compared to ibuprofen in osteoarthritis of the knee. Osteoarthritis Cartilage 2[1]:61-9, 1994).

Ipriflavone can be used as a *prostaglandin inhibitor*. Women also use it to decrease the incidence of osteoporosis. This medicine can actually stop bone loss. It can decrease the risk of bone fractures in females. This drug, like the other drugs that are *prostaglandin* inhibitors, can increase the blood-thinning activity of other drugs that you may be taking, such as Coumadin. It also can increase the effects of some asthma drugs such as theophylline, so avoid taking ipriflavone if you are using such medications. Side effects are mostly stomach upset. The average dose is 200 milligrams 3 times a day.

Procyanidolic oligomers are natural substances extracted from grape seeds. They are useful for their *antioxidant* effects. They can decrease arthritis pain. However, another important effect of this medicine is that it can decrease the effects of *nitric oxide. Nitric oxide* is released from cells in your bloodstream. *Nitric acid* essentially exists in a gas form to transmit pain impulses. There are no significant side effects associated with this drug. The daily dose of this drug ranges from 150 to 300 milligrams per day.

Cytokine inhibitors include the fish oils, as previously mentioned. *Cytokines* are chemicals produced in your bloodstream that enhance pain impulses. They contribute to the formation of substances that can destroy your joint linings if you have rheumatoid arthritis.

Substance P inhibitors include cayenne and ginseng. *Substance P* is a *neurotransmitter* chemical that can be associated with nerve pain, such as shingles. If you have shingles, you may want to consider using a *substance P* inhibitor.

Histamine can also provide you with pain relief. Histamine released from certain cells in your body can cause you to develop a rash, a headache, and itching all over your body. However, in extremely small doses, histamine may relieve your pain. There have not been any placebo-controlled studies to date that compare a histamine cream to a placebo cream. However, one animal study did conclude that morphine may exert its pain-relieving effect in the brain and spinal cord by releasing histamine into the central nervous system.

Hydroxytryptophan is an amino acid that naturally occurs in your body. It has been found to significantly decrease *substance P* formation. Because *substance P* may be involved in fibromyalgia, this medicine can improve your fibromyalgia pain. It also may helpful for the treatment of headaches, shingles, and neuropathic pain entities such as carpal tunnel syndrome. Nausea is a common side effect of this drug. You may also experience drowsiness, dry mouth, and stomach pain. In 1989, some people taking this drug developed joint pain, high fever, weakness in their arms and legs, and had shortness of breath. The Center for Disease Control concluded that the drug came from a Japanese manufacturer and was contaminated. Drug interactions reveal severe effects if a person is taking an antidepressant medicine from their doctor. You should not take this drug if you have Parkinson's disease and are not taking the drug Sinemet. Do not use this drug if you have scleroderma. This drug may also interfere with the effects of drugs that you may be taking for migraine headaches. Adults should take no more than 50 milligrams 3 times a day.

Cannabinoids are another natural substance for the control of pain. State legislation throughout the United States will eventually make a decision on the use of cannabinoids for medical purposes. Marijuana has been used since antiquity. In 1942, marijuana was reported to be a dangerous, harmful, and addictive drug. In 1970, marijuana was classified as a highly addictive drug with no accepted medical use. However, in 1996, voters in Arizona and California passed referenda to legalize marijuana for medicinal use.

To date, doctors are prohibited from prescribing marijuana for medical conditions. There has been a recent discovery of two cannabinoid receptors, CB-1 and CB-2. Now the scientific medical community is interested in this substance. Cannabinoids are now reported to have therapeutic value as pain relievers. This means that marijuana could help you with your pain in many situations. There have not been any controlled clinical trials for the use of this drug.

Cannabinoids do exhibit some anti-inflammatory properties. However, they are no more effective than the current anti-inflammatory medications available. If you suffer from pain involving your nerves, such as shingles or reflex sympathetic dystrophy, you may be able to note some pain relief with the use of marijuana. To date the safety and efficacy of marijuana has not been found. In 1997, the American Medical Association House of Delegates recommended to allow adequately designed controlled studies of cannabinoids with respect to their effect on pain as well as other illnesses. This recommendation was adopted by the AMA House of Delegates as a policy during the 2001 AMA Annual Meeting.

Acupuncture

Acupuncturists practice *alternative medicine* methods. Acupuncture is used in traditional Chinese medicine. It involves inserting fine needles into the body at specific points that have been found to be effective in the treatment of specific health problems. The purpose of acupuncture is to balance the body's flow of energies. Acupuncture can relieve pain, and those who perform acupuncture say it is able to restore health. Sometimes acupuncturists will burn herbs around a specific acupressure point for added relief.

Chiropractic Medicine

Chiropractic medicine has been around since 1895. It is the second largest health profession in the world and one of the fastest growing. Chiropractors are aware of the possible dangers posed by conventional medical procedures. Chiropractors have found a way to approach the healing of body ailments that uses the body's own healing abilities to restore health.

Chiropractic medicine is a science dedicated to the treatment of diseases by the manipulation of your backbone. Chiropractic medicine is based on the theory that your pain can be traced to incorrect alignment of your bones, which can cause pressure on nerves that can cause not only nerve pain but also muscle pain.

Chiropractic medicine emphasizes individual well-being, including having a healthful diet and using natural medicines. Chiropractic therapy can be extremely effective in the management of painful conditions of the spine. Chiropractors are not allowed by law to prescribe conventional medicines, but do recommend natural substances that can promote healing of the body and prevent illnesses.

Chapter 9
Using Topical Analgesics

Pain relievers that can be applied directly to your skin are available for the control of a variety of your pain syndromes. These topical pain relievers are a noninvasive and convenient method for delivering pain-relieving medication to you. This is especially important and beneficial if you are not able to take medications by mouth. Topical pain relievers include complementary and alternative medications as well as conventional medications.

In this chapter, you will learn about ointments, creams, gels, and skin patches that can help relieve your pain. Often this is more effective than oral medications because they will have less side effects and less drug interactions. Topical analgesics can be used to relieve minor pain from muscle soreness to major pain from cancer. While the stronger versions of topical analgesics are prescription-only, you can buy mild topical analgesics over-the-counter. Your doctor will be able to help you find the one that is right for you.

How They Work

Topical forms of analgesics, or pain relievers, have been used throughout human history. The use of ointments for medicinal purposes is mentioned in the Bible on many occasions. The purpose of a topical analgesic is to transmit a medication through your skin for the effect of pain relief. The amount of drug that actually gets through your skin is determined by the amount of pressure applied as you rub it over your skin, the area of your skin covered by the drug, the way in which the drug is dissolved, and the use of dressings over your skin. Analgesics are available in ointments, creams, and gels. They also may be placed in patches that may be applied to your skin.

A study published in 2002 revealed that 27 percent of doctors prescribed topical analgesics. They reported that 43 percent of their patients responded favorably to topical agents. The advantage of topical analgesics is that they can be placed on the skin over the site of your pain. When compared to oral medications, you will have a lower blood level of the drug and will have fewer side effects and fewer drug interactions.

Ointments

Ointments are semisolid preparations that melt at body temperature and spread easily. Ointments are not routinely used in the practice of pain medicine unless the ointment is specially compounded by a pharmacy.

Ointments are defined in three categories based on your skin penetration. One type of ointment does not penetrate beyond the external layer of your skin called the epidermis. Ointments of this class can be used for the treatment of sunburn. A second type of ointment penetrates to the internal layer of your skin called the dermis. The third type of ointment actually goes through your skin to the nerves and ligaments and in some instances into your bloodstream.

Substances applied on your skin can evaporate. You do not want your analgesic drug evaporating from your skin. Your pharmacist will add substances such as glycerin to the ointment to keep this evaporation from happening. Ointments can be prepared by your pharmacist or purchased over the counter or by prescription; ointments should be packaged in tubes. Some ointment preparations will contain absorption enhancers. Absorption enhancers make it easier for the drug to be absorbed through your skin. Azone and DMSO can both enhance the absorption of ointments through your skin.

Creams

Creams are opaque, thick, liquid substances that consist of medications dissolved in a cream base that usually vanishes through the skin. They are less of a liquid consistency than ointments. The term *cream* is used to describe a soft type of preparation that is less affected by your body temperature than ointments. The therapeutic difference between creams and ointments is that creams penetrate deeper than ointments.

Gels

Gels are a drug-delivery system that usually contain penetration enhancers and are usually used for administering anti-inflammatory medications. The anti-inflammatory medication must be absorbed through your skin to provide you with pain relief. Gels are useful treatment methods if you have arthritic and/or muscle pain. Gels usually are thicker than creams or ointments and are usually clear, unlike creams and ointments. The concentration of medication in gels is usually no greater than 2 percent. For example, lidocaine, which is a numbing medicine for the control of pain, is dispensed as a 2 percent gel. However, the cream is available in a 5 percent concentration. This is because medications are usually absorbed through the skin better if used in gel form. Gels usually have clarity and sparkle. They maintain their thickness even with an elevated body temperature. Some gels have been developed to be given nasally. Some drugs are absorbed better through the nose than through the skin. Gels are usually dispensed in tubes or squeeze bottles.

Skin Patch

Another delivery system for analgesics is a *transdermal* patch, which contains medication that is transmitted directly through your skin. A patch containing a medication is placed on your skin and remains there for a specified time so that the drug within the patch can be delivered through your skin to your bloodstream. Local anesthetics such as lidocaine, capsaicin cream, and fentanyl, a potent opioid medication, are some of the medicines that can be delivered through your skin using a transdermal drug delivery system. These patches should be applied only to areas on your skin that have no blisters or open areas such as a cut. The patches are made of adhesive materials. You should not use the patch if you are allergic to some adhesives. With respect to the patches, the amount of drug that is absorbed from the patch is directly related to the length of the application of the patch, as well as the area of your skin to which it is applied.

The advantage of the patch is that it gives you a continuous flow of analgesic medications. When you take a pill, after it leaves your stomach or intestine and enters into your bloodstream, you receive a high concentration of the drug initially. As the drug is distributed to other tissues in your body, your blood level concentration of the drug decreases. Once your body breaks down the drug, you will no longer have an analgesic affect of that particular drug. However, when using a patch, you will have a continuous release of the drug from the patch into your bloodstream. You will have constant pain relief without the peaks and valleys of the drug concentration in your bloodstream associated with oral medications.

Prescription vs. Nonprescription Creams

Topical analgesics represent a promising area for future drug development. Their use has grown to a $150 million dollar industry. You should occasionally ask your doctor for any new developments in the field of topical pain relievers.

Women use these medications more than men. However, there have been no good studies comparing the effects of topical analgesics on men as compared to women. As new topical analgesics are being developed, it is anticipated that a gender analysis will be a part of the topical analgesic drug study.

Nonprescription Creams

Natural compounds such as herbs or leaves and roots can also be used to treat your pain topically.

Aloe vera can be used to decrease your pain if you have sunburn. Use of this natural topical product for the treatment of various medical conditions was discovered in 1935. This drug is effective for the treatment of skin inflammation as well as minor burns. There are no side effects nor are there any known drug interactions.

Capsaicin is a drug that has been extensively studied in both the clinical and laboratory settings. Capsaicin is the active component of chili or red peppers. Capsaicin can be put on your skin over your joints if you have joint pain. The capsaicin first stimulates the small pain-transmitting fibers by depleting them of the neurotransmitter *substance P.* After the *substance P* has been depleted, you will have a block of the pain fibers that cause burning pain sensations. Observations in Hispanic individuals demonstrated that they did not have mouth or stomach pain after ingesting red peppers. The reason is the depletion of the *substance P* in the nerve endings in these areas following continual exposure to red peppers.

Substance P also is present in your joints throughout your body. For this reason, capsaicin can be an effective pain reliever for the treatment of pain associated with osteoarthritis and rheumatoid arthritis. It may take a week for you to feel the pain-relieving effects of capsaicin. As substance P is being depleted from your nerve endings, your nerve endings still manufacture substance P. As a result, it will take several days to deplete enough of the substance P to provide you with pain relief. Once you discontinue use of this cream, your nerves will replenish substance P and your pain may return.

Some studies have shown that if you have a *neuropathy* related to your diabetes you could have significant pain relief with topical capsaicin. Some pain-medicine physicians have used topical capsaicin to relieve the pain associated with shingles. You may have a brief burning sensation following the use of capsaicin. You should be warned to avoid contact with your eyes and genital areas. It is recommended that you use rubber gloves when applying the capsaicin cream. You should use the capsaicin cream no more than three times a day. Various concentrations of capsaicin exist. Begin with a small concentration that contains 0.025 percent capsaicin. You may eventually increase your capsaicin dose to 0.075 percent capsaicin.

Menthol is an oil that is one component of peppermint oil. This oil in a cream base can significantly decrease your pain. When you place a menthol preparation on your skin, the menthol will feel cold to your nerve endings. While you feel the cold, your pain-stimulating nerves will be depressed. Following the initial cool sensation, you will feel a period of warmth. Menthol products can be used for the treatment of pain associated with arthritis, muscle pain, and tendonitis.

Application of a menthol-containing cream may be of benefit to you if you suffer from tension headaches. It can be rubbed around the neck muscles just below the skull. It can be an extremely effective method for the treatment of your headaches.

Allergic reactions with menthol have been reported. It is recommended that you test a small amount of menthol on your skin before applying it extensively to assure yourself that you are not allergic it. You should not use the menthol preparation more than three times a day. Do not use a heating pad or a cold pack over the area of your skin where the menthol substance was placed.

Some *natural herbs and vegetables* can be used as a topical analgesic. One example is an onion. It is reported by some doctors that spreading the juice of a sliced onion over one of your painful areas could reduce your pain. A tincture can be made by putting 100 grams of minced onions in 30 grams of ethanol for a 70 percent solution. There are no hazards or side effects associated with the topical administration of an onion. However, frequent contact with the onion over time could possibly lead to an allergic reaction.

Poplar tree bark can also be used for relieving your pain. The bark is dried and placed in capsules or chemicals are extracted, for example, as in a tea. The bark can be used for control of your pain over your joints or nerves or if you have rheumatoid arthritis. You should not use the bark if you are allergic to aspirin. When externally applied using the poplar bark and leaves, you should use no more than five grams of the drug per day.

When using these topical natural products, you must follow the directions for the use of these medicines that are contained either on the outside of the package or from an insert that may be placed in a box that holds a tube of any of these substances. You should remember that although these are natural products, they can have side effects like any other medication. You may want to discuss the use of these remedies with your doctor or pharmacist. To date there are no significant drug interactions reported with these natural topical agents.

Prescription Creams

Another topical medication used to prevent pain is *EMLA cream*. It is used as a numbing agent more than it is used for reducing pain. This is a cream consisting of lidocaine and prilocaine, which are both numbing agents. This local anesthetic combination is packaged in tubes. There is also an EMLA cellulose disc that can be applied over your painful area.

The purpose of this medication is to provide pain relief over the area of the skin. It is used in children to reduce the pain of starting intravenous lines. Some pain-management doctors advocate its use to decrease the pain associated with reflex sympathetic dystrophy or the pain associated with shingles. This cream should be placed on an intact skin area. The EMLA should be applied under a bandage for at least 60 minutes to provide relief over the painful area of your skin. This cream is not recommended if you have an allergy to lidocaine or prilocaine. If you have the blood disorder methemoglobinemia, you should not use this cream. You should not exceed the recommended dose prescribed by your physician.

The problem with this cream as opposed to the Lidoderm patches is that it does provide pain relief for your skin. This means that you have a block of all sensation in the skin treated with this cream. You should avoid causing any trauma to the area, including scratching your skin or rubbing or exposing your skin to extreme hot or cold temperatures until you have complete return of sensation to your skin. It is recommended that you not use this medication if you are taking heart medication. The local anesthetics in this cream can interact with some heart medicines.

There appear to be no gender-specific differences between men and women when using this cream. If you develop a rash with use of this cream, you must stop using it. There have been reports of blistering on skin following application of the EMLA cream. You may experience itching as well. The problem with this topical analgesic is that it is hard to control and regulate the dose of medication that you receive. You must refer to the insert supplied by the drug company. This can be found in the box that contains the tube of the cream.

Another analgesic cream that is available is a combination of *methyl salicylate and menthol*. This is a cream that is effective for the temporary relief of arthritis and pain in your muscles. You should not use this medicine if your skin is sensitive to the oil of wintergreen. You should apply this cream around the sore areas on your body. You should not apply this cream more than three times a day. Do not place this cream over areas of the skin that are broken because it will cause extreme discomfort to that area.

Steroid creams are sometimes used for the treatment of joint pain. Topical steroids are anti-inflammatory agents. Pramoxine hydrochloride is a topical anesthetic agent that sometimes is combined with steroids to attempt to manage pain. This cream provides a temporary relief from pain. You should not use this cream if you are allergic to any of the substances in the cream such as the steroid or the pramoxine. If you develop a rash or blistering, you must stop using the cream. You should not use this cream more than three times a day. Furthermore, do not use this steroid preparation for more than five days. Do not reuse this cream until you have discussed the situation with your doctor.

Nonsteroidal anti-inflammatory agents (NSAIDS) that are commonly taken by mouth for the treatment of bone, joint, and muscle pain may be placed into a cream by your pharmacist. For these drugs to give you pain relief, they must penetrate your skin and enter your bloodstream. These creams should not be used more than three times a day. Side effects with the nonsteroidal anti-inflammatory creams are the same as with the NSAIDs taken by mouth. However, the side effects of the topical NSAIDS are less than the oral NSAIDS. The side effects of any NSAID can include stomach upset and allergic reactions. If the dose is high enough, it could affect your liver and kidneys.

These NSAIDs can be very effective for the management of your pain when applied over your skin. The use of a ketoprofen gel and a diclofenac gel, both NSAIDs, were compared at painful sites in a four-week study. The ketoprofen gel gave positive results for the treatment of knee pain and was shown to be better at relieving pain than the diclofenac gel. If you have joint pain, you may want to discuss these facts with your pain-medicine doctor or orthopedic doctor. Aspirin creams also may provide you with some pain relief when applied over your painful joints or muscles.

New research is being done into the topical administration of *amitriptyline* and *ketamine*. Ketamine is a potent analgesic that can cause you to hallucinate if the dose is too high. A study in animals has used both of these agents together to treat pain in the laboratory setting.

Amitriptyline, which is an antidepressant, has recently been shown to have pain-relieving properties when applied topically. Amitriptyline cream may be advantageous if you do not want to take amitriptyline pills by mouth. The amitriptyline cream will not help you if you are suffering from significant depression, but can be helpful in decreasing your pain. Some people complain of being tired while taking amitriptyline. However, amitriptyline can contribute to pain relief in fibromyalgia and the topical application may be a way of avoiding significant side effects that can be associated with oral use. There is ongoing research in this area. You may want to keep informed of the research on both of these drugs through the National Library of Medicine website at www.nlm.nih.gov.

Current research is being done at a cancer center using a combination of *lidocaine and morphine* administered topically. This combination showed greater pain-relieving effects than the topical opioids or topical local anesthetics by themselves. Studies demonstrate a potent interaction between the morphine and the lidocaine that can offer potential advantages in the clinical management of your pain if it is severe. Again, follow the development of this drug combination. This combination is currently only under investigation for cancer patients.

New Horizons in Topical Analgesics

Another way of delivering medication is through a patch placed on your skin over the site of your pain. Research is promising in the area of skin patches that relieve pain. Because analgesic patches have fewer side effects and fewer drug interactions than some oral medications, you may find that a patch will work better for you. If you think a skin patch analgesic would help you, be sure to discuss your options with your doctor.

The Fentanyl Patch

The *transdermal Fentanyl patch* system has become popular since it was introduced in the 1980s. This strong *opioid* medication was used initially for cancer pain management and then for noncancer, chronic pain management. The fentanyl is able to penetrate your skin easily. Fentanyl is 70 times more potent than morphine. It produces less histamine release from cells in your bloodstream and causes less itching than morphine. The fentanyl patch is primarily used for chronic or cancer-related pain. A fentanyl patch can be used for most moderate to severe pain syndromes.

In the fentanyl patch, the medication exists as a gel in a drug reservoir. Between this reservoir and your skin is a release membrane that has various-size holes that regulate the amount of fentanyl that is delivered to your skin. The larger the size of the holes, the more fentanyl that is distributed to your skin and eventually through your skin. The adhesiveness around the patch keeps it in place. When the fentanyl patch is placed on your skin, the drug diffuses through the holes in the release membrane to the surface of your skin. It then goes to the outer layer of your skin and is deposited in a storage area. From the storage area, it is gradually absorbed into your bloodstream. This is the reason that it takes at least an hour before the fentanyl has begun to enter your bloodstream. You will probably not notice any pain-relieving effects from this drug delivery system for about six hours. The patch is usually removed every three days. After the patch is removed, you will still have some drug that remains in the storage area under your skin. If you remove the patch and do not replace it, you will still receive Fentanyl for hours after the patch has been removed.

Fentanyl patches come in different concentrations. The concentrations correlate with the area of the skin to which they are applied. The effectiveness of the patch is not affected by placing it on your chest, your back, or your upper arm. An increase in temperature will cause the medication to be rapidly delivered from the patch to your bloodstream. Your skin's thickness also can affect the amount of fentanyl that is absorbed through your skin. The thicker your skin, the slower the rate of delivery of the fentanyl will be. The patch should not be applied over broken skin because the blood level of fentanyl can be significantly raised. The patch can cause a decrease in breathing and even death if you receive a significantly high dose of the fentanyl.

If you have significant vomiting associated with your severe pain, you cannot keep oral medications in your stomach. Therefore, they are not absorbed into your bloodstream and you receive no pain relief from the medicine. If this is the case, consult with your doctor about possibly using the fentanyl patch for pain control. There is no upper limit as to the number of fentanyl patches that can be worn at one time. Some cancer patients require more than one patch at a time. Side effects of the patches containing fentanyl include nausea, constipation, and sleepiness. Be aware that the patch can cause reactions to your skin related to the adhesive used in the patch. If you notice an irritation on your skin related to the patch, stop using the patch. If you have difficulty with the patch sticking to your skin, you can secure the edges of the patch with adhesive tape. You should not use the fentanyl patch if you are allergic to adhesives.

Occasionally, you may require medication for breakthrough pain, an episode of temporary pain, if you do something to aggravate your chronic pain syndrome. For example, if you are using the patch for chronic pain and you go into your garden and do lifting, pushing, or digging, you may cause the onset of temporary pain on top of your chronic pain. At that time, an oral medication can be taken for treatment of your breakthrough pain.

With respect to gender specificity, the fentanyl patch appears to work just as well in men as it does in women. The fentanyl patch has been successful for the management of cancer-related pain and chronic pain syndromes and has paved the way for further research into the utilization of other *opioid* drugs for the management of chronic pain.

The Lidoderm Patch

Another popular patch that is readily available by prescription from your pain-management doctor is the lidocaine-containing patch called *Lidoderm*. The Lidoderm *transdermal* drug-delivery system exerts a significant amount of its pain-relieving effects by releasing a small amount of lidocaine into your bloodstream. There is also an effect on the nerves under your skin that are transmitting pain. This patch is used for the treatment of postherpetic neuralgia, a long-lasting pain that is a result of shingles. Approximately 1 million people develop shingles every year. Twenty percent of these individuals will develop post-herpetic neuralgia, which is an extremely painful syndrome.

The U.S. Food and Drug Administration has approved the use of the Lidoderm patch for the treatment of the severe pain following the onset of shingles. Shingles is an infection caused by the chicken pox virus. You may have had chicken pox as a child. However, the virus remains inactive in your nervous system for many years. At some time in your life, this virus can become reactivated and travel via nerves to certain areas of your skin, causing you to have severe pain. When the virus reaches your skin, you may develop blisters that can be severely painful as well. After the blisters have disappeared, you may have persistent pain. This pain is call postherpetic neuralgia. You may feel as if your body is on fire in the areas affected by the postherpetic neuralgia. Your skin may become extremely sensitive to touch. In many instances there is no cure for this pain. Often your doctor will try to treat the symptoms of your pain to provide you relief. The Lidoderm patch has been demonstrated in clinical studies to significantly decrease pain following the outbreak of shingles.

The Lidoderm patch contains 5 percent lidocaine. The lidocaine essentially does not reach your bloodstream like fentanyl does in the fentanyl patch delivery system. The lidocaine penetrates your skin just enough to reach the nerve endings that are transmitting your pain. As a result, there are minimal side effects from the use of this patch other than from the adhesive layer of the patch. The amount of the lidocaine that is absorbed from the Lidoderm is related to the length of application over your skin. The patch should be used for 12 hours over your painful area and then removed for 12 hours. If an irritation or a burning sensation occurs around the adhesive aspect of the patch, you should discontinue use of the patch. None of the patches mentioned in this chapter should ever be reused.

The Lidoderm patch has a polyester felt backing covered with a polyethylene film release liner. Prior to applying the patch on your skin, the release liner must be removed. Be aware that the patch does contain methylparaben, which is found in many suntan lotions. Do not use the Lidoderm patch if you have allergies to any suntan lotions that contain this chemical.

There does not appear to be any gender specificity related to the lidocaine in the patch. However, the incidence of shingles is higher in women than it is in men. You should not use the Lidoderm patch if you are using a heart drug to control your heartbeat. Even though the amount of lidocaine that you can absorb is small, it can interfere with some heart medicines. If you are using heart medications, discuss any potential drug interactions with you doctor. If you become lightheaded following application of the patch, you must stop using the patch immediately.

The Clonidine Patch

Clonidine is another *transdermal* medication. This patch is applied weekly to an area of your skin. The clonidine patch inhibits the release of norepinephrine, which is a pain transmitter. The clonidine patch is also used for the treatment of hypertension. If you have neuropathic pain (pain from a nerve that is diseased) or reflex sympathetic dystrophy, the clonidine patch may provide you with significant pain relief. It also can be successfully used if you have pain following shingles.

The application of the clonidine patch can be most useful for pain associated with a nerve injury or inflammation of a nerve. A new formulation of a topical clonidine gel will be available soon for the treatment of reflex sympathetic dystrophy and post-shingles pain. However, the clonidine transdermal drug delivery system is the only system currently available. The clonidine patch will not completely relieve your pain if you have reflex sympathetic dystrophy or post-shingles pain, but it can significantly decrease the burning component of your pain. The patch comes in different doses. The usual dose is the 0.1 milligram patch that is administered weekly.

Chapter 10

Realizing the Effects of Physical Therapy

Physical therapy is an important method that can be used to help manage your pain. A physical therapist can make you feel better when you hurt. If you have ever hurt your back while working, experienced tension headaches, or had a whiplash injury, you may benefit from seeing a physical therapist before you simply take a pill.

Before seeing a physical therapist, first talk to your doctor. Your doctor will tell you whether physical therapy treatments can benefit you.

This chapter will educate you on what to expect from visits to a physical therapist, how your doctor and physical therapist will work together to help relieve your pain, different physical therapy regimens for men and women, and physical therapy exercises you can do on your own to alleviate your pain.

What to Expect from a Physical Therapist

Physical therapists are highly trained individuals who will obtain a medical history from you and perform their own type of examination on you. Your physical therapist will decide what treatment is best for you based on your overall health. Your physical therapist will emphasize to you that you yourself are a major component in your rehabilitation and in the management of your chronic pain. Your physical therapist also will train you to avoid future re-injury and/or a recurrence of your pain problems. An example of how to avoid injury in the workplace is by keeping your back straight and bending your knees when lifting.

Not only is a physical therapy evaluation a planned treatment course for your pain, you also will receive an education on future injury prevention using hands-on treatment and verbal education. If you were injured in your workplace, your physical therapist will tell you how to avoid further injury there. You may also be placed in what is called a work-hardening program. This program duplicates your regular work duties and helps increase your muscles' strength and endurance so that you can return safely back to work, hopefully without further injury.

Your physical therapist will emphasize flexibility exercises to you and show you how to do them. You have to be able to move your joints without stiffness and pain. Furthermore, your physical therapist will work with you on your endurance and strength. Most important, your pain management treatment will be addressed. Your physical therapist will tell you how to deal with your ongoing pain and emphasize to you that you should try to minimize drug therapy. Your therapist will attempt to get you back to normal daily activity as soon as possible in a safe manner. You do not want to return to activity too soon following the onset of sudden pain because you could re-injure yourself or cause yourself a worse injury. For example, a physical therapist can help you prevent a work re-injury by strengthening both your back and leg muscles.

Your First Visit

When you see your physical therapist on your first visit, you should expect the therapist to obtain a detailed medical history from you. To provide you adequate treatment, your therapist will want to know your complete medical history as well as your pain history. For example, if you have a history of angina, your therapist will not overly stress you during exercise-related treatments because this may cause an increase in your heart rate and chest pain. If you have had surgery or have been involved in a motor vehicle accident, it is important that you tell your therapist while he or she is taking your history. Your therapist will become familiar with your pain history as well as your current pain complaints. Your history will give the therapist important information about your pain syndrome, its prognosis, and the appropriate time that you will be under the physical therapist's treatment.

Your therapist will also assess your behavioral response to your pain associated with your injury if you were injured in an accident or at work. Or if you have arthritis, your therapist will evaluate your pain input and behavior response to the arthritic pain. For example, your therapist will note if you grimace when you move your joints. You should inform your therapist about any previous therapies that you have had for control of your pain, including injection therapies with steroids.

Your therapist may additionally want to ask questions about your social history and family history if they may be relevant to your condition. If you have back pain or neck pain, for example, a family history of rheumatoid arthritis is important for the therapist to know. A family history of some pain causing diseases can increase your chance of developing pain. You should not be reluctant to give your therapist your age. Many conditions occur within certain age ranges. Osteoarthritis and osteoporosis are known to occur in an older population. Your therapist must know your occupation. If your job involves heavy physical labor, for example, you may be prone to overstress of your back muscles. Tell your therapist when the pain gets worse during the day or notify your therapist if you have increased pain with certain activities. With this information, your therapist can direct an appropriate therapy program for you.

If you have had a similar pain syndrome before your most current pain syndrome, again tell your therapist. If the intensity, duration, and frequency of your pain are increasing during therapy, your therapist may want to send you back to your doctor. This is an indication that you are becoming worse with respect to what is causing your pain.

For example, if you sustained a severe back injury years ago, a less traumatic back sprain may require longer and more intense physical therapy than in a situation where you had no previous back injury.

You should try to remember where your pain was when you first noticed it. Was the pain originally in your back and then later it moved to your leg? This may indicate a disc rupture. If your pain has moved or spread since you first noticed it, be sure to tell your therapist. Tell the therapist what exact movements worsen your pain. Even pain with bowel movements can be an important history fact. A disc rupture can be associated with back pain during the act of defecation. If your pain is worse in the morning and becomes progressively better during the day, this may be an indication that you have arthritis. Your therapist will need to know this information in order to prescribe the proper treatment for you.

Providing a good medical history to your therapist will make it much easier for the therapist to prescribe the proper method of treatment for your pain. You should write down all important information about yourself prior to your first therapy visit. Your therapist will need to know if your pain is in your bones, muscles, nerves, or all of them together. If the pain is in your bones, the pain is usually confined to that particular bone. If your pain is in a nerve, the pain will usually go down your arm or leg from where the therapist is pressing on your spine or neck. If your pain is in your muscles, your physical therapist will note that those muscles will contract more. Your therapist will examine the range of motion of your joints, including the range of motion of your neck and lower back. If you have a history of dizziness or fainting, tell your therapist before you begin an exercise program. A history of dizziness would alert the therapist to do less vigorous therapy.

You should expect your physical therapist to look you over. Your physical therapist will record how well you move as well as your posture. Your willingness to cooperate with your physical therapist also will be noted. Your therapist will evaluate how you walk. Your muscle size will be observed for unevenness between the right and left sides of your body from your neck down to your feet. This is because muscles can shrink in size from injury and may need more intense physical therapy.

The color of your skin will be noted. Sometimes if you have arthritis, there may be redness about your joints. Your hair pattern in your arms and legs will be evaluated. If you have decreased blood flow, there may be a loss of hair on your skin. Movements of your joints, neck, and lower back will be done to see how flexible you are. Any movements that are painful will be recorded and then will be addressed during your therapy session. Your therapist will decide whether heat or cold could help you with your range of motion or decrease your muscle spasms, which in turn will help decrease your pain.

Your physical therapist's examination will emphasize the joints of your body. The examination by your therapist will probably be more thorough than the examination by your doctor with respect to joint movement. On examination, your therapist will try to determine what movements worsen your pain. As you can see, the examination by your physical therapist can be very extensive. Your physical therapist will examine you for paralysis or a loss of your reflexes in your arms and legs. Any shrinkage of the muscle in your arms and legs will be addressed. For example, if you have decreased muscle size in your thigh, your therapist will target this area to increase strength and muscle mass. Your therapist will, furthermore, examine you for any loss of sensation in your arms and legs. For example, if you have loss of sensation in your right shoulder, your therapist will be careful not to apply heat on this area for any significant length of time. A heating pad could cause the burning of your skin if you are unable to detect the sensation of heat about your shoulder.

Becoming Part of the Team

After your therapist has examined you, the therapist may call your doctor to recommend any further laboratory tests or x-rays. After the history and physical examination has been completed, your physical therapist will determine what is causing your pain problem and will design a treatment program for you based on these findings. You will be treated as a complete individual, not just a pain symptom. If your assessment was not done thoroughly, your treatment regimen may not help you with respect to your pain syndrome. If you are experiencing significant pain during your therapy, immediately notify your therapist. One goal of physical therapy is to identify the cause of your pain with an attempt to treat the cause of your pain syndrome.

In addition to rehabilitating you following your injury or illness, your physical therapist will attempt to correct any mechanical flaws in your body that could lead to further injury, such as your posture. Your therapist may do a muscle and joint stabilization program to increase your strength and flexibility. For example, if your lower back muscles or stomach muscles have become weak you will need to do vigorous exercises that give your back stabilization, which means that your back (including your discs and joints) will not move when you move. This stabilization will decrease your pain.

You, on the other hand, must always feel that you are a main component in your rehabilitation. If your therapist gives you exercises to do at home, follow the instructions on how to do them and do them on the prescribed schedule. Try and take charge of your pain.

Because you will be working closely as a team member with your physical therapist, you must choose a physical therapist that you feel most comfortable with. Your physical therapist will treat you with exercise and strengthening techniques, but also may complement your therapy with whirlpool baths, paraffin baths, or other methods such as using electrical current. Heat packs can provide you with surface heating, which may reduce the pain in some surface muscles in your back, arms, or legs. Ultrasound is a deep application of heat. This method can relax your deep muscles. Elastic exercise bands and medicine balls may be used to increase your arm and leg strength. The elastic bands can be used to increase your strength, and the medicine balls can be used to increase your range of motion and your flexibility as well as your strength. Some physical therapists use traction for the management of your pain. Traction on your neck or back can increase blood flow to the injured area of your back. However, if the traction does significantly increase your pain, you must immediately notify your physical therapist. Your physical therapist may instruct you in stretching exercises to be used at home. You must be diligent in doing these exercises provided for you.

Remember that physical therapists are highly trained individuals. Each state requires that a physical therapist pass a licensure exam after graduating from an accredited physical therapy program. Some physical therapists have Master's degrees as well as Ph.D.s in physical therapy. Most physical therapists will be glad to give you a resumé of their credentials. It takes an abundance of hard work to become a physical therapist, and they are proud of their credentials. Therefore, you should not feel timid in asking for them.

Different Regimens for Men and Women

Women can have very different fitness and training needs than men. Be aware that the muscle and bone development of adolescent girls is different from that of adolescent boys. A woman's nutritional requirements change with each phase of life. Proper nutrition is crucial to achieve proper hormone balance. For example, be aware that osteoporosis in adult women can be a result of poor nutrition. Women are more prone to fad dieting and eating disorders. If you have a problem with your diet or have an eating disorder, tell your doctor. A woman's muscle mass in many instances will be less than that of a man, and a woman may have more body fat. Physical therapy is not performed in a cookbook fashion. This is the reason that physical therapy has to be tailored for you as an individual. Because of these gender differences, a physical therapy evaluation is important before initiating an exercise program for you.

Physical therapists are trained to address a woman's health care before and after pregnancy. A therapist can help you with incontinence, vaginal and pelvic pain, pre- and post-delivery muscle and bone pain, and sacroiliac joint pain. The sacroiliac joint is a joint between your back bone and your hip bone. Many times during and after pregnancy, the ligaments in this joint become loose and cause chronic joint pain. Your physical therapist can work on strengthening the muscles around your pelvis and also provide you with a Velcro belt to stabilize your joints until they become stronger again. Because of the hormones that are released during pregnancy, the joints in your spine and pelvis may become loose. These hormonal effects and the looseness of the ligaments and joints make it easier for you to deliver your baby. These hormonal changes are natural protective mechanisms in your body. Be aware of these hormonal changes and realize that these changes ultimately cause you to have back and joint pain. Hormonal effects in a woman may be a cause of breast cancer. Women who have had radiation treatment for breast cancer may experience declines in their immune system function. Aerobic exercise programs given to you by your physical therapist can lessen the decline in your immune system function. Moderate-intensity aerobic exercise during radiation treatment for breast cancer is undergoing further study and does appear to be promising. Women undergoing radiation therapy for breast cancer can become tired easily and their mood can become depressed. It has been shown in studies of women undergoing radiation therapy for breast cancer that moderate-intensity aerobic exercise can improve both their mood as well as lessen their tiredness.

Knee injuries are becoming more common in women athletes. As more women participate in sports, more studies are being conducted into the injuries they suffer. The anterior cruciate ligament in a woman's knee has been shown to have a much higher rate of injury as opposed to a man's. It may be related to the looseness of ligaments, depending on the hormone levels of a woman at the time of injury. Furthermore, a woman's strength may be less than a man's, and other body structure differences can make a woman more prone to this type of injury than a man. Before engaging in sports, women must be preconditioned with muscle-strengthening programs. Physical therapists are a part of this program. Following an anterior cruciate ligament injury, there are no differences between men and women with respect to post-injury rehabilitation.

You must remember that women as opposed to men have a higher percentage of body fat and a smaller muscle mass. The metabolism of a woman can be less than that of a man. These differences in body composition have implications for gender specificity in the muscles and bones of women. These differences affect the way a physical therapist addresses pain syndromes in a man versus a woman. Also remember that men still have more physically demanding occupations and recreational activities. These differences are changing but still exist, which will affect the way in which a physical therapist manages your pain complaints.

Women are more likely to use different methods in physical therapy than men, including relaxation, heat or cold packs, and massage. However, the effects of massage and heat and cold therapies can change for women sensitive during their menstrual cycle. If you consider all the factors mentioned in this chapter, you can see that a physical therapist should use a different approach for both men and women. Therapies should be determined based on gender specificity so that the wide array of methods offered can be selected based on each person's diagnosis, age, and gender rather than at random.

Therapy Exercises

Remember that you, your physical therapist, and your physician make up a pain-management team and that it is important for all the team members to be aware of any new pain problems. If certain exercises that you are doing do not provide you with pain relief, ask your physical therapist to recommend some other exercises or range-of-motion methods that you can do at home or at work.

Physical therapists can help you decrease your muscle tension. Your therapist can also educate you on how to decrease muscle tension yourself. Most muscle tension is related to the stress of everyday life. As you know, it is impossible to decrease your discomfort associated with stress when the stress does occur. While flying on an airplane, you may experience stress when the plane bounces around in turbulent weather. You may experience stress in your job if you have to make a presentation in front of a group. The muscles in your body naturally tense up when you are stressed. When you experience stress, your body has a protective mechanism that increases your muscle tightness. This is an early part of the fight-or-flight response to stressful situations. A generic example of fight-or-flight is perhaps a rattle snake encounter in which you may either try to kill the snake (fight) or run away (flight) because of your fright or fear.

This fight-or-flight response can be helpful for your protection if you are threatened. However, when your muscles stay contracted, the blood flow to your muscles decreases. This cuts off the oxygen supply to your muscles. Without oxygen, your muscles begin to hurt. Your muscles are trying to tell you that something is wrong. When you are under stress, the muscles around your ribcage become contracted and you don't breathe as deeply. At this time you may want to concentrate and take a deep breath to increase the oxygen into your bloodstream so that your muscles may have adequate oxygen.

Stretching Exercises

Why take pain-relieving medications if you can do some simple stretching exercises to decrease your pain? All pills can have one or more side effects. Your therapist will show you stretching exercises that will be safe for you to do based on your overall health. You may want to do these exercises periodically throughout the day. Do stretching exercises in the morning and before you go to bed at night.

Hot and Cold Therapy

Remember that you can use heat packs or cold packs in addition to stretching to relieve your pain. If you have an acute injury, you can use a cold pack for 10 to 12 minutes to decrease tissue swelling following the injury. You can take a package of frozen food out of your freezer and apply it over your area of pain. You should wrap the frozen food package in a towel to prevent a cold injury to your skin.

You should not use cold packs if you have chronic muscle spasm pain. The cold can decrease the blood flow to the muscle and in turn decrease oxygen, which may increase your muscle contraction and worsen your pain. For chronic muscle or joint pain, use a heat pack. Be careful not to burn your skin with a heat pack. Wrap the heat pack in a towel to prevent a heat injury to your skin. While using heat or cold packs, remember to breathe deeply. Take a deep breath in through your nose and hold it for several seconds and then blow out through your nose. Also remember to oxygenate the injured area every four or five minutes by removing the hot or cold pack.

Learn to manage your pain with breathing and exercise techniques. Pregnant women have been shown to decrease their labor pain by doing certain breathing exercises. However, if your pain remains severe and constant, or if you develop numbness and weakness in your arms and legs, you must notify your doctor.

Relieving Headache Tension

If you have a headache, you may want to do some exercises yourself before seeking medical attention. It is too easy to take a pill and hope that it relieves your pain. Instead, you should learn to control your pain. As you feel your symptoms coming on, try to take control of your headache immediately. If you are under stress, the muscles in your neck and at the base of your skull become tense. This tension can cause you to have a headache.

If you spend a long time over your computer with your neck in a forward bent position, this can stress the muscles in your neck and cause muscle tension headaches. Your head weighs about 10 pounds. So when your head is in a forward position, it is similar to placing a 10 pound bowling ball at the end of your neck. This increased weight pulls your neck and tightens your neck muscles.

Be sure to properly support your head. Your head is like a golf ball on a tee. It needs support. Your muscles and the discs between your neck bones have to bear the extra stress placed on your neck and back if you have poor posture. Hold a bowling ball out directly in front of you and observe how fast that your arm becomes tired. Now imagine what stress your neck experiences to hold your head in an upright position.

The next time you are in front of your computer, pay attention to your head and neck position. If your head has been in an abnormal position for a long time, you may need to do range of motion exercises. Simply repositioning your head in a neutral position will not relieve your pain. When you are standing, sitting, or driving, remember that your head is a 10-pound weight at the end of your neck. You must attempt to keep your head in line with your neck as much as possible.

Here are some helpful headache exercises for you to try when you begin to experience a headache. These exercises will take your neck through its normal range of motion (the degree of movement of a joint or tissue). Be sure that you do not force your range of motion. If your pain increases, stop the range-of-motion exercises. If you have rheumatoid arthritis of your neck, you do not need to do these exercises:

1. Put the palms of both of your hands at the top of your forehead. Your fingers will be on your scalp. Massage your scalp in backward and forward motions 5 times to relieve tension in the muscles over your scalp.
2. Use the index (pointer) fingers of both hands and make circular motions to massage the area about 1 inch above your eyebrows 5 times.

3. Bend your head down and place your chin on your chest 5 times.
4. Take a deep breath through your nose and exhale through your nose 5 times.
5. Look up to the ceiling and bring your head as far back as you can. Hold this position for 2 to 3 seconds and repeat it 5 times.

Neck Pain Exercises

Neck pain is a common occurrence in almost everyone. Be sure that you always use proper posture techniques. Also pay attention to your neck position when you are using a telephone. Deep breathing before and after completing your exercises is important. If you feel that your neck is stuck or "catches" in a certain position when doing exercises, that cause may be related to a joint in your neck. Be sure to notify your doctor or physical therapist immediately. The bones in your neck and back stack on top of each other like Lego blocks. Sometimes these joints can get out of position, especially if you slouch over a computer all day. Your physical therapist may be able to help you with this misalignment of your neck. The following exercise may help relieve some pain as soon as you begin to feel it in your neck. If any of these exercises cause you to have pain, you must stop the exercises and range-of-motion maneuvers. Be sure to take a deep breath before you begin and after you finish the exercises:

1. Begin with your head in a neutral position. Now bend your neck down and put your chin on your chest, hold if for 2 to 3 seconds and then bring it back up to a neutral position. Repeat this exercise 5 times.
2. Turn your neck to the right and hold that position for 2 to 3 seconds. Then slowly turn your neck to the left and hold that position for 2 to 3 seconds. Repeat this exercise 5 times.
3. Starting from a neutral position, bend your neck to place your right ear on your right shoulder and hold the position for 2 to 3 seconds. Then slowly bend your neck the other direction and place your left ear on your left shoulder and hold the position for 2 to 5 seconds. Repeat this exercise 3 to 5 times.

Back Pain Exercises

Pain in your lower back is very common. The vast majority of people who go to a pain-medicine doctor have pain in their lower back. Eighty percent of people living in the United States will experience back pain in their lower back at some point in their lives. Stress in your life can be a cause of significant back pain because it tightens your back muscles.

Throughout your spine there are a large number of bones that are separated from one another by discs that work as shock absorbers. There are small joints that exist as one bone stacks on top of the other, which is similar to the principle of a Lego block. These joints throughout your back are called facet joints. Between the two bones, a small joint is formed which allows your back bones to have smooth spinal movement. This is the maneuver that enables you to bend forward, bend backward, and twist to the right and left sides. There are holes in each bone that allow the nerves in your spine to go to your arms and legs and occasionally to your internal organs. Your spine is kept in place by the muscles in your lower back, which enables you to maintain your posture as well as give you stability in your back when you move. Ligaments attach the bones in your back, neck, and mid-back to each other. Your ligaments and muscles are necessary to give your back stability and to enable you to position your spine correctly.

If you slouch or have bad posture, these elements of your back can become out of alignment. Your muscles then can pull to one side and stretch on the opposite side of your back. Remember, if you slouch over a chair for a long period of time, your spine is going to adapt to these positions. Just changing your posture, therefore, will not relieve you of your pain. If you sit hunched over a desk all day, your ability to stand or sit upright will be compromised. Slouching puts more pressure and stress on the discs of your back than any other posture. When you are sitting for any length of time, you should stand for 10 minutes each hour to take the pressure off the discs in your lower back. You might be wondering how the average office worker gets the boss to agree to this. Try discussing options with your human resource risk management personnel—some companies require this.

If you sit in an abnormal position for a long length of time over months and years, the joints in your back that fit together like Lego pieces wear away, the joints calcify, and the alignment of your spine becomes abnormal. When this happens, the bones and joints can press down on the nerves going to your arms and legs and cause you pain. Note your position now while you are reading this book. Are you sitting up straight? When sitting for any length of time, put a pillow behind your back in the lower part of your chair to relieve some of the stress on your back.

Whenever you feel any twinge of back pain, stand and face the wall directly in front of you and do the following range-of-motion exercises:

1. Keep both feet straight pointing toward the wall. Place both hands over your lower back with your fingers pointing down to the floor. Bend slightly backward and stretch as far as you can go. Bend backward until your face is pointing directly to the ceiling and hold the position for 2 to 3 seconds. Slowly return to the upright position. Repeat this exercise 5 times, beginning each time with a deep breath in and ending the exercise with a deep breath out.
2. Begin in an upright position. Bend forward at the waist and go forward as far as you can and then stop. Hold this position for 2 to 3 seconds. Repeat this exercise 5 times and be sure to use deep-breathing exercises.
3. Stand straight facing the wall. Bend your waist to the right and hold this position for 3 seconds. Slowly return to an upright position again. Then bend to the left as far as you can and hold this position for 3 seconds. Repeat this exercise 5 times.
4. Sit on the edge of your chair. Place your knees as far apart as possible. Reach down between your legs and grab your ankles. Now try to pull yourself down even further. Hold this position for 2 to 3 seconds and repeat it 5 times.

Be sure to begin and end each exercise with deep breathing. If any of these exercises increases your pain, stop doing them immediately and notify your doctor or physical therapist. If these exercises provide you with significant relief, your physical therapist may give you even more exercises to strengthen your back and help preserve your range of motion.

Good posture is important to help prevent back pain. You should adjust your chairs and car seat to keep your mid-back in a straight position. If you sit in an improper position, such as bending over a computer, you may injure the area where your ribs attach to your breastbone. This can cause you to have an aching chest pain, which you may confuse with a heart attack. It is important that you always attempt to sit up straight.

You should look at your mid-back in the mirror. Do you have an "S" shape in your mid-back? If you slouch at your desk with your spine directed to one side, it can make you lopsided and cause scoliosis. Scoliosis is the curvature in your mid-back. A muscle imbalance either above or below the curve in your back can cause scoliosis. If you have any type of curvature in your back, concentrate on keeping your mid-back straight. Here are some exercises to help you with this type of situation. Be sure to use a proper breathing technique before and after each exercise:

1. Begin sitting up straight. Put your palms behind your head. Now bend your mid-back backward. Hold the position for 2 to 3 seconds and repeat it 5 times.
2. Sitting up straight once again, cross your arms in front of your chest. Turn your upper body to the right and hold this position for 3 seconds. Now rotate your body to the left and hold the position for 3 seconds. Repeat this exercise 5 times.
3. Finally, stand up straight. Place your hands together and hold your arms over your head. While facing a wall in front of you, bend to the right as far as you can. Hold this position for 3 seconds. Come back to a straight position and bend to the left and hold the position for 3 seconds. Repeat this exercise 3 to 5 times.

Chapter 11
Trying Alternative Therapy

You don't have to rely simply on the use of traditional medicine to treat your pain. There are many other options for you to try, including chiropractic therapy, reflexology, massage, acupuncture, and even aromatherapy. These methods often can be less expensive than traditional medicine. As with any type of treatment, be sure to speak with your health-care provider to make sure you understand the type of treatment you are considering and to see if it will be the most beneficial for relieving your pain.

Some alternative medicine practices and herbal medications were mentioned to you in Chapter 8. This chapter will go over some of those more in-depth for you. You will learn again about chiropractic therapy with more detail on how it works, its benefits, and what your chiropractor can do for you. You will also learn about hot and cold therapies, electric therapy, traction, reflexology, massage, aroma therapy, and acupuncture.

Don't be afraid to seek out other forms of treatment. Remember, this is your pain and it is up to you to help yourself try to relieve it.

Chiropractic Therapy

Chiropractic therapy was established as a profession in 1895. It is now the second-largest primary health-care field in the world. You may be scared of the dangers and side effects of pills and procedures that may lead you to seek out chiropractic therapy. Chiropractic therapy as a profession emphasizes your body's natural health abilities. Many people associate chiropractic therapy with only back and neck pain. However, chiropractic therapy has been shown to be safe for the treatment of headaches, carpal tunnel syndrome, and pain in your arms and legs.

Chiropractic medicine can improve your body function and enhance your body's healing powers. Some chiropractors emphasize a healthful lifestyle, a healthful diet, and stress reduction. They will educate you with respect to your lifestyle at each visit. Many times your doctor will refer you to a chiropractor or physical therapist if you have neck and back pain. In many instances your doctor will refer you to a chiropractor, who often works together with a physical therapist working at their clinic. Both of these professions can help you with your chronic pain.

How Chiropractic Therapy Works

At one time *conventional medicine* practitioners viewed chiropractic care as quackery. Now chiropractic therapy enjoys wide acceptance by *conventional medicine* practitioners. Some chiropractors have been appointed to workmen's compensation boards. Some are even on staff at hospitals. Some chiropractors work closely with pain-medicine doctors. Following injections into the small joints in your back, a chiropractor may come to your hospital to adjust your back and realign your spine. This is less painful to you because you are numb following an injection and it makes it easier for your chiropractor to adjust your spine.

Chiropractors are involved in sports medicine. They provide medical expert testimony with respect to whiplash injuries and other injuries of the spine in courtrooms. Be aware that the relationship between chiropractors and medical doctors has improved over the past decade. Do not be alarmed if your doctor recommends a referral to a chiropractor.

The definition of chiropractic therapy is the correction of problems that exist in your spinal column. This enables your body to function at its peak level without medications, surgical procedures, or steroid injections. In 1999, more than 25 million Americans were treated by chiropractors. Not only do chiropractors take care of back injuries, they also can help you with your neck, hip, leg, ankle, foot, arm, and hand pain. Most back and neck pains are the result of mechanical disorders in your spine.

It has been shown that people treated with chiropractic medicine recover faster than nonchiropractic-treated patients. The problem with chiropractic medicine is that it has been maligned for a long time in the United States. However, it is now widely accepted. In Canada, which is under a national health-care system, chiropractic care is included among treatment methods that are reimbursed by the national system. If you have a back injury caused by a twist or turn, you may want to go to a chiropractor. If you have a back injury and need strengthening exercises, your doctor may refer you to a physical therapist.

Chiropractic medicine focuses its attention on the relationship between the structure of your spine and how it affects your nervous system. You have 24 back bones and 31 nerves that come off of your spinal cord. The nerves come out of a hole in the bones called a foramina. If your spine is not in alignment due to slouching or poor posture, this can cause some of your nerves to be pressed on by your spine. Your chiropractor will adjust your spine to remove any spinal abnormalities to reduce pressure off of the nerves in your arms and legs.

The bones in your back form a protection for the spinal cord. Be aware that the nerves coming off of the spinal cord can go to your organs and glands as well as to your muscles, bones, and nerves in your arms and legs. Your brain, which functions as a computer, sends electrical impulses that essentially regulate all of your bodily functions. When your spine is not aligned correctly, it can cause you tension in your muscles that will in turn affect your nervous system. Compression on your spine and the nerves that come off of your spinal cord can cause you significant health problems and pain.

If your neck and back are not in alignment, your neck and back will have a decrease in their range of motion. This will make you feel stiff. It also can cause you to have muscle spasms, pain, and even headaches. Be aware that blood vessels also run next to nerves that go to your arms, legs, and organs. If your spine is not aligned, you can possibly compress some of these blood vessels, which will make your arms and legs become cold. Therefore, the goal of chiropractic therapy is to correct the misalignment throughout your spine to allow your body to restore itself. Chiropractic therapy gives you a chance to control your pain while emphasizing better health.

Chiropractors complete six to seven years of college, including postgraduate study. There are 17 accredited chiropractic colleges in the United States. Chiropractors complete two years of undergraduate courses before going to chiropractic school. Chiropractors must pass a national exam and obtain a state license just like your regular medical doctor before they can practice.

Benefits of Chiropractic Therapy

The early Egyptians practiced spinal manipulation. However, in 1895, the founder of chiropractic medicine, Daniel Palmer, was a student of both physiology as well as anatomy and studied the effect of spinal manipulation on neck and back pain. The overall goal of chiropractic medicine is to treat the cause of one's pain as opposed to just treating symptoms.

You do not have to wait until you have pain to seek chiropractic help. Periodic chiropractic adjustments can prevent everyday wear and tear on your joints and ligaments throughout your spine. Your chiropractor will emphasize increases in motion around your neck and back. If you receive regular chiropractic care, you may have better long-term relief with this method as opposed to *conventional medicine* methods.

Be aware that chiropractic medicine is safer than *conventional medicine* in the fact that no narcotics, muscle relaxants, and other potentially addicting drugs are prescribed by chiropractors. All drugs can have some side effects as well as cause some allergies. It has been shown that only sixty percent of people with back pain actually receive relief with surgery. As a result of these findings, you may be interested in chiropractic medicine to help you relieve your pain.

Many reports indicate that chiropractic medicine results in high patient satisfaction. According to the National Library of Medicine website, www.nlm.nih.gov, studies reported that this is due to the hands-on application of a chiropractor as opposed to a *conventional* medical specialist. You may be afraid that if a chiropractic physician manipulates your neck or back that you may become paralyzed. The chance of these occurrences is extremely rare. Remember, if you have a steroid injection in your neck or back, there is a small chance that you could become paralyzed as well. Studies have also shown that chiropractic medicine is cost-effective.

Be aware that some chiropractors limit their practice to your spine. Other chiropractors emphasize not only spinal manipulation but treat arm and leg pain and provide nutritional counseling as well. Often chiropractors will use traction, cold packs, electrical stimulation, ultrasound, and cryotherapy to help control your pain. These methods are similar to those used by physical therapists. If you aren't familiar with cryotherapy, it is the application of cold packs to your tissue—the cold decreases tissue swelling and decreases pain fiber nerve ending sensitivity. Some chiropractors can even perform acupuncture and recommend herbal medicines. Make sure you talk with your chiropractor before beginning treatment to see if he or she can provide you with the right type of therapy to best help you control your pain.

What Your Chiropractor Can Do For You

Your first visit with a chiropractor will result in a complete medical history as well as a complete examination of your spine. Your chiropractor will tell you what the goals of chiropractic medicine are. Your chiropractor will feel the entire spinal region to detect any misalignments throughout your spine. Your chiropractor will most likely take an x-ray and possibly even an MRI of your spine. After this has been accomplished, your chiropractor will recommend a treatment course for you. Your chiropractor will explain to you the purpose of manipulative therapy. Your chiropractor may even do a manipulation of your spine on the first visit. It is difficult to estimate how many treatments you will need before your pain has been significantly decreased. Following your care, your chiropractor will re-evaluate your progress from time to time. After your spine has been misaligned for any length of time, your body may have a tendency to resume that misalignment again. Therefore, periodic visits with your chiropractor are recommended.

Your chiropractor can treat you for neck and back injuries. Some chiropractors also treat carpal tunnel syndrome and sports injuries that limit your range of motion. You may seek a chiropractor if you are pregnant and have pain in the joints of your back and hips during pregnancy.

You may want to have your spine aligned on a regular basis. This is called preventive medicine. This keeps the spine from going out of alignment. Your chiropractor will address your posture with you and your posture during your awakening days and your posture around your home doing regular activities of daily living. You may want to see your chiropractor every six weeks for preventive purposes.

Remember that steroid injections are not permanent and the effects only last from weeks to months. Chiropractic manipulation can be utilized for the rest of your life. There is a limit to the amount of steroids that you can receive in a year and there is also a limit to the amount of medications that you can take. Remember that all of these methods can have potential side effects.

There are three degrees of ligament or muscle injuries that you should be aware of. An injury to a muscle is called a *strain,* whereas an injury to a ligament is called a *sprain.* If you sustain a grade I soft-tissue injury, this means that the fibers of your muscle and ligaments remain intact. If you have a grade II injury, this is more serious and the fibers of your muscle or your ligaments are partly torn. If you sustain a grade III injury, the fibers of your muscle or your ligaments are completely ruptured or torn. At this time, your arm, leg, shoulder, hip, or knee has essentially no functional use. Grades II and III injuries need to be addressed by an orthopedic surgeon. Your orthopedic surgeon may have to suture your ligament together if you have a severe sprain.

Hot and Cold Chiropractic Therapies

After your chiropractor has diagnosed your degree of injury or the cause of your back or neck pain, your chiropractor may treat you with the following methods: cryotherapy, paraffin baths, hydrocolator packs, and whirlpool baths. Infrared lamps and ultraviolet light can also be used to treat your pain with these methods that release heat. Ice and cold water are used to treat swelling in your arms and legs after an injury. If you have arthritis or chronic pain, heat is used to increase blood flow to the painful tissue. The heat can relax your muscles as well. If you have pain that is immediately under the skin, called *superficial pain*, an infrared heat lamp can be used to treat your pain or to relax the upper muscles in your neck and back. The heat can increase the blood flow in the skin and superficial muscles. The superficial heat can also relax some of the muscles immediately under the skin. Superficial infrared heat can relax your muscles.

Another superficial method of treating your pain is cryotherapy, which uses ice packs, cold sprays, cold whirlpools, or even ice massage to your body. The cold will decrease the blood flow to your muscles and skin. The purpose of the reduction in the blood flow to these tissues is to decrease the swelling that follows an acute injury to your tissues. Cold can decrease pain transmission to your nerves. Cold spray has been used to treat the pain associated with muscle pain syndromes. If your health-care provider leaves cold over your tissue for more than 15 minutes, the blood vessels in this tissue may get bigger, which in turn will increase the blood flow to this tissue. This may be of benefit after your swelling has decreased with the initial application of the cold methods. You must be aware that cold can decrease the speed of nerve conductions. Therefore, cold will decrease the amount of pain impulses that reach your spinal cord and ultimately the pain impulses that go to your brain.

Cold methods should be used within the first 72 hours following an injury to your tissue. You should not use cold for more than 15 minutes at a time. You can repeat the cold applications every two hours if necessary. Here are a few types of cold therapy you can try at home:

- You can use a package of vegetables, holding the frozen package against your areas of pain to decrease your pain.
- You can have someone put ice in a plastic bag and massage your neck or back if you have had a recent injury to your neck or back. The ice massage should be done in a rotating pattern.
- Cold sprays can be used to decrease your muscle spasms. After your muscle has been sprayed with the cold spray, the muscle should then be massaged.
- Cold whirlpools can be used for any swelling in your arms or legs following an injury. The water temperature should be about 60 degrees, and your treatment time should not exceed 15 minutes.

There are also some heat methods you can try yourself to help relieve your pain:

- Take a hot shower or a hot bath, directing the water over your painful body areas.
- Moisten a towel and warm it in the microwave. You might need to wrap another towel around the hot towel to prevent a burn to your skin. Apply it to your painful area for 10 to 15 minutes.
- If you have pain in your hands or feet related to pain syndromes such as arthritis, a superficial heat method that is frequently used is a paraffin bath. During this treatment, you place your hands or feet in melted paraffin wax. You then remove your hand or foot from the paraffin and allow it to cool. Repeat this procedure 8 to 10 times. This method can help you with movement of your fingers and toes as well as your wrist and ankles. The treatment time should be about 15 minutes.

You can also consider alternating heat and cold every two to four hours for pain relief.

Ultraviolet light is not frequently used for the management of pain. However, people with back pain have gone to tanning booths and related that they have had relief for up to 24 hours after leaving the ultraviolet booth.

Deep heat is another form of heat therapy that can be used to manage your pain. The use of ultrasound heat is common in both chiropractic medicine as well as in physical therapy. This deep heat can provide significant pain relief and is used to treat a wide range of disorders, including bursitis and deep muscle spasms. Ultrasound consists of sound energy. You are unable to hear the sound emitted from the ultrasound machine. The ultrasound device gives off sound waves to your body. The sound waves will get the molecules of your tissue to vibrate. The vibration creates friction between the molecules of your tissue and the friction is converted into heat. This type of heat goes deep into your body and can provide you with better pain relief than superficial heat such as warm baths and showers. The ultrasound energy can penetrate about 2 inches into your body. The ultrasound will allow nutrients to go into your nerve and muscle cells. Overall, ultrasound will increase your circulation in many situations and provide you with pain relief. Deep-heat therapy as well as superficial heat therapy should not be used if you have had a recent injury within the past 72 hours. The duration of your treatment is about six minutes.

Another procedure used along with the deep-heat therapy is phonophoresis. During this procedure, medications are driven under your skin to a depth of about 2 millimeters. Phonophoresis is ultrasound mixed with steroids or numbing medicine such as lidocaine. The purpose of the phonophoresis is to apply the medication at the area of your pain. All the ultrasound treatments can be used in muscle pain as well as tendonitis and bursitis.

Diathermia is also another deep-heat method. This type of heat can use microwave energy waves. This device can provide heat to your deeper muscles which can relax your muscles as well as increase the blood flow to your deeper muscles to give you pain relief.

Electric Therapy

Electricity can be used to treat your pain syndrome as well. Over the years, many claims have been made for the therapeutic application of electrical current for the treatment of some pain syndromes. Electrical current is applied to your body by placement of electrodes, which are patches with adhesive that stick to your body. The current is directed over the painful areas of your body. Electrical current can vibrate the molecules of your tissues similar to ultrasound therapy. The vibration produced by friction between the molecules of your tissues will increase your tissue temperature. As a result, heat is produced. As electrical current passes through your tissue, some nerves are excited while others are not.

It has been shown that electricity can stimulate tissue growth and repair and is sometimes used by orthopedic surgeons to stimulate bone growth following bone surgery. Sometimes stimulators can be placed following orthopedic surgery to enhance bone growth. Theoretically, the electrical current should speed up your healing time.

A popular electrical current emitting device that is used frequently in pain medicine by *conventional* physicians, chiropractic physicians, and physical therapists is the *transcutaneous electrical nerve stimulator (TENS)*. A TENS unit applies electrical current to your body through electrodes that are adhered to your body. The TENS unit is used for pain control. The power source is battery operated. TENS unit therapy became popular in the late 1960s and early 1970s. The use of a TENS unit for the treatment of your chronic pain syndrome if you have neck, back, arm, and leg pain is well documented.

A TENS unit has an amplitude knob that lets you control your pain relief. These TENS units are about the size of a pager. The TENS unit patches can be placed over your muscles or nerves for the management of pain both in your muscles as well as the nerves in your arms and legs. You can use a TENS unit for the control of your pain long-term without any significant side effects. Some people have allergic reactions to the adhesive in the patches. There are nonallergen patches that can be purchased. A TENS unit can reduce your pain as well as your stress. However, you should still strive for proper body mechanics and posture. You must remember that a TENS unit is only treating your symptoms. You are in charge of the cause of your pain. If your pain is related to poor body posture, strive to correct this problem.

Iontophoresis is the use of an electrical current to drive medications through your skin. Different medications can be applied through your skin to decrease your pain. Not only is electrical current used for pain relief, it can also speed up your tissue healing.

Traction Therapy

Traction is another method that is frequently used by chiropractors and physical therapists. Traction involves mechanical forces that separate adjacent body parts away from each other. If you have problems with a disc in your neck or back, traction can separate the bones in your back and increase your blood flow to your injured tissue, which can speed up healing. If traction causes you worsening of your pain, you should inform your health-care provider so that the traction can be immediately discontinued. Because of the differences in muscle mass between men and women, the amount of traction applied will differ between men and women. If you have a ruptured disc in your neck or back, traction can help heal this painful entity.

Reflexology

Reflexology is another method used in nonconventional medicine practice to decrease your pain. Reflexology relieves muscle stress and relaxes your muscles through the application of pressure on specific areas of your feet. Reflexology has been used for thousands of years in mideastern countries. In the early twentieth century, a doctor mapped the foot areas that related to areas of the body that affected different medical conditions. This doctor divided the body into 10 zones and labeled parts of the foot that he believed controlled each zone. Gentle pressure on an area of the foot would generate not only pain relief but healing in general in the defined zone. These areas of pressure in your feet are called *reflex points*.

The philosophy of reflexology is that your body contains an energy field. When your energy field is blocked, you develop pain and/or illness. Stimulation of your foot and the nerves that end in your feet can unblock the energy flow and, therefore, increase energy to various parts of your body and promote healing as well as decrease your pain. It is also believed that stimulation of your feet can release the natural pain killers in your body called *endorphins*. Reflexology treatment sessions can last from 30 to 60 minutes. Usually you will receive a four-week treatment program. You can learn to do reflexology maneuvers yourself. Unfortunately, there is no state licensure nor is there any specific training to become a reflexology specialist.

Reflexology can be used for the management of your back pain. Reflexologists believe that nerve endings in the feet have inner connection throughout the spinal cord and brain to reach all areas of the body. The problem with reflexology is that it has not been scientifically studied and still remains an unproven treatment regimen for the management of your pain.

According to some reports on the NIH and NLM alternative medicine websites, reflexology reduces symptoms associated with female premenstrual syndrome. A study that has recently been published reported that women suffering from breast cancer pain have had a significant decrease in their pain following reflexology treatment. Migraines are more prevalent in women than in men. Reflexology has been reported to be effective for the management of some people who are suffering from migraine headaches.

Massage Therapy

Therapeutic massage can significantly help you control your pain, especially if you have muscle spasms. Massage can decrease your stress as well as decrease your headaches and pain associated with whiplash injuries. Massage therapy promotes generalized body relaxation. Massage is the application of touch to your muscles or ligaments that does not cause your tissue to move or change position of a joint. Massage therapy can decrease your lower back pain as well as your neck pain. It also has been effective to reduce pain associated with sciatica. Massage therapy can decrease the pain associated with your headaches and can relieve your muscle spasms.

There are different types of massage therapy. The Swedish massage is the most common form of massage therapy in the United States. Swedish massage works on the superficial layers of the skin as well as the superficial muscles of your body. Swedish massage promotes relaxation and improves circulation in your superficial muscles. Another type of massage is deep-tissue massage. This is more direct pressure on the deeper muscle layers of your body. Deep-tissue massage is highly effective for the treatment of lower back pain. Sports massage combines Swedish massage with deep-tissue massage. This type of massage therapy can decrease your pain following a vigorous athletic workout. It may not be a good idea to use therapeutic massage if you have certain forms of cancer, heart disease, or some infectious diseases. If you have these conditions, massage therapy could cause some spread of your tumor if done over your tumor. Talk with your doctor before beginning massage therapy if you have any of these conditions.

Women are more willing to use massage therapy. This finding should suggest that men may benefit from massage therapy if they were encouraged to use it and if they were educated in this method. Menstrual status can affect the effectiveness of massage when it is used for pain relief.

Aromatherapy

Another method to help you with your pain is aromatherapy. Women have a better perception of smell than men. Therefore, women are more likely to use aromatherapy because they have better results from this method. For hundreds of years, oils extracted from plants have been used to relieve pain. During your first session with an aromatherapy specialist, the specialist will select the oil that is appropriate for relieving your pain. You may have a treatment for up to nine minutes. Aromatherapy stimulates pleasure centers in your brain from nerves in the nose that senses smell. Aromatherapy can be used to improve your quality of life and provide you with some relaxation. It has been used for pain management during childbirth. It can be used if you have arthritis, back pain, neck pain, and other chronic pain syndromes.

Aromatherapy is reportedly effective for the treatment of muscle pain as well as pain that originates from your nerves. You should not use any of the aromatherapy oils if you are allergic to the herbs from which the oils were derived. If you have trouble breathing, you should not use aromatherapy. Some aromatherapy can cause drowsiness. Sage, rosemary, and juniper oils may increase uterine contractions if you are pregnant. You should not use these oils during pregnancy. Essential oils such as clove, cinnamon, and thyme can have anti-inflammatory properties and are useful in decreasing your pain if you have arthritis. Aromatherapy can be used in the following preparations: nose drops, air sprays, steam tents, candles, and drops in your bath.

Aromatherapy is rarely practiced by *conventional* medical doctors in the United States. However, in France, aromatherapy is practiced by medical doctors. Studies are still being conducted on this method. To date there are no state licensing boards for practitioners of aromatherapy.

Acupuncture Therapy

Acupuncture is another popular method that can be used for the treatment of your pain. Acupuncture can decrease both your pain as well as your stress. Acupuncture originated in China more than 5,000 years ago. Acupuncture is based on the belief that your health is determined by a balanced flow of vital life energy referred to as chi. There are 12 major energy pathways in your body called meridians. Each meridian is linked to a specific internal organ. There are more than 1,000 acupoints within the meridians of your body. Stimulation of these meridians enhances the flow of your vital life energy. Needles are inserted just under your skin to stimulate these meridians and provide you with pain relief. It is believed that acupuncture releases the body's own chemicals that relieve pain, called endorphins and enkephlins. These two chemicals are your body's natural pain-killing chemicals. Acupuncture can decrease the production as well as the distribution of substances that cause pain nerve impulses to go to the brain. Acupuncture, therefore, can decrease your need for conventional pain pills. Acupuncture has been demonstrated to decrease muscle-tension headaches.

When you see your acupuncturist, you will be asked to fill out a medical history form. You will then be interviewed by your acupuncturist. After your examination, your acupuncturist will place 10 to 12 needles in any of the 1,000 acupoints throughout your body depending on your pain complaints. The needles are small. Acupuncture is essentially painless. You must tell your acupuncturist if you are experiencing any pain during the procedure. Some treatments performed by your acupuncturist may only last several minutes, whereas other procedures can last up to 45 minutes. Instead of needles, some practitioners apply pressure to your acupoints for pain control.

In 1997, the U.S. Food and Drug Administration classified acupuncture as an actual medical device. It has also been classified as a safe method. In 1997, the National Institutes of Health endorsed acupuncture for postoperative pain, dental pain, tennis elbow, and carpal tunnel syndrome. In the United States, people make approximately 10 million visits per year to acupuncturists.

The World Health Organization has reported that acupuncture can treat migraine headaches, trigeminal neuralgia, sciatica, and arthritis. Acupuncture also can be used to treat fibromyalgia, neck pain, and back pain.

Acupuncture is now being accepted by *conventional* medical practitioners. More than 30 percent of all *conventional* medical schools include reference to acupuncture as an accepted scientific method that can be used in the health-care system. Acupuncture predates Western civilization. Acupuncture, which is used more often in women, is continuing to be studied by the scientific community.

In some states there is no licensing required to be an acupuncturist, whereas other states limit the practice to medical doctors and chiropractors. In some states acupuncturists are considered primary health-care professionals and may see you without your doctor's referral. Some states require that an acupuncturist graduate from an approved school and pass a state licensing examination. To find physicians that practice acupuncture, you can go to the website www.medicalacupuncture.org. Furthermore, the American Association of Oriental Medicine has a website, www.aaom.org, which is a national trade organization of acupuncturists who have met acceptable standards of competency. This organization can provide you with the names and locations of competent members of this organization in your community.

Chapter 12
Understanding Neck Pain

At any given time, neck pain affects 10 percent of the general population in the United States. Neck pain is a frequent reason why patients seek medical attention. A reported survey of 10,000 adults in the United States discovered that 34 percent of responding individuals experienced neck pain during the previous year of the survey. Chronic neck pain was reported in 17 percent of women and 10 percent of men in a similar study. Another study evaluated 8,000 adults, and chronic neck pain was identified in 13.5 percent of female respondents as compared to 9.5 percent of males.

Neck pain can range from mild discomfort to severe throbbing and is experienced by everyone at some point in their life. This chapter will teach you how your neck and spine work together and what parts of them can cause your pain. You will also begin to understand neck injuries more, learn how it affects men and women differently, and how you can prevent some neck injuries.

Your Neck and Spine

Most of your neck pain is self-limited and does not usually require seeing a doctor for the management of your pain. However, if you have serious cervical spine problems such as that seen in rheumatoid arthritis, notify your doctor if you have the sudden onset of significant neck pain that does not go away within two or three days. Neck pain is caused by conditions that compress nerves or irritate the outer part of discs that are cushions between the bones in your neck. Ligaments in the front and in the back of your bones in your neck can cause pain because they have many pain fibers within these ligaments. These ligaments are called the anterior and posterior longitudinal ligaments. (L.G.F. Giles and K. Singer. *Clinical Anatomy and Management of Cervical Spine Pain*. n.p.: Butterworth-Heinemann, 1998)

Where the bones of your neck stack on top of each other like Lego blocks, they form a joint called a facet joint. The outer capsule of this joint has a rich supply of pain fibers. The outer capsule holds the top and bottom of the facet joint together not unlike a clamshell. If this capsule is pulled or stretched by an injury, the parts of the joint loosen making the joint unstable. This instability can cause spine pain. If your neck becomes misaligned, you can also develop significant neck pain. Over time, the bones and joints in your neck can wear out as well. This is called degenerative disc or joint disease or in medical terms is called osteoarthritis. The disc between your bones can rupture. Your facet joints in your neck can deteriorate and be a cause of your chronic neck pain. Your neck muscles can become tense and cause you neck pain.

There are seven separate bone segments in your neck. These bones are held together by ligaments and stack on top of each other and form joints with the analogy of joints formed by Lego blocks. The lining of these joints can wear out. These joints contain a lubricating fluid that helps you turn and move your neck up and down. These joints in your neck not only limit your neck motion but also allow your neck to move in many planes. Try and put your ear on your shoulder. You facet joints limit your movement so your neck will not bend too far. The muscles and ligaments in your neck can have many pain nerve endings. These nerves transmit pain impulses following trauma or if you slouch and have poor neck posture. Irritation or injury to muscles or ligaments in your neck as well as the discs and joints in your neck can cause you to have neck pain.

The bones in your neck protect your spinal cord and the nerves that come off of your spinal cord. The nerves that come off of your spinal cord pass through holes in the bones in your neck. If these nerves are compressed by narrowing of the hole where the nerve exits from the bone in your neck, it can cause you to have significant pain. If the nerve is compromised by bones in your neck, you can have weakness as well as pain in your arms. (L.G.F. Giles and K. Singer. *Clinical Anatomy and Management of Cervical Spine Pain*. n.p.: Butterworth-Heinemann, 1998)

You should see that there are many causes of neck pain because there are many structures in your neck and each of these structures have pain fibers and one or all of them can cause you to have neck pain. Neck pain can come not only from the degeneration of discs in your neck or the degenerating facet joints in your neck, but also can arise from infections or tumors of structures in your neck.

Neck pain in general does not occur as often as lower back pain. Therefore, the overall cost of neck pain to society is much less than that of lower back pain. There are fewer work days lost and less medications prescribed in patients with neck pain as opposed to lower back pain. Your head weighs between 10 and 12 pounds. The bones in your neck are relatively small in comparison to your head. Your neck muscles are necessary to hold your head in a proper position. Your neck muscles must be strong to hold your head up. Try holding a bowling ball vertically for as long as you can. You will notice that your arm muscles get tired easily. The same analogy is true with respect to your neck muscles tiring from holding your neck up.

If you experience stress in your neck, it can cause you to have not only neck pain but also the headaches. Headaches may begin in your neck and go to the top of your head. At times if your neck is tense you can have difficulty turning it. If you are beginning to experience neck pain, evaluate your posture both sitting and standing in the mirror. Poor posture can lead to muscle spasms as well as dislocation and misalignment of your facet joints. If you have the onset of numbness of your arms, notify your doctor immediately. You must also be aware that nerves in your neck that come off of your spinal cord also can cause pain elsewhere in your body. The pain that is perceived elsewhere that comes from your nerves in your neck is called *referred pain.* For example, pain in your shoulder may be referred from nerves in your neck.

The bones in your neck that are called vertebral bodies contain many pain fibers. Each bone is wrapped by a tissue called a periosteum. If you fracture one of the bones in your neck, you can have severe pain. The tissue wrapper around your neck bones can be injured. The fracture of a bone in your neck can cause abnormal stress to the ligaments, muscles, and joints around the fracture as well as injury to your periosteum. Osteoporosis, which is a weakening of your bones with a loss of your bone density, can cause small, tiny fractures in the bones of your neck and in turn can be a cause of your pain. Osteoporosis can be a source of severe neck pain.

Discs are cushions between the bones in your neck. These discs act as shock absorbers in between your bones. The cushions are important because without them your neck bones would stack on top of each other. Remember the periosteum and the pain fibers contained in the periosteum? Without these cushions you would have terrible pain.

In the very center of your disc in your neck is a thick fluidlike substance called a nucleus pulposus. This fluid ball is surrounded by an outer tough fiber called an annulus. Annulus is Latin for "outer ring." A fluid nucleus acts as a ball bearing when you bend your head forward and backward or from side to side. It also is a ball bearing when you rotate your neck. The annulus around your disc acts as a ligament that prevents your neck from having excessive motion. Otherwise your bones would sit on a fluid-filled ball. (L.G.F. Giles and K. Singer. *Clinical Anatomy and Management of Cervical Spine Pain.* n.p.: Butterworth-Heinemann, 1998) You can imagine that your neck would not be very stable. Excessive motion in your head and neck would make you function as a Slinky toy. Your annulus at its outer layer has many pain fibers.

To find out if your pain is coming from the disc in your neck, a doctor can place a needle in your disc. After the needle has been properly placed, fluid can be injected into your disc. If the injected fluid into your disc reproduces your neck pain, this is a good indication that your disc in your neck is the cause of your pain syndrome. If your pain is from your disc you will need physical therapy to strengthen the neck muscles which hold your discs in place.

Understanding Neck Injuries

Neck pain makes up a significant portion of the complaints confronting your doctor as well as your physical therapist and your pain doctor. Your insurance carrier also can be affected by your neck pain complaints because tests commonly used to diagnose your neck pain, such as an MRI, can be expensive. Furthermore, your workmen's compensation carrier can be involved in your neck pain complaints if your problem is work related. For example, if you have a job that requires you to repetitively look at the ceiling, which happens if you are a painter, your job may be a source of your neck pain.

Research continues to be done to identify what happens to your neck tissues that are or can be involved in your pain complaints. The tissues that are identified with your neck pain are being identified in laboratory research, which helps scientists further understand the causes of your pain. Magnetic resonance imaging (MRI) and computerized tomography (CT) scanning can help your doctor identify any bone or disc abnormalities that may be a source of your neck pain. Be aware, however, that an abnormal imaging study does not necessarily mean that you will have neck pain. It is possible that you can have a ruptured disc in your neck and you may not experience any neck pain.

After the cause of your neck pain has been identified, a precise and therapeutic method can be used to decrease your pain. These studies, however, do not eliminate the need for your doctor to take a thorough medical history from you and to do an extensive physical examination on you as well. Remember that your neck has many structures that can cause you to have pain. Your doctor will attempt to reproduce your pain symptoms by having you do a specific movement or position to observe the impact on your pain perception. Your health-care provider will then compare the findings on your examination with your medical history and then with your x-ray, MRI, or CT scan.

Your Neck and Discs

There is a normal C-shaped curve in your neck. Your neck bones form a C curve with the C part of the curve located in the middle of your neck. The C curve is called a lordosis. The curve is sharper at the lower level of your neck. The curve in your neck determines your posture. If you have a neck injury, the muscles in your neck may pull your neck in a straight line and the curve is obliterated. If you have an x-ray following an injury, your doctor will note that your neck is straight as opposed to being curved. Your neck supports your head. Your brain controls most of your total body functions. If your neck becomes lopsided, you can compress a nerve that goes to one of your organs and could affect the function of one of your organs. For example, a spinal cord injury could affect your diaphragm and make it difficult for you to take a breath. Your head always needs to be supported in the proper position to allow you to have normal motion.

The discs in your neck have a normal blood supply when you are a toddler until you become a teenager. These discs are nurtured with oxygen and sugar in your bloodstream until your blood supply shuts off, which occurs when you reach adolescence. Your blood vessels essentially become obliterated at this time. By your 30s, the discs in your neck have no blood flow. Therefore, the nutrition to your discs must come from the ends of the bones in your neck. The bones in your neck are like sponges soaked with your blood. Pressure gradients will provide your discs with nutrition. Your disc essentially acts like a sponge and takes the blood that it needs from the bones in your neck. When your disc eventually begins to lose fluid, it will deteriorate. The very center of your disc, called the nucleus pulposus, is 80 percent water. Substances in this liquid environment can attract fluid into your discs to keep your discs well hydrated. Eventually this hydration will dry up. As you get older, the ends of your neck bones calcify. When this happens, less blood flow is available for your discs as the blood cannot get out of your vertebrae to hydrate your disc. Your disc will essentially dry out. Your disc becomes wafer thin and does not provide you with a nice cushion. As a result, you will begin to experience some degree of neck pain. One way to slow it down is to exercise, stop smoking, and watch your posture.

The outer ring of your disc, called the annulus, will contain the nucleus pulposus within its structure. Think of this anatomy as a jelly doughnut. The jelly in the doughnut is held in place by the outer doughnut ring. Be aware that a basic law of physics states that the nucleus pulposus, which is a liquid, cannot be compressed. Therefore, any pressure applied to your disc at any point can cause the nucleus pulposus to spread outward and even rupture through the outer annular ring. As an example, you can compress a foam pillow to make the pillow smaller during compression. But, compressing a liquid will not decrease its size (volume). Your disc jelly will not become smaller in its dimensions under pressure. Consequently when this liquid mass is attempted to be compressed, it will push through the outer ring of your disc.

When this happens, you suffer what is called a disc herniation or rupture. The nucleus pulposus material contains acids. When this disc material does come out of the annulus, the surrounding tissues can become swollen and red from the acidic liquid. This is the reason that your doctor may do a cervical epidural steroid injection on you. The purpose of this method is to decrease the swelling of your tissue and nerves caused by the acidic nucleus pulposus contents. The acid will make your nerves extra sensitive to irritability, which will cause you to experience pain.

Your Neck Ligaments

In front of the bones in your neck is a ligament that runs vertically. In the back of the bones in your neck is another ligament that also runs vertically. These ligaments are called longitudinal ligaments. These ligaments run all the way from the base of your skull to your lower back and contain many pain fibers. The ligament in the back of your bones limits your ability to bend your head forward. If you bend too far, the ligament transmits pain signals to your brain telling you to stop this movement. The front ligament and the joints in your neck keep you from bending your neck backward too far. Sometimes your neck can be bent backward following a whiplash injury and can cause you significant pain.

To better understand the concept of a whiplash injury, consider that your head is like a bowling ball attached to a flexible whip called your neck. At the time of an accident your bowling ball flies away from the traumatic event but fortunately or unfortunately it is still connected to your neck. This connection causes your neck and head to snap like a whip which can cause an injury not only to your neck but also to your brain.

Not only does your neck go forward and backward, it also rotates to the right and the left. You also can place your ear toward your shoulder, which is called lateral flexion of your neck. When you have neck pain, inform your health-care giver as to what movement or movements cause you to have neck pain. Remember to keep a pain diary. When you bend your head forward, your discs can be compressed. This also occurs when your neck goes backward. However, forward movement of your neck can cause your discs to rupture. This is sometimes caused in motor vehicle accidents if your vehicle strikes an object from the front. This can cause your neck to bend forward, which in turn can compress the nucleus pulposus in your disc and can cause a disc herniation.

If you run your fingers along the center of the back of your neck, you will feel bony objects. If you look at someone from behind, you will notice an area that sticks out from their neck in the center. These bony prominences are called spinous processes. The one that sticks out the most is the bony prominence of the seventh cervical vertebra. In between these spinous processes are ligaments that hold the spinous processes together from top to bottom. These ligaments keep your head from going too far forward. An injury can disrupt or tear these ligaments, which can cause you to have pain. Always remember that pain can be a warning to you and can be a protective mechanism for you telling you to decrease your movement. The joints in your neck that are called facet joints will keep your neck from going backward too far.

Your Spinal Cord and Nerves

The holes in the bones in your neck allow the nerves from your spinal cord to come out and go to your arms, legs, and organs. If your neck bends too far forward, this can cause you an injury to the nerves coming out of these holes. Excessive movement of your head can cause you to have significant pain. You are probably aware that if you sustained a blow to your head and if your neck bends to far toward one of the sides of your body, the holes on the side where the head bends will be closed. This can cause you to have a nerve injury because the closed hole can compress one of your nerves coming off of your spinal cord. On the opposite side, the holes where the nerves emerge from your spinal cord will be opened. When your head is thrown to the side, as frequently happens when you suffer a whiplash injury, the side on which the head is thrown to can compress the facet joints on that side of your neck. On the opposite side the facet joints are opened. Either of these maneuvers can cause you to have a facet joint injury and can cause you to suffer significant pain. The capsule that encloses your facet joint contains many pain fibers. Excessive strain of this capsule will cause you to experience pain. The pain tells you not to move your neck any more because of the chance that you could cause a worse injury. Your muscles tighten up to prevent you from moving your neck. Remember that pain is a protective mechanism.

Your spinal cord and the nerves that come off of your spinal cord can be sources of neck pain. When you bend your head forward or bend your head backward, your spinal cord will move up and down a short distance because it is somewhat elastic. This means that the nerves that go through the holes in your neck bones also move along with spinal cord movements. If the holes in your neck bones decrease in diameter as is seen in arthritis, movement of these nerves across a small hole can cause irritation in your nerves and make them swell and become extra sensitive to irritability. You can then experience pain in your arms. Occasionally, if you have arthritis, the small bony growth that forms anywhere around the holes in the bones of your neck can irritate or compress one of your nerves. This bone growth is called an osteophyte. Osteophytes themselves are not painful. However, when they brush over your nerves or ligaments, they can cause you to have neck pain. Osteophytes, if they occur, are usually pointed. If one of your nerves brushes up against one of these osteophytes, or if the osteophytes compress your nerves, you may experience mild to moderate pain.

Steroid injections in and around your nerves can decrease the swelling of the nerve and decrease your pain. Sometimes your doctor may give you oral steroids. The problem with oral steroids is that they can cause you to have significant weight gain. The injection places a tiny amount of steroids at the area of your pain. Oral steroids have to go to your stomach and pass out of your gastrointestinal system to reach your bloodstream. The total amount of the steroid that will reach your swollen nerves will vary. This is why pain-medicine doctors advocate the use of special needles to place steroids at the level of your nerve swelling. The amount of drug placed at your nerve is more reliable than that given by mouth.

Blood vessels run vertically up your neck toward your brain. A neck injury with compression can occasionally decrease the blood flow to your brain. If your neck is bent backward for a significant length of time, you could possibly lose consciousness. This can be seen occasionally in a syndrome called a beauty shop syndrome. In people with a poor blood supply to their brains, such as an elderly person, a prolonged extension of the neck could cause that person to have a stroke. This posture could also cause you to rupture your discs in your neck.

Your Neck Muscles

The muscles of your neck can be a source of your pain. The neck muscles are probably the most common cause of your neck pain. There are two groups of muscles in your neck. There is a group that bends your head forward, and there is a group of muscles that extends your head backward. Most of the muscles in your neck are located toward the back of your neck. These are the muscles that bend your head backward. If you have poor posture, the muscles in the back of your neck can become longer or can become shorter. When this happens, the short muscles in your neck lose blood flow, causing you to have pain.

If you are at work and have poor posture, persistent compression of your neck muscles can cause pain. The muscles in the front of your spinal cord bend your head forward. The muscles under the base of your skull and above your mid-back pull your head backward. A strain of any of these muscles can also cause you to experience neck pain. If you slouch over a computer or workbench, you may compress your neck muscles and shorten them. Your neck will eventually conform to this posture. This is the reason why you have to have good posture. The muscles in your neck need to be strong to protect the nerves coming off your spinal cord from injury due to excessive head movement, which happens in a whiplash injury. Major muscles that pull your neck backward are located just under the base of your skull, and another group is located right above your lungs. The muscles that pull your neck forward are located in the front and middle of your neck.

The muscles in the base of your skull can compress a nerve that comes off of your spinal cord and travels to the top of your head.

This is called the occipital nerve. If this nerve is compressed by a tight muscle, you can develop a headache called an occipital headache. If you put some heat over the muscle that is compressing this nerve, it can relax the muscle and relieve your headache.

Posture can cause you to have numerous orthopedic problems in your neck. Poor posture changes your tissues, bones, ligaments, and muscles. Poor posture can weaken the discs in your neck. Your posture can be influenced by work demands. If you have to paint overhead daily, you may develop weakness in the discs in your neck that could eventually rupture. Be aware of what tissues cause you to have neck pain. Your cervical disc is a common cause of neck pain. The anterior longitudinal ligament in front of the bones in your neck contains many pain fibers. The posterior longitudinal ligament also has pain fibers.

Assessing Your Neck Pain and Diseases

The nerve roots coming off of your spinal cord that run through the holes in your neck bones can also be a source of your neck pain. Coverings of the facet joints in your neck called facet joint capsules can be a source of your pain as well. As previously stated, your neck muscles are a common cause of your pain. To properly assess your pain, your health-care provider will obtain a medical history from you and do a physical examination on you as well. Because there are so many structures that can cause pain in your neck, your health-care provider will try to isolate the tissue or tissues that contribute to your pain syndrome. This is not a precise science and x-rays, CT scans, and MRIs may need to be performed by your doctor following your history and physical examination. Sometimes laboratory tests taken from your blood are needed to rule out rheumatoid arthritis, which can cause significant neck pain.

Electromyography and/or nerve conduction tests consist of needles placed in the muscles and nerves of your upper arms and legs. The electromyography study can enable your doctor to determine if you have compression of one of the nerves that goes from your spinal cord to your fingers. Another way of diagnosing your pain is for your doctor to inject a numbing medicine in each of your tissues to see if your pain can be decreased. This series of injections can help to diagnose the cause of your pain.

When you become older than 35 years of age, you may develop degenerative disc disease in your neck. Degeneration of your neck is called spondylosis. Degenerative disc disease of the cervical spine causes more neck pain and upper-extremity nerve pain than does a disc herniation. Men have a higher incidence of cervical spondylosis than women. In one study, the evidence of spondylosis was noted to be 60 percent in women but 80 percent in men. These findings were before the age of 49 years. However, at age 70 or greater there was a 95 percent incidence of degenerative disc disease in men and women. With degenerative disc disease, your disc becomes narrow. Think of a normal disc as a jelly donut; a degenerated disc is more like a thin communion wafer.

Diagnosis of spondylosis is made by x-ray but also can be seen on an MRI. Degeneration of your disc can cause calcification of the ends of your neck bones. As stated previously, there is decreased blood flow to your discs following puberty. Your discs normally obtain blood from the spongy vertebral bodies. However, if the end plates are calcified, your discs cannot receive hydration and nutrition. As a result, your discs essentially dry out, also called dessication. At this time, the outer ring of your disc called the annulus, can deteriorate. Cracks can occur in the outer ring allowing the acidic center of your disc to leak out. This leakage can cause irritation of your nerves, ligaments, and muscles. Epidural steroid injection therapy can sometimes decrease your pain if you have leakage of acidic material from your disc. Epidural injection is placement of a needle into a space in your neck that surrounds your spinal fluid.

If you do develop degenerative disc disease of your neck, which most of us do when we are over age 50, you can have decreased range of motion around your neck. The decreased range of motion around your neck is an early indication that you are developing degeneration of the discs and joints in your neck. You will have trouble turning your head and attempting to look behind you. Looking up or down can also be difficult as well as painful. Attention to your neck posture and doing daily range-of-motion exercises for your neck can reduce the progression of degenerative disc disease involving your neck. For example, move your neck up and down, put your ears on your shoulders, and turn your head to the right and left as far as you can.

Sometimes you can have neck pain without having any problems with the bones, joints, and ligaments of your neck. If you have neck pain that is made worse with swallowing, you may have an inflammation of your esophagus. Pharyngitis sometimes can cause pain in your neck and throat. Mumps have been reported to cause neck pain as well. If your thyroid enlarges, it can be a source of neck pain that is made worse with swallowing. If you have inflamed tonsils, you also may have neck pain.

Some neck pain is made worse by chewing. A fracture of your lower jawbone can be a source of neck pain. Your temporal mandibular joint (TMJ) is a joint that separates your upper and lower jaws. TMJ problems can cause neck pain that is made worse with chewing. Tumors around your lungs can cause referred pain to your neck. Angina (heart pain) that occurs if you are having a heart attack can have pain referred to your neck as well. Referred means that the pain is felt at a location away from the source of your pain.

If you have a severe state of contractions of a muscle in your neck, you may have severe pain. This prolonged contraction of a neck muscle is called torticollis. This usually occurs on one side of your neck. Your head is usually twisted to one side with your chin pointing to the opposite side. Torticollis usually results from disease or an injury to your brain or spinal cord. Injuries to the muscles of your neck can also be a cause of torticollis as well. Sometimes an injection of botulism toxin into your muscles can provide temporary relief.

The causes of your neck pain are many and are varied. Your health-care provider must have thorough knowledge of the anatomy of your neck. You must also provide your health-care provider with a complete medical history as well as tell them about any similar previous pain in your neck. Try to remember which methods decreased your pain and which movements made your pain worse.

Because other medical diseases can cause neck pain, tell your doctor if you have had a recent sore throat. Remember that pharyngitis can cause neck pain. If you do have a significant pharyngitis, you may require antibiotic therapy. If you have normal mechanical pain, you may need physical therapy or chiropractic therapy. In most instances, you should avoid using a neck brace, because chronic use of a neck brace can make your neck muscles weak.

Neck Pain Among Men and Women

Women have more neck pain than men. The incidence of neck pain increases with age. Whiplash injuries can cause neck pain as well and are more common in women than in men. Furthermore, repetitive activities in a workplace setting can be a source of neck pain.

Unfortunately, you can have neck pain for a long time. It is not self-limiting as some other types of pain syndromes are. Neck pain is a symptom of problem processes going on in your neck.

Did you know that women are more prone to develop neck pain than men? Scandinavian research has reported that neck pain occurs half as often as lower back pain. A study in Finland reported that neck pain can occur in 9.5 percent of men, whereas it occurs in 13.5 percent of women. Reports in the United States also reveal that neck pain occurs more frequently in women than in men. Older patients, both men and women, have a higher incidence of neck pain. People who have mentally and physically stressful jobs are more prone to have neck pain as well. The reason why smokers have increased neck pain has been studied. Cigarette smoking stops the formation of bone. Smoking interferes with the repair of fractures involving your neck bones. The mechanism of association between smoking and neck pain is still being studied.

Women are more prone to neck pain because they have smaller necks and it makes them vulnerable to the onset of pain. Remember that the neck must hold a 10- to 12-pound head. A smaller neck receives more stress from the head than a larger neck. It has also been hypothesized that men are more stoic than women and do not report their neck pain as often as women. Because of their smaller necks, women are more prone to suffer severe whiplash injuries than men. Not only do men have larger necks than women, but the overall body mass of the neck is more than a woman's.

Be aware that women can suffer neck injuries in beauty parlors and hair salons. As mentioned earlier in this chapter, you could have a stroke if your arteries are clogged with fat and calcium and if you extend your neck backward for a long length of time. When you bend your head backward into a sink to have your hair washed, the angle of the compression of the neck sometimes causes a disc in your neck to rupture. Some people also pass out when their head is bent backward because of compression of arteries that go to the brain that are present in the back of the neck.

Studies in women who have chronic neck pain have shown that women respond positively to strength and endurance training, which can significantly decrease their pain. Strength training is emphasized for the rehabilitation of women with neck pain. A physical therapist can tailor a proper strengthening program for you.

A study published in January 2003 said that women complain of a greater intensity of neck pain than men. This same study said that women were more prone to use narcotic medicines if they had even minimal psychological stress compared to men. Because of the differences in muscle mass and neck size between men and women, physical therapy and chiropractic therapy programs must be tailored specifically to each gender and each person's complaints. It appears that gender specificity with respect to neck pain is currently being well addressed.

Preventing Neck Pain

The slender column of your neck is the most vulnerable part of your spine. Your mid-back and lower back are protected by more tissue mass. You must keep your muscles strong. Your physical therapist or chiropractor can give you sets of exercises to safely do to strengthen your neck muscles. (B. Goldberg. *Alternative Medicine, The Definitive Guide*. Berkeley: Celestial Arts, 2001)

To prevent neck pain, you must move your neck. You should do the range-of-motion exercises defined in Chapter 10 on physical therapy. Your facet joints are designed to provide your head and neck with movement. The joints get nutrition through movement. If you have experienced neck pain before, complete range-of-motion exercises with your neck. For example, move your head up and down followed by attempting to place your ears on your shoulders. These maneuvers will provide increased blood flow to your facet joints.

Remember that sitting in a position over a desk or work table for a long time can cause you to have pain. Not moving your head and neck can cause you pain. When you do not move your neck, the lubricant in your facet joint can dry out. When this occurs you will have difficulty moving your neck. When you are working at a computer, remember to keep your eyes looking straight ahead. This will keep your neck in proper alignment. When you are sleeping, you must not place your head on a big, fluffy pillow. This could cause your neck to become misaligned. Large, foam-filled pillows are not good for your neck. There are pillows available that are made specifically for neck comfort. You may be interested in purchasing one of these pillows. If you are riding in a vehicle, you should raise your head rest to the position that meets the back curve of your skull to help prevent whiplash. If you have an onset of pain, you may want to take a long hot shower, letting the shower water bathe your neck.

This method may provide you with pain relief if your pain is not from a recent injury. If have had a recent injury, you should apply ice packs on your neck pain. You should wrap ice or a package of frozen vegetables in a towel. Press the cold substance to the painful area on your neck for about 10 minutes. You should not let the cold packs numb your neck.

You should also remember that strenuous working postures can cause you to have significant neck pain. For example, if you paint frequently overhead, make sure that you take a break every hour or two and do range-of-motion exercises for your neck. You must remember that high levels of psychological stress in your workplace can also contribute to your neck pain. If you are in a stressful situation at work, talk to your supervisor to see if there is something that can be done to lessen your stress level.

Treatment for Neck Pain

Treatment of neck pain for men and women will be determined on an individual basis by your doctor or therapist. Be sure that you follow the doctor's or therapist's instructions carefully so that you do not injure yourself further. If your pain does not get better during your treatment, be sure to discuss this with your doctor or therapist so that he or she can perform further examinations and discuss other treatment options with you.

For Men

Treatment of neck pain for men will often consist of heat therapy, rest, neck exercises, and pain medications.

- If your pain, such as that from an injury, has just occurred, you can apply cold to the area for 5 to 15 minutes every 2 hours for the first day or two. Do not use cold therapy after this time, unless instructed to do so by your doctor.
- If possible, use a heating pad for 15 minutes a day, 4 to 5 times per day. Be sure not to use the heating pad while you are sleeping.
- Rest your neck for two to three days if possible to keep from doing excessive bending and turning. This will help your muscles heal and keep them from further stress.
- Take any prescription medications prescribed by your doctor.
- Perform neck exercises as described in Chapter 10. Use these exercises to strengthen your neck muscles and improve your pain symptoms.
- See a chiropractor to help relieve the pain in your neck.

For Women

Treatment of neck pain for women will often consist of heat therapy, rest, neck exercises, and pain medications.

- If your pain, such as that from an injury, has just occurred, you can apply cold to the area for 5 to 15 minutes every 2 hours for the first day or two. Do not use cold therapy after this time, unless instructed to do so by your doctor.
- If possible, use a heating pad for 15 minutes a day, 4 to 5 times per day. Be sure not to use the heating pad while you are sleeping.
- Rest your neck for two to three days if possible to keep from doing excessive bending and turning. This will help your muscles heal and keep them from further stress.
- Take any prescription medications prescribed by your doctor.
- Perform neck exercises as described in Chapter 10. Use these exercises to strengthen your neck muscles and improve your pain symptoms.
- See a chiropractor to help relieve the pain in your neck.

Chapter 13
Understanding Back Pain

You could be experiencing pain in your back as a result of injury, stress, poor posture, or even aging. Many people experience back pain, and there are treatment methods available that could help ease that pain. It is important to note that the onset or worsening of back pain can be prevented by utilizing proper posture techniques and performing stretching exercises.

This chapter discusses what causes back pain, how it can be prevented in some instances, and how to best treat your type of pain.

Causes of Back Pain

Do you know why lower back pain is so common? Our backs are made up of a large number of bones called vertebrae that are separated from one another by discs. These discs act as shock absorbers. Between each bone in our spine, the bones stack on top of each other like Lego blocks and form joints called facet joints. The purpose of the bones in your spine is to protect your spinal cord from injury. There are foramina, which are holes in each vertebra. The nerves off of your spinal cord go through these holes and go to your arms, legs, and organs within your body. Your spine is kept in place by muscles in your back that maintain your posture. Your muscles also make your back stable during movement. You have many muscles in your back. Any one of these muscles can cause you to have lower back pain. In addition to muscles, you have ligaments that attach each bone in your spine to both the one above and the one below. Ligaments are also necessary to give your back stability. Your ligaments contain pain fibers and can be a source of your back pain.

Most of your lower back pain and any associated disability associated with your lower back is usually mechanical in nature. This means that there is usually an abnormal alignment of your bones and/or joints that can cause you to have significant lower back pain. You have five bones in your lower back that are called lumbar vertebrae. Your spine functions to support you when you are standing, walking, bending, pushing, and pulling. Your back must perform repetitive tasks on a daily basis without failure. Occasionally your spine can falter. At that time, the cause of your pain needs to be diagnosed. The tissues that are causing your pain in your back need to be identified. Your health-care provider will do a physical examination on you after you give them a detailed history of the onset of your pain. They will then do an examination on you to isolate the cause of your pain. After this has been done, you will be prescribed the appropriate therapy to begin to decrease your lower back pain.

Most of your everyday back pains are not serious. (W.H. Kirkaldy-Willis, et al. *Managing Low Back Pain*, New York: Churchill Livingstone, 1992) Your back pain is most probably related to a muscle strain or a ligament sprain from doing an activity that you are not used to doing. You should never ignore your back pain. You should be concerned if your back pain goes into your legs. If your back pain is associated with weakness of your legs or numbness or difficulty walking, you need to see a doctor. If you have damage to your spinal cord, you may become paralyzed. If this happens, you may lose all control of your bowel and bladder. If you lose control of your bowel and/or bladder you need to immediately see your doctor.

Back pain is the most expensive and common industrial- or work-related injury. (W.H. Kirkaldy-Willis, et al. *Managing Low Back Pain*, New York: Churchill Livingstone, 1992) Back pain is the most common cause of disability for workers younger than age 45. In 90 percent of working people, back pain limits working activity for usually less than 30 days. Five percent of people who have back pain have weakness, loss of sensation, or loss of reflexes in a leg. Two percent of people with back pain may end up needing surgery. Back pain is the most common cause of activity limitation in the working population between ages 18 to 55 in the United States. Back pain is responsible for 15 percent of work absenteeism in developed countries. Approximately 5 percent of the workforce is disabled by back pain yearly. (T. Herrington, L. Morse, Occupational Injuries: Evaluation, Management, and Prevention, n.p.: Mosby, 1995) Attempts to prevent back pain have not been proven to be effective.

In 1990 in the United States, there were 15 million office visits to doctors for lower back pain. This accounts for approximately 3 percent of all visits to doctors. The number of visits to chiropractors was even greater. The rates for surgery in the United States have increased over the past 20 years. (W.H. Kirkaldy-Willis, et al. *Managing Low Back Pain*, New York: Churchill Livingstone, 1992)

The rate of surgery for back pain in the United States is greater than in most other countries. The reason for this finding is probably due to the large number of surgeons in the United States when compared to other countries.

Following the onset of back pain, there can be a recurrence of lower back pain in a person within 1 year and a 75 percent recurrence in a person's lifetime. Sixty-five percent of patients usually recover from an episode of back pain within six weeks. (W.H. Kirkaldy-Willis, et al. *Managing Low Back Pain*, New York: Churchill Livingstone, 1992)

At 12 weeks, 85 percent of those with back pain are essentially pain free. If you have pain for more than 12 weeks, it is unlikely that you will receive significant relief of your back pain. If you have been off of work for more than 26 weeks, you will probably not be able to return back to work. Studies have shown that if you have been off of work for 104 or more weeks, you will not return back to work. If you receive compensation from a workmen's compensation insurance carrier or compensation following a motor vehicle accident, your chances of returning to work are significantly decreased.

Lower back pain is the cause for approximately 20 percent of all industrial injuries. Back pain amounts to 50 percent of the cost of all work-related injuries. Only 10 percent of the injuries account for 80 percent of the total cost due to disability. If you are over 50 years of age, you can expect to have problems with your back and also have limitations in your activity due to back pain. Back pain from heavy physical work is common by age 50. Back pain is an unavoidable part of your life. If you do a job that requires physical labor, you can expect to have back pain when you are 50 years of age or older. (T. Herrington, L. Morse, *Occupational Injuries: Evaluation, Management, and Prevention*, n.p.: Mosby, 1995) Even people who have not done heavy physical work can begin experiencing increased back pain by age 50. (W.H. Kirkaldy-Willis, et al. *Managing Low Back Pain*, New York: Churchill Livingstone, 1992)

You should realize that it will be difficult to decrease your back pain if you have become inactive. For this reason, you should do aerobic exercise to prevent back pain. You also can use exercise to treat back pain. The muscles in your back must be strong in order to support your back. This is the reason that you must do regular exercise activity.

Your Spine and Discs

Be aware that your spine can cause you to experience back pain in many ways. (N. Bogkuk. *Clinical Anatomy of the Lumbar Spine and Sacrum.* New York: Churchill Livingstone, 1999) You may have suffered minor or major trauma to your back. You may have a job where you must do repetitive lifting or twisting. This can injure your back as well as your discs. If you have a job where you sit all day at a computer desk or at a work table and you slouch, your back can become misaligned. You may have suffered sports injuries to your back. If you enjoy gardening, you can cause yourself to have back pain if you are doing a considerable amount of digging or lifting. If your back is not conditioned and strong, try to avoid heavy lifting and strenuous recreational activities.

Your lower back is made up of five bones called lumbar vertebrae. (N. Bogkuk. *Clinical Anatomy of the Lumbar Spine and Sacrum.* New York: Churchill Livingstone, 1999) The lower part of your back below these bones is called the sacrum. It is made up of five fused bones. Your pelvis anchors here. Your tailbone is called a coccyx. If you sit in a chair correctly or in the seat of your car correctly, you are keeping all of these bones properly aligned. Each bone then bears the full weight of the bone above it. It is reported that proper alignment of your back can help build bone mass. This is important if anyone in your family has a history of osteoporosis.

The figure that follows shows the lumbar vertebrae, vertebral disk, spinal nerve, hip bone, head of femur, and sacrum. These are common areas associated with back pain. You can see how a misaligned back could pinch nerves and cause you to feel pain.

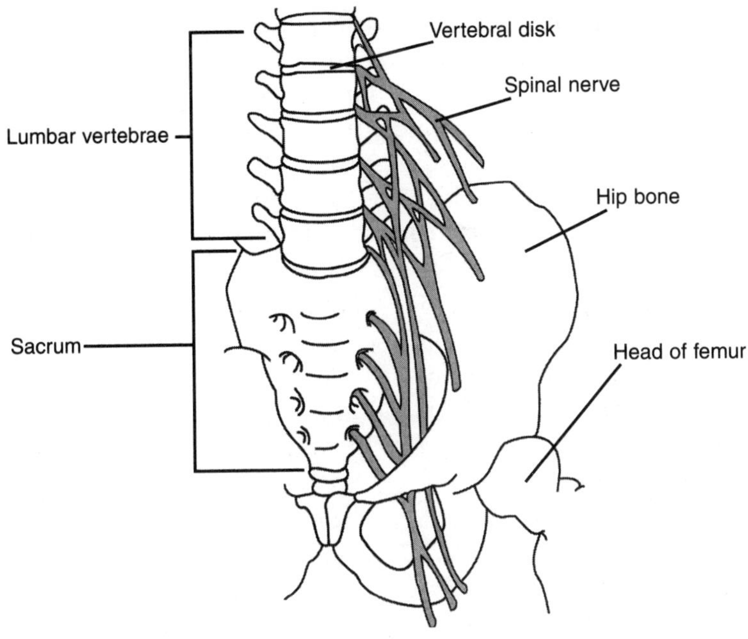

Your spinal column.

How Discs in Your Back Can Cause Pain

Cushions that are called discs are located between the bones in your back. These discs are prone to injury as well as to wear and tear. As you grow older, your discs lose their elastic properties and they become thinner and can become wafer thin. As the discs in your back decrease in height, your overall height decreases. If you are over 40, you may have noticed that you are beginning to decrease with respect to your height. As your discs begin to shrink, pressure from the bones above and below can cause your discs to press outward. This is called a disc bulge. Sometimes a disc bulge can press on one of your nerves. A disc bulge is not a disc rupture. However, a disc bulge can press on one of your nerves coming off of your spinal cord and can cause you significant pain. If your pain persists and you develop numbness, you may ultimately have to have surgery to remove a portion of this bulge off of your nerve.

In the very center of your disc is a thick liquid. Liquids cannot be compressed. If you bend a certain way or attempt to lift a heavy object in an awkward position, the fluid inside of your disc can burst through the outer ring of your disc. This is called a disc herniation or rupture and can cause you significant pain. The liquid material that bursts outside of your disc is highly acidic. This acid content can cause your nerves, your ligaments, and your muscles to become swollen and inflamed and you can develop severe pain.

Most of the origins of your back pain discussed are mechanical in nature. However, injuries to your discs between your back bones can cause you to have pain. Remember that your discs are made up of cartilage. Your cartilage is elastic and functions as a cushion between your back bones. These discs absorb the impact of your body motion.

As discussed previously, your discs have a liquid in the center. You should also remember that liquids cannot be compressed. (N. Bogkuk. *Clinical Anatomy of the Lumbar Spine and Sacrum*. New York: Churchill Livingstone, 1999) Therefore, if you bend and twist while lifting a heavy object, you put intense force on these discs. The liquid forces your discs to bulge out and then can rupture. If your discs put pressure on the nerves going to your leg, your leg may become numb or you could develop a foot drop. You must seek medical attention if this happens. When your doctor examines you, you may have no reflexes in your leg on the side of your pain.

When you become over age 50, the liquid center of your discs, called the nucleus pulposus, becomes dry and less elastic. When you are young, the nucleus pulposus is like glue just out of a tube. When this glue becomes dry, it is definitely less elastic. The liquid center of your disc does the same thing. At that time, pressure on your discs can cause them to protrude and cause your discs to keep protruding until they may become compressed around one of the nerves going to your legs. When this happens, it can compress your nerve. If your leg becomes numb and weak, you will probably become a candidate for surgery. You will need consultation with a neurosurgeon or an orthopedic surgeon.

Discography is a way of diagnosing whether or not you have disc-related pain. An MRI and CT scan can show a disc herniation. However, these imaging studies cannot define pain. A discogram is an injection of material into your disc. The pressure in your disc is then measured. You should have a relatively high pressure when material is injected into the center of your disc. If your disc leaks, the leakage of the acidic nucleus pulposus can cause you to have pain. When your nucleus pulposus leaks out of your disc it hardens just like glue out of its tube.

Sciatica Pain

You may have heard friends or relatives complain of a term called sciatica. Sciatica is a pain that is felt in your back and the outer side of your thigh, leg, and foot. It is usually caused by degeneration of one of the discs between your back bones. When the disc protrudes laterally off to the side, it can compress the nerves in your lower back. Usually the last two or three nerves are compressed on the side of your pain. The onset of sciatica can be sudden. Furthermore, it can be brought on if you are performing an awkward lifting position or if you are doing a twisting movement such as raking the leaves.

People who have sciatica usually have stiff backs and have pain when they attempt any movement. You may have numbness in your leg as well as weakness associated with your sciatica. Bed rest for 24 hours may decrease your pain. If you have significant weakness and pain, nonsteroidal anti-inflammatory medication can help. If this medication does not provide you with relief, your pain-medicine doctor may want to inject the sciatic nerve with some numbing medicine and a steroid. If you still have pain after conservative treatments have been done, a surgeon may need to do a surgical procedure to get either a muscle or disc off of your nerve to relieve your pain.

Your Sacroiliac Joint

Where your backbone and pelvis meet, they form a joint called the sacroiliac joint. (N. Bogkuk. *Clinical Anatomy of the Lumbar Spine and Sacrum*. New York: Churchill Livingstone, 1999) Your sacroiliac joint can be a source of your back pain. This joint has a thick capsule that has strong ligaments both in the front and the back of your joint. Other ligaments also help to form and support this joint. The joint is C shaped. As you become older, the cartilage that attaches to your pelvic bone degenerates faster than the cartilage in your sacrum. As a result this joint can become unstable. It can be a cause of your pain as well. Related to hormone changes that occur during pregnancy, the ligament becomes loose. This is the reason that many pregnant women experience pain in their sacroiliac joint that can last after the birth of their baby until the ligament becomes stronger.

Sometimes the pain from your sacroiliac joint can cause pain to go down your leg. You may notice pain in your back when you roll over in bed or when you get out of a car. Furthermore, you can have pain when you go up or down steps. If the muscle over your sacroiliac joint is tender, it can cause you to have pain. Diagnosis of this problem can be done by examination. A bone scan is helpful in diagnosing sacroiliac arthritis. During this procedure, a very small dose of a radioactive dye is injected into your veins. After the radioactive dye has had time to go to your joints, pictures are taken with a camera of your sacroiliac joint. If you have arthritis, there will be darkened areas in your joints that will show up on the scan.

Usually plain x-rays are not sufficient to diagnose problems with your sacroiliac joint. The treatment of this problem consists of physical therapy. A type of Velcro belt called an SI belt can be used to hold your joint in place. If you have no relief from these methods, your pain-medicine doctor can inject a steroid and local anesthetic into your joint under x-ray needle guidance. These methods should rid you of your pain. If your pain does persist, destruction of the nerves that goes to your joint can be done with either heat or cold. This is called a rhizotomy. Occasionally, a surgeon may have to stabilize your joint surgically. Nonsteroidal anti-inflammatory medications can also be very helpful for the management of pain in your sacroiliac joint. Because the pain involves a joint, muscle relaxants may not be of any benefit. If you have a disc herniation, the disc herniation can be diagnosed by a CT scan or an MRI.

Exercising Your Back

A normal spine that has been maintained with exercise, proper posture, and range-of-motion exercises enables you to bend and rotate your back without pain. Chapter 10 describes some range-of-motion exercises for you to do. These exercises will help you maintain adequate range of motion for your back. These movements can also help increase blood flow to your discs. Increased blood flow can encourage your discs to heal and can even prevent scar tissue from forming around your nerves that were temporarily injured. In some instances, you may need to seek chiropractic therapy to realign your back. If the bones in your back are properly aligned, your nerves should be able to transmit normal impulses to your muscles to allow your muscles to function in an optimal fashion. If there is some entrapment of your nerves, or pressure on your nerves by adjacent body structures, your nervous system cannot function properly.

You must discuss exercise programs with your doctor. No matter what your age and what your health condition is, there should be some exercise that you can do. You should be able to do the range-of-motion exercises that have been described in this book as well. Even if you do not suffer from back pain, you should follow the recommendations in this chapter to prevent the onset of the pain in your back. If you engage in a healthful lifestyle, this lifestyle could lower the chance of you having a disc herniation.

Disc ruptures or herniations are just like heart attacks. It takes time for the conditions to become right for you to have a disc herniation or a heart attack. The arteries in your heart build up substances called plaque over time. If you are doing some type of physical exertion such as shoveling snow, you may have a heart attack. People who smoke and eat a diet that is high in some fats are prone to have a heart attack. The incident of shoveling snow can push your heart over the edge. The same is true with back pain. If you are overweight and don't exercise and don't use proper posture, your back and discs will become progressively weaker. You will then be prone to a disc rupture if you go out and shovel snow.

The weakness in your discs does not just happen over night. This weakness progresses over time due to the lack of activity as well as other factors. (W.H. Kirkaldy-Willis, et al. *Managing Low Back Pain*, New York: Churchill Livingstone, 1992) This is the reason why you need to maintain a healthful lifestyle that includes exercise. Preventative pain medicine is just as important as the treatment of pain problems.

Osteoarthritis

You can lose muscle strength all over your body as you age. Ligaments can become lax and weak and your joints can become stiff from degeneration. The discs in your back can lose fluid and become wafer thin. (W.H. Kirkaldy-Willis, et al. *Managing Low Back Pain*, New York: Churchill Livingstone, 1992)

Changes in the architecture of your discs and joints due to wear and tear is called osteoarthritis. This is the most common form of arthritis and it affects approximately 21 million Americans. Arthritis can cause the diameter of your spinal column to decrease. Your spinal column is hollow in the center. Your spinal cord runs vertical within the hole in the spinal column.

If you begin to experience osteoarthritis, the hole in which the spinal cord is placed can narrow and can eventually put pressure on your spinal cord, which can cause you to have significant pain. The holes in the bones in your spine allow your nerves from your spinal cord to go to your arms, legs, and organs. These nerves can cause pain in your extremities or organs. However, these nerves also can control muscle movement in your arms and legs. With osteoarthritis, the holes in which your nerves emerge from the spinal cord can decrease their diameter. When this happens, one or more of your nerves can be compressed, which can cause you pain, numbness, and weakness.

Osteoporosis

After the age of 30, your bones gradually lose calcium. (W.H. Kirkaldy-Willis, et al. *Managing Low Back Pain*, New York: Churchill Livingstone, 1992) The loss of calcium can decrease your bone mass, especially in your vertebral bodies. This is called osteoporosis. Osteoporosis is seen more commonly in women than men. In females, the loss of the female hormone called estrogen, which occurs at menopause, will accelerate this bone loss. The loss of calcium in bone mass in your vertebral bodies can collapse them and cause a fracture of your vertebrae. These fractures are called compression fractures. The height of your vertebral bone decreases. Osteoporosis can be very painful. Some doctors are now putting a hardening substance into the bones of the back if patients have osteoporosis and have compression fractures. This technique is referred to as vertebroplasty.

Muscle Tension and Spasms

In addition to degenerative changes in the back and joints as being common causes of back pain, the most common cause of back pain is muscle tension in the lower back. Approximately 80 percent of people living in the United States will experience one incident of an aching back at some time in their lives. (W.H. Kirkaldy-Willis, et al. *Managing Low Back Pain*, New York: Churchill Livingstone, 1992)

Be aware that stress plays a major role in the origin of your lower back pain. If you are frightened or nervous, your muscles become tense. When your muscles tighten, the tightness of the muscle can progress to muscle spasms where the muscles contract and pull. You should know that the muscles in your back are not under your control when they become tense. However, you can control the relaxation aspect of your muscles to decrease your spasm and decrease your pain. Deep-breathing exercises can help you with respect to pain in your lower back.

If you play tennis or golf, the muscles on one side of your back can become short while those on the other side become long. Tennis and golf rotate your spine in one direction in a repetitive fashion. If you sleep on one side most of the time, the muscles on that side of your spine shorten while the muscles on the other side of your spine lengthen. The muscles that are lengthened can become weak while the ones that are shortened can become tight.

Have you ever slipped on the ice and landed on your buttocks? If this has happened to you, the muscle in your lower buttocks called the piriformis muscle can spasm or can even shorten, which compresses your sciatic nerve. Injection of a local anesthetic into the muscle can relieve your pain. If your pain returns, botulism toxin (Botox), which can relax your muscle for up to three months, may be effective when followed by stretching exercises by your physical therapist. Only rarely does a surgeon have to operate on your piriformis muscle if you have persistent sciatic pain. Sometimes chiropractic therapy can offer you a conservative alternative for the treatment of your sciatica. Your chiropractor can treat you with methods such as heat and electrical current to decrease your need to take a pain pill.

Posture

Misalignment of your back due to poor posture or other mechanical strains such as slouching in a chair can cause you to have back pain. If you sit over a computer desk with your back rounded, your muscles are going to adapt to that position. Often the muscle fiber length will change to conform to your improper position. When this happens, your spine is going to adapt to these positions as well. You must remember that hunching over a desk or slouching in a chair can press some muscles and elongate other muscles. Also, tendons, joints, and ligaments that support your back are affected. Some of the ligaments are stretched while some are compressed. When you slouch or when you sit rounded over, you can compress some of the facet joints while opening other facet joints.

Anatomically speaking, you must remember that your lower back supports your body. Your lower body extends from your ribcage to your pelvis. Not only does your lower back include muscles of your lower back, it also includes muscles around your stomach. Muscles in your back, including the muscles around your stomach, attach the front of the spine to the hips. At the attachment of the hips, the muscles are anchored. Persistent slouching will eventually affect your posture. When your posture causes your back to be misaligned, you will develop pain.

The figure that follows shows the skull, cervical vertebrae, thoracic vertebrae, lumbar vertebrae, and sacrum. Notice how this back is in correct alignment. It is important that your back remain in correct alignment to reduce the risk of you feeling pain. The vertebrae and sacrum are common areas for back pain.

As previously mentioned, the discs in between the bones in your back can be a source of back pain. Again, you must be aware that slouching puts more excessive pressure and stress on your discs than does any other posture. Slouching can, therefore, decrease the blood flow to your discs and cause your discs to lose their height and begin to calcify, which is called degeneration. This condition can cause you chronic pain. Slouching in a chair and at a desk also can cause you to have chronic pain by compressing the nerves that come off of your spinal cord and go to your legs.

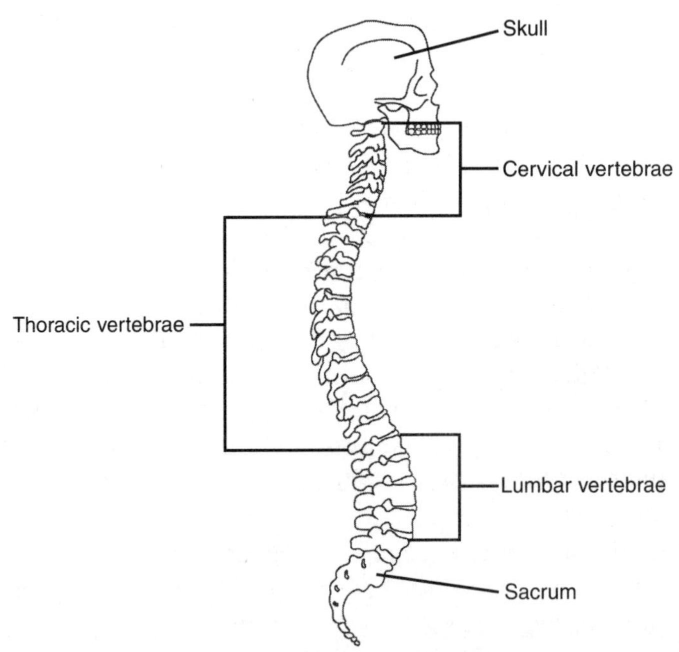

Proper spine alignment.

Your lower back has a natural C curve at the lower end of your back. This normal curve is called a lordodic curve. Chronic slouching can straighten this normal C curve in your back. This misalignment will affect your discs, muscles, ligaments, and joints. Look at your posture in your mirror. If your posture is abnormal, you must correct it. If you cannot do it yourself, you may want to visit a chiropractor or physical therapist to help you with this problem.

Aging

Be aware that as you age one of the first consequences of aging is unfortunately in your discs. (W.H. Kirkaldy-Willis, et al. *Managing Low Back Pain*, New York: Churchill Livingstone, 1992) Before your hair turns gray or before you lose hair and develop wrinkles, changes usually occur in one of both of the two lower discs in your lower back. These are the last two discs in your back.

The lower discs in your lumbar spine essentially do not have a blood supply from arteries to your disc after age 12. The blood supply of your discs must come from the ends of your vertebral bodies. Most of the oxygen and sugar that goes to your discs comes from the ends of your vertebral bodies. Your discs need these nutrients.

After your discs have begun to age, the joints in your vertebral bodies will degenerate. Remember that your bones stack up on top of each other and that the back of your bones form joints with the bones above and below your discs. As your disc narrows as a result of degeneration, the space between your discs narrows. Not only do you decrease your height, you also compress your discs. This compression causes your discs to wear out faster.

The facet joints in your spine work to stabilize your spine. As your joints deteriorate, you will lose motion as your age increases. For some reason, the development of loss of lower back range of motion is slower in women than in men.

Bone Slippage

Spondylolisthesis can be another cause of your back pain. (W.H. Kirkaldy-Willis, et al. *Managing Low Back Pain*, New York: Churchill Livingstone, 1992) This occurs when one of your bones slips upon the one below it. This is usually hereditary in origin. However, when one bone slips over the other, it can cause pain in your facet joints and sometimes it can compress the nerves coming off of your spinal cord going to your legs. Usually surgery is not needed for this slippage. Your pain can be controlled with NSAIDs. Occasionally a steroid injection into your epidural space or a steroid into your facet joint can help to control your pain. Sometimes chiropractic therapy can help you in the management of your pain with this syndrome.

Current Back Pain Research Findings

With respect to gender specificity, sacroiliac joint pain, which can cause significant pain in your back, is common in women during pregnancy and is a result of increased hormones secreted by a woman's body during pregnancy. We also have stated that with aging, women experience less pain initially than men. Osteoporosis, however, is more prevalent in women and can be a significant cause of chronic back pain. Compression of the bones in the lower back can cause fractures and is more common in postmenopausal women because their hormones have significantly declined after menopause. (R. Melzack and P. Wall, *Handbook of Pain Management a Clinical Companion of Textbook of Pain*, New York: Churchill Livingstone, 2003)

Not only does gender affect the incidence of back pain, but age in gender also can affect the incidence of back pain. For example, it was published in 1988 that back pain prevalence was higher among women than men at younger ages, but around age 45 the rate for back pain among men exceeded that of women. When people reach 65 years of age or over, the incidence of back pain was similar for both men and women. It is interesting to note that there is a decrease in the prevalence of back pain in women between the ages of 70 to 79. (R. Melzack and P. Wall, *Handbook of Pain Management a Clinical Companion of Textbook of Pain*, New York: Churchill Livingstone, 2003)

In 1994 a study of back pain patients was done by a female investigator. She found that there was increased body awareness and depression associated for women but not for men. She concluded that it is more socially acceptable for women to admit pain and depression than men. She concluded that women have a greater perception of their symptoms and body awareness than men. She also concluded that there is a fundamental difference in the psychosocial profile of men and women. According to published reports, a combination of estrogen/progestin significantly decreases back pain and disability in premenopausal women who have a decreased bone density in the vertebrae of their lumbar spine.

Also be aware that the irritable bowel syndrome, which is more prevalent among women than men, is commonly associated with an increased incidence of back pain in women. The exact reason for this is unknown. It may be a hormonal effect or a lack of a hormonal effect on the inflammatory chemicals in the female body that causes the incidence of lower back pain. Research continues on the causes of lower back pain and why lower back pain appears to be greater in women than in men overall. (R. Melzack and P. Wall, *Handbook of Pain Management a Clinical Companion of Textbook of Pain*, New York: Churchill Livingstone, 2003)

Groups of people are currently being studied in rural as well as urban areas. Other factors such as obesity, smoking, and alcohol consumption are being studied. The goals of these studies are to attempt to prevent back pain and, if it occurs, to lessen the symptoms in both men and women.

Another recent study was done looking at women who had back pain. The selection of patients was between 25 to 45 years of age. This was intended to eliminate women with menopause-induced alterations of their bodies. Results of the study in women only revealed that the lifetime prevalence of back pain was 35 percent in farmers, 32 percent in manual workers, 28 percent in housewives, 26 percent in nurses, and 15 percent in clerks. The most prominent risk factor for lower back pain in this group was stooping. Remaining in a sitting or stooped position for more than four hours daily was a clear risk factor. The same occupational risk factors similarly affect men.

Did you know that menstrual periods in women can trigger back pain? Even pregnancy can increase a woman's vulnerability to the onset of lower back pain. About 50 percent of pregnant women develop pain in their lumbar spine and hips during their pregnancy. (R. Melzack and P. Wall, *Handbook of Pain Management a Clinical Companion of Textbook of Pain*, New York: Churchill Livingstone, 2003) You should now be aware that it is normal for you to have back pain as you age. You must try and minimize your pain. You should do range-of-motion exercises, take vitamins regularly, and if you smoke, you must stop.

In Germany, in men, back pain was the most frequent cause of absence from work. (W.H. Kirkaldy-Willis, et al. *Managing Low Back Pain*, New York: Churchill Livingstone, 1992) In women it was the second most common reason for absence from work. The frequency of back pain in men was higher than the frequency of back pain in women.

It can be concluded that not all back pain is gender specific. However, this chapter has presented instances where hormones do affect back pain, especially in women. The incidence of lower back pain in men is usually from an injury, whereas in women it can be from repetitive movements. The main triggers for the onset of lower back pain in women are the result of carrying heavy objects periodically.

Treatment for Back Pain

Studies have demonstrated that in certain parts of the world back pain is considered a normal part of life. It is, therefore, less debilitating. In Japan, for example, few individuals complain of back pain when compared to the United States. As a result, disability related to back pain is less.

It was reported before the 1990's (is felt) that previous treatments for your back pain included rest. (W.H. Kirkaldy-Willis, et al. *Managing Low Back Pain*, New York: Churchill Livingstone, 1992)

Rest causes problems in that the muscles in your back that are weak are not being strengthened. It was thought at one time that you should have rest to allow recuperation of your back pain. Back rehabilitation now involves increasing activity and strengthening the muscles in your back.

Following an injury, you may rest for one to two days. However, after this time you need to get active and begin doing range of motion about your back. If you injure your knee, your doctor will begin knee-strengthening exercises. Therefore, the same applies to your back. If you injure your back, the muscles that hold your back in position need to be strengthened. Inactivity weakens these muscles. Lower education levels, smoking, obesity, and inactivity contribute to the prevalence of back pain in the United States.

Treatments for your lower back pain can include physical therapy and chiropractic therapy. As mentioned previously, nonsteroidal anti-inflammatory drugs can decrease the swelling in your tissues as well as in your nerves to decrease your pain. Muscle relaxants on rare occasions can be of benefit to decrease your pain. However, if your pain is related to muscle tension, heat and range-of-motion exercises can be extremely beneficial.

If you have muscle tension back pain, only after conservative measures have failed should you take a pill to relax your muscles. You will know if you have muscle tension pain by touching your muscles around your area of pain. If your muscles are tight, this is a good indication that your pain is at least in part related to muscle tension.

If you are under stress at work or at home, attempt to alleviate your stressful situations. Remember that chiropractic therapy can also be an alternative method to significantly decrease your lower back pain.

If all conservative methods fail to provide you with pain relief, injections of numbing medicines and steroids can be performed in your muscles, your epidural space, around your nerves going to your spinal cord, and even in your facet joints. If you have compression of your nerves, sometimes surgery can provide you with benefit. A new procedure called intradiscal electrothermal annuloplasty can be done to relieve your pain on occasion. This procedure consists of placing a catheter in your disc. The catheter has two electrodes which can heal your disc and keep disc material from leaking from your disc.

A back brace can sometimes be used to decrease your pain. However, the problem with the back brace is that you lose range of motion around your spine. You should know that range of motion around your facet joints helps get nutrients to the joints. It is important to have nutrients in your joints to help form a lubricant within the joint that allows the joint to move freely. Furthermore, if you use a brace long term it can decrease the strength in your muscles that holds your back in a vertical position.

Treatment of back pain for men and women will be determined on an individual basis by your doctor or therapist. Be sure that you follow his or her instructions carefully so that you do not injure yourself further. If your pain does not get better during your treatment, be sure to discuss this with your doctor or therapist, so that he or she can perform further examinations and find a different treatment method.

For Men

Men are more likely to have back pain associated with heavy lifting and muscle strains. Treatment will often revolve around heat therapy, rest, and using muscle relaxants.

- If your pain, such as that from an injury, has just occurred, you can apply cold to the area for 5 to 15 minutes every 2 hours for the first day or two. Do not use cold therapy after this time unless instructed to do so by your doctor.
- If possible, use a heating pad for 15 minutes a day, 4 to 5 times per day. Be sure not to use the heating pad while you are sleeping.

- Rest your back for two to three days if possible. This will help your muscles heal and keep them from further stress.
- Take a prescription muscle relaxant such as Flexaril as prescribed by your doctor.
- Perform back exercises as described in Chapter 10. Use these exercises to strengthen your back muscles and improve your pain symptoms.

For Women

Women often experience back pain due to poor posture and pregnancy. Hormones play a large part in the types of back pain that women experience.

- Make sure that your shoes fit properly and do not cause your back and spine to become misaligned.
- If your back pain is caused from pregnancy, try to find a comfortable resting position and get as much rest as possible.
- If your pain, such as that from an injury, has just occurred, you can apply cold to the area for 5 to 15 minutes every 2 hours for the first day or two. Do not use cold therapy after this time unless instructed to do so by your doctor.
- If possible, use a heating pad for 15 minutes a day, 4 to 5 times per day. Be sure not to use the heating pad while you are sleeping.
- Rest your back for two to three days if possible. This will help your muscles heal and keep them from further stress.
- Take a prescription muscle relaxant such as Flexaril as prescribed by your doctor.
- Perform back exercises as described in Chapter 10. Use these exercises to strengthen your back muscles and improve your pain symptoms.

Chapter 14
Understanding Whiplash

Whiplash injuries can be a devastating experience. If you have ever had a whiplash injury, you probably realize how incapacitating these injuries can be. In 1990 in Quebec, Canada, a group of scientists, including doctors, reviewed the scientific literature and made public policy on the prevention and treatment of whiplash injuries. (W. Ackerman and M. Ahmad. "Whiplash Injuries," *Current Review of Pain* [1999]: 406-410) They described the magnitude of the problem of whiplash injury and presented some strategies to address this entity effectively. The cost of treatment for whiplash injury is high and continues to rise. The problem is that there is considerable inconsistency concerning diagnostic criteria for the diagnosis of whiplash injury.

In this chapter, you will learn about how whiplash occurs, other problems associated with whiplash injury, how a diagnosis of whiplash is made, instances in which depression may occur, and various treatment methods for whiplash injuries. If you think you have suffered from a whiplash injury, be sure to see your doctor right away. There are other serious conditions associated with some whiplash injuries that need immediate medical attention.

The Physics of Whiplash

The term "whiplash injury" was initially described in 1958 by Dr. H. Crowe. (W. Ackerman and M. Ahmad. "Whiplash Injuries," *Current Review of Pain* [1999]: 406-410) Whiplash was described as a sudden speeding up or slowing down of the neck that results in a lashlike effect. Your head weighs anywhere from 10 to 20 pounds and sits on a relatively small neck. If you are hit from behind, your body speeds up. Your head is left behind. As your body speeds up, your head falls backward, causing trauma to your neck. In 1958 it was reported that if you had a whiplash injury you could have symptoms that could last for several years. The term "whiplash" has become a medical and legal term, as well as a social dilemma. Be aware that the term "whiplash" is not a medical diagnosis. It is a result of muscle, ligament, and joint trauma to your cervical spine.

Sometimes your spinal cord can be affected. Whiplash by definition does not include a bone fracture or a disc location of the bones in your neck or a rupture of one of the discs in the neck. (W. Ackerman and M. Ahmad. "Whiplash Injuries," *Current Review of Pain* [1999]: 406-410) The mechanism of a whiplash injury is a result of a sudden speeding up or a sudden stoppage of your head and neck with respect to your body. The motion of a whiplash injury results in the extensive bending backward of your neck or an excessive forward bending of your neck. Motor-vehicle accidents account for more than 90 percent of all whiplash injuries. However, sports injuries also contribute to whiplash injuries. Be aware that rear-end collisions account for 88 percent of whiplash injuries. Less than 10 percent are from side-to-side collisions. With this in mind, you should properly position your head restraint on your seat so that you have protection where your head and your neck meet. Put the top of the restraint where the top of your neck meets your head.

The classic description of whiplash injury is where you are a driver or passenger in a vehicle that is struck by another vehicle. You are sitting in a vehicle that is stationary and it is hit from behind. When this event occurs, it causes a rapid acceleration of your body. Your head is left behind relative to your body. At that time, your head and neck bend backward. The degree of this extension of your neck can be limited with the headrest. Without a headrest, your head could extend to your upper mid-back. An injury of this type could cause excessive trauma to your spinal cord. Following this initial head and body movement, the remainder of your body is held by your safety belt or will hit the steering wheel. At this time, your head and neck bend forward. Your chin can hit your breastbone. Your breastbone limits the degree of forward neck bending.

If you or a friend have suffered a whiplash injury, you need to be aware that the degree of damage to a vehicle involved in the motor-vehicle accident bears little relationship to the size of the force applied to your neck, head, and the remainder of your body. (W. Ackerman and M. Ahmad. "Whiplash Injuries," *Current Review of Pain* [1999]: 406-410) Be aware that injuries in which your neck is bent backward usually result in more trauma to your neck than injuries that cause your neck to bend forward.

The very medical definition of whiplash injury is controversial. The essential element involved in a whiplash injury is that the injury takes place in a motor-vehicle accident or in a sports injury. Your head is subject to acceleration forces that result in the bending of your neck. You may have backed into a sign at the grocery store, for instance. If your neck did not bend, you did not have a whiplash injury by definition. Neck pain can follow a front or back collision. So to have a whiplash injury, you must have an injury followed by neck pain. A definition of whiplash injury includes injury to one or more elements of your neck that arises from forces applied to your head in the course of an accident and that results in your perception of neck pain. (W. Ackerman and M. Ahmad. "Whiplash Injuries," *Current Review of Pain* [1999]: 406-410)

Trauma to the muscles of the neck as well as the facet joints contributes to the whiplash syndrome. Whiplash is now defined as a neck muscle injury as a result of a hyperextension and/or a hyperflexion injury without head contact trauma, post traumatic amnesia, or fractures of the cervical spine.

The incidence of whiplash injuries is 3.8 injuries per 1,000 people in the United States. Of these injuries, 20 percent of people develop symptoms in their neck. Note that the incidence in women is 14.5 whiplash injuries per 1,000 women. In Switzerland, it is interesting that the incidence of whiplash injury is 0.44 per 1,000 people. (W. Ackerman and M. Ahmad. "Whiplash Injuries," *Current Review of Pain* [1999]: 406-410)

Just because you have suffered a whiplash injury does not mean that you are going to have chronic neck pain. Remember that most patients recover from whiplash injuries. Studies done in 1990 indicated that of those patients who do recover do so in the first two to three months after an injury. In other words, your neck pain will resolve in the first few months or it may persist indefinitely.

The mechanics of whiplash injury have been studied using a trauma sled. Human cadavers were placed in trauma sleds using computer probes to record degrees of trauma to the neck at different speeds and high-speed cameras recorded neck movement. (W. Ackerman and M. Ahmad. "Whiplash Injuries," *Current Review of Pain* [1999]: 406-410) The conclusion from the study was that a whiplash injury causes your neck to form an S-shaped curvature with your lower neck bent backward and your upper neck bent forward.

If your vehicle is involved in a front-end collision, your neck can bend forward. When this injury happens and when your neck goes forward, the ligaments in the back of your neck are stretched and sprained. The degree of stretching depends on the force of acceleration of your head forward. The muscles in your neck can also suffer a severe strain. The discs between the bones in your neck can be compressed, and the joints that are in the back of your neck also can be compressed. The facet joints in your neck can be fractured.

The following figure shows the muscles and bones in your neck that are involved in a whiplash injury.

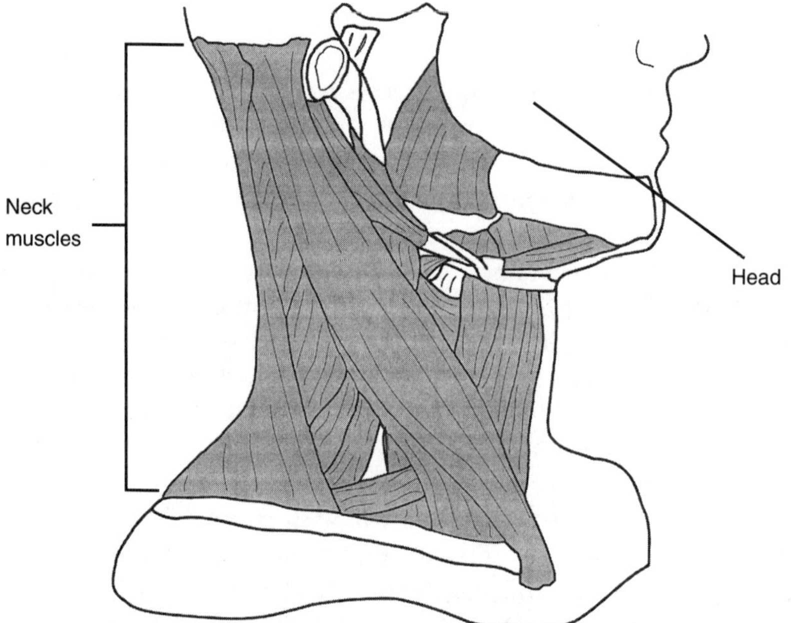

The muscles and bones involved in whiplash injury.

At the time of impact to your vehicle, it is pushed forward. Immediately following an acceleration of your vehicle, your trunk and shoulders accelerate forward. At this time, your head has no force acting upon it. It remains still in space. Your shoulders then travel forward under your head. When this happens, your head begins to bend backward. After your head is thrown backward just like a whip, your head then accelerates forward. Your neck acts as a lever to effect the forward bending of your neck as well as the backward bending of your neck. The forces involved with respect to your head movement are significant.

If at the time of vehicle impact your head is slightly rotated, a rear-end impact will cause your head to rotate further as well. When this happens, you not only have a forward and backward movement of the neck but also a rotary movement of your neck, which can injure the capsules of your facet joints and also injure the discs and ligaments in your neck. After an injury of this type, the structures in your neck are more susceptible to becoming injured again. This is the reason that after a whiplash injury you need to eventually have physical therapy to strengthen the muscles in your neck.

You may have been involved in a front-end collision. With respect to frontal impact injuries, the frontal impact rapidly stops your vehicle. Your body continues forward until you decelerate, caused by your seat belt or if you hit the steering wheel or dashboard. Your head continues to move forward until your neck stops the forward movement of your head. At this time, you may sustain an injury at the joint where your head attaches to your neck. After this movement occurs, your neck recoils with a whiplike effect and your neck is pulled backward. (W. Ackerman and M. Ahmad. "Whiplash Injuries," *Current Review of Pain* [1999]: 406-410)

Studies in mathematical models have demonstrated that a frontal impact injury can also cause your head to rotate. You can have a neck injury in the absence of a head injury. So now you understand that in a motor-vehicle accident your neck is subject to excessive backward bending, excessive forward bending, as well as rotation of your neck to the right and left. If you are hit from the side, your neck can flex to one side or the other or possibly even both sides. If you are hit on the driver's side of your vehicle when you are driving, your head may flex to hit the driver-side window and then whip to the opposite side causing injuries to muscles, ligaments, and joints in your neck. If you are involved in a motor-vehicle accident, try to remember what happened to your neck at the time of the injury. This is extremely important information for you to give to your doctor, chiropractor, or physical therapist.

If you suffer a whiplash injury, your spinal cord may be stretched. Your spinal cord may be bruised as well, which can cause you pain that should resolve over time. Sometimes, the area where the nerves from your arms or legs attach to your spinal cord is traumatized. An area where your nerves meet your spinal cord is called a dorsal root ganglia. This ganglia can be stretched and/or bruised and can cause you to have pain in your neck and arms for a significant length of time.

When the tissues and nerves in your neck are stretched or compressed, tissue damage occurs. This event excites your pain fibers in all of these tissues, which increases their firing rates. Rapid, repetitive, firing rates of pain impulses in your neck could cause changes in your spinal cord. Your spinal cord usually filters out some pain impulses. However, following an injury, to tell you that your body has been injured, your spinal cord may not filter out many of these pain impulses, which is a warning to you that you have sustained an injury. You may develop muscle spasms at this time. Your body is trying to tell you to slow down and decrease some of your activities. You must remember that pain in your body is your body's way of telling you that something is wrong and is advising you to take it easy.

Other Problems Related to Whiplash Injury

As stated previously, whiplash injuries can traumatize your muscles, facet joints in your neck, and ligaments in both the front and the back of the bones in your neck. Disc ruptures in your neck have also been reported. You must remember that there are other structures in your neck besides discs and ligaments. You have an esophagus and an airway that can be traumatized as well. As your neck excessively bends forward and backward, arteries in your neck that go to your brain can be compressed. This is the reason why you could lose consciousness following a whiplash injury. You could also sustain a concussion, which is a bruise to your brain tissue as a result of trauma to your brain. You can even develop a temporal mandibular joint (TMJ) dysfunction.

Following a sudden neck movement, you may develop symptoms of a whiplash injury. (L. Barnsley, S. Lord, and N. Bogduk. "Clinical Review: Whiplash Injury," *Pain* 58 [1994]: 283-307) The cardinal manifestation of a whiplash injury is pain in your neck. Most often your pain is perceived over the back of your neck and is usually described as dull and aching. Movement worsens your pain. If you have had a significant whiplash injury, you may complain of neck stiffness as well as restricted movement about your neck. The pain in your neck may radiate to your head, shoulder, or arm.

Whiplash injuries do not affect genders equally. Women appear to experience whiplash injuries more often than men. Studies done in 1995 related that women experienced more whiplash injuries than men because they have slimmer and less-muscular necks. As a result, women are less able to resist the damage in acceleration forces of the head that are generated at the time of motor-vehicle impact. Another reason for gender differences between men and women with respect to whiplash injury complaints is that women are more likely to seek medical attention. (L. Barnsley, S. Lord, and N. Bogduk. "Clinical Review: Whiplash Injury," *Pain* 58 [1994]: 283-307) Women are also more likely to be sent to medical specialists for complaints of their pain. Women are more prone to respond to their injuries in a way that aggravates their conditions. Sometimes women may be more subject to external stress that can make it more difficult for them to cope with their whiplash injury pain. For example, external stresses like difficulty with a supervisor at work or spousal problems can worsen a whiplash injury complaint. Further research is being done on the gender differences with respect to people presenting to doctors with whiplash symptoms.

Hurting Your Joints and Discs

If your neck is thrown backward too far, both muscles and ligaments in the back of your neck as well as the front of your neck can be injured. Your esophagus, the muscles in the front of your neck, and your discs are at a risk of injury. In the back of your neck, the spinous processes (the parts of your neck bone that are in the center of your neck and stick out from the back of your neck) can be fractured, and the joints in your neck can be fractured and/or misaligned. If your neck if thrown forward in an injury, you run the risk of injuring the discs in your neck as well as the bones in your neck. Furthermore, your facet joints can be stretched if thrown forward. The muscles in the back of your neck can be injured, too.

The facet joints in your neck may be significantly damaged if you suffer a whiplash injury. (L. Barnsley, S. Lord, and N. Bogduk. "Clinical Review: Whiplash Injury," *Pain* 58 [1994]: 283-307) These joints can easily be fractured. A case of a single severe arthritic change in a cervical facet joint was noted after death in a person who had neck pain for many years following a whiplash injury. The pain persisted and became severe, causing the person to become depressed and commit suicide. The single isolated facet joint that was traumatically injured was found on examination after death.

The discs between the bones in the neck are often injured in a whiplash injury. The outer ring of the discs can be torn. The discs could be separated from the bones in the neck. Furthermore, fractures at the ends of the bones in the neck have been reported and can cause significant pain. A whiplash injury can cause the discs in the neck to degenerate as well as the joints in the neck. The injury accelerates the degeneration of both the discs and the facet joints. If your neck extends too far backward, the liquid nucleus pulposus in the center of your disc can burst through your disc after being compressed by your extended neck.

Studies have shown that approximately 60 percent of whiplash injury pain can come from your facet joints. (L. Barnsley, S. Lord, and N. Bogduk. "Clinical Review: Whiplash Injury," *Pain* 58 [1994]: 283-307) This information was noted following a study in which different structures of a patient's neck were injected with local anesthetics to determine the exact cause of a patient's neck pain following a whiplash injury. Injections of local anesthetics in other structures in the neck can confirm the cause of your neck pain. Other structures causing your neck pain are muscles and ligaments. These structures can be injected with local anesthetics mixed with steroids. This combination of drugs injected into your joints may stop your pain. If the pain goes away after injecting these structures (guided by x-rays), the exact cause of your pain can be diagnosed.

Muscle Tears and Sprains

Muscle tears and sprains have been documented and noted since these types of injuries were published in 1976. (L. Barnsley, S. Lord, and N. Bogduk. "Clinical Review: Whiplash Injury," *Pain* 58 [1994]: 283-307) Muscle tears have been visualized on ultrasound examinations. Animal studies have been done simulating whiplash injuries. Partial and complete tears and hemorrhage have been noted. If you have a bleed into your muscles following trauma, these areas can calcify and contract your muscles. Scar tissue can form within your muscles as well. These changes can cause trigger points in your neck and shoulders. Trigger points are areas on your body that when pressed (as during a doctor's examination) cause you pain. These trigger points can be one of the most common causes of chronic pain if you suffer a forward bending of your neck followed by a backward bending of your neck. If you have a trigger point, there is a palpable band noted under your skin. This band is a ropelike consistency to the touch.

Ligaments in your neck and other soft tissues may be damaged following a whiplash injury. If you sustain a ligament injury of your neck, it is difficult diagnosing this type of injury. In animal experiments, tears of the ligaments in the front of the neck bones have been reported. The ligaments in front of your neck bones attach to the discs between your vertebrae. If you sustain an injury to your ligament, you may also sustain a disc injury.

Bone Fractures

The top two bones of your neck (C1 and C2) enable your head to rotate and look up and down. A fracture of either or both of these bones can cause death or cause you to have a serious neurological injury. Some individual have become quadriplegic as a result of an injury to one or both of the first two vertebrae in the neck. The first two bones in your neck provide you with a wide range of rotational movement about your neck. The two bones are connected by ligaments. If your ligaments have been damaged, your head in relation to your neck may become overly mobile.

As stated previously, parts of the bones in your neck can fracture at the time of a whiplash injury. Sometimes the fractures in your vertebrae are missed. Sometimes compressive forces on your cervical vertebrae can compress your vertebral bones downward. This is called a compression fracture.

Brain Injuries and Headaches

Your brain can be injured at the time of a whiplash injury. As your head is being whipped around, your brain can be traumatized as your brain hits the inside of your skull. You can suffer a concussion. You may have headaches for months following an injury. Unfortunately, some brain injuries may go undetected.

Following neck pain, headaches are the most frequent complaint following a whiplash injury. The pain typically begins at the base of the skull. It then progresses to the top of the head. Sometimes the pain can go to the temples on either side of the head. If you have sustained a concussion, you may have a headache as well. Most headaches following a whiplash injury are from soft tissues in the neck. If you have sustained a whiplash injury, you may complain of difficulty with your vision. You may have problems focusing your eyes. Sometimes the nerves that go to your eyes from your brain can be damaged. Sometimes the arteries that go to the back of your brain where you actually see objects can be temporarily blocked as your neck is whipped about at the time of impact. This can cause you to have temporary loss of some vision.

Neuropsychological tests following whiplash injury revealed deficits in areas of attention, concentration, and memory. (L. Barnsley, S. Lord, and N. Bogduk. "Clinical Review: Whiplash Injury," *Pain* 58 [1994]: 283-307) It is possible that if you have decreased attention and memory that it may be due to the severity of your pain as opposed to a direct brain injury. Studies using CT scans and MRI studies in patients who have had whiplash injuries disclosed no significant pathology. Brain wave studies have been done. It has been estimated that approximately 50 percent of patients following a whiplash injury have abnormal electroencephalograms (EEG).

TMJ Injury

The joint in your jaw that enables you to open and close your mouth is called the temporal mandibular joint (TMJ). Injuries to your temporal mandibular joint may occur during a whiplash injury. The exact mechanism regarding how the temporal mandibular joint is injured in a whiplash injury remains to be studied. It is believed that the maxilla (the upper jaw bone) compresses with the mandible (the lower jaw bone). This sudden compression can injure the temporal mandibular joint. As a result, you may have difficulty opening and closing your mouth and may have chronic pain in this joint. For more information, see Chapter 22 on facial pain.

Dizziness, Weakness, and Numbness

You may suffer prolonged dizziness following a whiplash injury. (L. Barnsley, S. Lord, and N. Bogduk. "Clinical Review: Whiplash Injury," *Pain* 58 [1994]: 283-307) The exact mechanism by which dizziness occurs following a whiplash injury remains speculative. Again, it is thought that the arteries in the neck that go to the brain are irritated, which compromises the blood flow to the brain. A decrease in the blood flow to the brain can cause people to have disturbances in balance and equilibrium. You may notice weakness in one of your arms or both of your arms following a whiplash injury. As your neck is thrown about at the time of vehicle impact, your neck bones can compress one of the nerves exiting from the holes in your vertebrae. This nerve compression can cause irritation in the nerve. These nerves go to the muscles in your arms. As a result of nerve compression, you may develop weakness in your arms. If this happens to you, some people may think that you are pretending to be ill or in pain. However, these symptoms are transient symptoms and will usually resolve.

There is no good diagnostic test to demonstrate that you did have a temporary nerve compression at the time of your neck injury. Furthermore, if you sustained a muscle injury and have muscle pain, that particular muscle will be weak. Sensation of tingling and numbness in your hands can occur following a whiplash injury. These symptoms can be attributed to nerve compression similar to the weakness that you could experience. These symptoms usually resolve quickly in one to two months and are usually of no long-term consequence. You may suffer from a loss of concentration as well as memory disturbances following a whiplash injury.

Depression Occurrences Related to Whiplash

Some studies published during the past decade have noted psychological factors in whiplash patients. (L. Barnsley, S. Lord, and N. Bogduk. "Clinical Review: Whiplash Injury," *Pain* 58 [1994]: 283-307) If you have severe persistent pain, over time you may develop psychological symptoms such as depression. A whiplash injury may cause you to have abnormal psychological distress.

Sometimes the public's perception of a whiplash injury is an injury that enables the injured individual to collect a lot of money as a result of the injury. This concept is frequently depicted in cartoons. Another aspect that you should be aware of is called "litigation neuroses." With respect to this aspect, it is hypothesized that people will complain of exaggerated pain and injury in order to secure financial gain. However, studies have demonstrated that the duration of pain following a whiplash injury is independent of litigation. It is interesting to note that in one study of whiplash patients, after monetary settlement 88 percent of these patients recovered and had no residual symptoms. (L. Barnsley, S. Lord, and N. Bogduk. "Clinical Review: Whiplash Injury," *Pain* 58 [1994]: 283-307) A problem exists in that there is no real evidence that pretending to be ill or in pain with the hopes of being awarded a large settlement in a court of law contributes in any significant way to the natural history of a whiplash injury. Most whiplash injuries can cause you to have real tissue trauma with chronic pain as well.

After a Whiplash Injury

What are the chances that you will resolve your neck pain following your whiplash injury? The chance that you will recover fully is called your prognosis. Studies have shown that an increase in age and an injury-related decrease in attention and memory as well as the severity of your initial neck pain are predictive of symptoms that will last beyond six months. If you had a history of degenerative disc disease in your neck prior to your injury, for instance, your prognosis for resolution of your pain is poor. Older people do worse after whiplash injury. As stated earlier in this chapter, women have a worse prognosis because of their thin necks and lack of muscle girth. In most people, however, neck pain resolves over time.

Diagnosing a Whiplash Injury

You may be wondering how your doctor will be able to diagnose a whiplash injury. In most instances, x-ray studies of the cervical spine as well as MRI studies and CT scans taken immediately after a whiplash accident are generally of no use. (L. Barnsley, S. Lord, and N. Bogduk. "Clinical Review: Whiplash Injury," *Pain* 58 [1994]: 283-307) These imaging studies usually only reveal an evidence of a preexisting degenerative disc or joint disease. The most common abnormal x-ray finding is straightening of the normal curve in your neck. Remember the C curve that was mentioned earlier? When your muscles go into spasm, you will have straightening of the curve in your cervical spine. It is rare for an x-ray to reveal a bone injury such as a fracture.

CT scans or MRIs are usually done if a significant injury is suspected by the doctor examining you, who is usually an emergency room doctor. If it is suspected that you may have an undiagnosed bone fracture, your doctor may order a bone scan. Only 2 percent of plain x-rays of the neck following trauma to the cervical spine revealed any significant injury. A CT scan can show neck bone dislocations as well as misalignments and fractures but do not demonstrate soft tissue injury. The MRI is useful in assessing soft tissue injury as well as injury to your bones. Soft tissue is any tissue in your body with the exception of bone.

Your MRI imaging should be carefully examined for any soft tissue bleeding as well as ligament tears around your spine. If you suffer an injury to one of the nerves in your neck, electromyography may be helpful in diagnosing a nerve injury. This test is usually done if you have a normal MRI but have complaints of weakness and numbness in your arms.

Treatment Exercises for Whiplash Injury

Treatment of your whiplash injury should be personalized specifically for you. Personalization is necessary because of the variation in symptoms as well as the degree of severity of soft tissue injury. In other words, you may have a worse injury than another individual who has a whiplash injury. A soft cervical collar to keep your head in a neutral position should not be used more than three days following your injury.

Range-of-motion exercises around your neck should be started beginning the third day and progress to neck-strengthening exercises. Active range of motion by you should start as soon as you can tolerate it. This means rotating your head from side-to-side as well as up and down. Your chiropractor or physical therapist may do passive range-of-motion exercises with you. This means that your health-care provider will move your neck while you attempt to relax it. Heat therapy may increase your range of motion but should not be used immediately after your injury. Cold therapy, such as ice packs, may reduce swelling in the muscles and tissues around your neck. *Transcutaneous nerve stimulation (TENS)* may help you decrease your pain symptoms so that you may not need to use pain pills. Attempt to resume your normal activity as soon as possible. Studies have demonstrated that you can benefit significantly if you begin to move as soon as possible following your injury.

Be educated with respect to your injury and what tissues have been injured. You must clearly understand the goals of your treatment in the control of your pain. Education helps you plan realistically for your future and provides you with a sense of pain control. You must understand that pain does not equal harm. If you do not use your neck following your injury, you may decondition your muscles. These muscles may increase tension and cause you muscle pain. Try to avoid neck collars and pain pills. Be advised as to what activities will worsen your pain, such as heavy lifting and maintaining prolonged postures at work or over a computer desk.

Medications to Control Pain from Whiplash Injury

Sometimes you need medications to control your pain. Drugs, however, have a limited role in the management of whiplash injury pain. Drugs, especially narcotic drugs, have a significant potential for misuse and can have potential adverse side effects. Sometimes your doctor may overuse medications because your doctor is uncertain how to ease your pain. Realize that pain pills have their greatest application immediately after injury. Nonsteroidal anti-inflammatory drugs can provide you with pain relief as they decrease swelling in your tissues. However, long-term use gives you a risk of ulcers.

Muscle relaxants may or may not help you with muscle spasms. You should apply cold to the injured muscles after the injury and heat after five days. Remember that narcotic pills can cause you to become tolerant or addicted. Long-term narcotic use is usually discouraged. Studies have shown that morphine could reduce pain following whiplash injury but did not improve function. *Never* take a narcotic medication for your mood enhancement. Antidepressant drugs can help you to rest. Proper sleep is important in your healing process and allows your body to build up chemicals that can decrease your pain. Sometimes following an injury and if you have associated chronic pain, you can become depressed. Antidepressant medications may not only decrease your pain, they may also decrease your depression if you have developed depression post-injury.

Muscle pain is a common source of pain following a whiplash injury. (L. Barnsley, S. Lord, and N. Bogduk. "Clinical Review: Whiplash Injury," *Pain* 58 [1994]: 283-307) This pain should be treated either with hot packs, cold packs, or with steroid injections. Your pain-medicine doctor can inject your painful muscle areas with a local anesthetic that will numb your muscle and relax it. A steroid may also be injected that will decrease the inflammation in your muscle. This is usually followed by a cold spray on the muscle and a stretch of the muscle by a physical therapist or a chiropractor.

Sometimes cervical epidural steroid injections decrease neck pain. "Epi" means around and "dural" means the area that surrounds the fluid that surrounds your spinal cord. (L.G.F. Giles and K.P. Singer. *Clinical Anatomy and Management of Cervical Spine Pain*. New York: Butterworth-Heinemann, 1998.) This epidural space may become swollen following an injury. If your doctor injects a small amount of steroid into the area, your pain may be significantly reduced. If you sustained a disc injury in your neck following a whiplash injury, sometimes leakage of this disc material may form small scars in your epidural space, called adhesions. An epidural steroid injection can break up some of these adhesions and decrease the swelling in the nerves. (L. Barnsley, S. Lord, and N. Bogduk. "Clinical Review: Whiplash Injury," *Pain* 58 [1994]: 283-307)

If you have headaches that begin in the base of your skull, the nerve coming out of this area to the top of your head can be treated with local anesthetic and steroid. This nerve is called the occipital nerve, and the name of the headache is occipital neuritis.

Sometimes the joint between the top two bones of your neck can become compressed and injured. (L.G.F. Giles and K.P. Singer. *Clinical Anatomy and Management of Cervical Spine Pain*. New York:

Butterworth-Heinemann, 1998.) The administration of a steroid into this joint can provide you with significant pain relief as well. Most of the injections mentioned should be done with x-ray needle guidance. As previously mentioned, the facet joints in the neck may also be injured. Injection into the joint itself or injection of the nerve that goes into the joint may decrease your pain. Injection into any of these joints may provide you with good pain relief; if the pain returns, however, surgical removal of the nerve to this joint can be done with either heat or cold application. This procedure is called a facet joint rhizotomy.

If you do not have significant pain relief with the previously mentioned methods, sometimes a psychological evaluation along with a method such as biofeedback help you deal with your pain. Do not be offended if your doctor refers you to a psychologist. A study in 1998 concluded that those who suffered a whiplash injury with headaches may also suffer psychological distress from the chronic pain. Your pain from whiplash injuries may be considered by some people, including doctors, to be of a psychological origin. However, you now know that various soft tissue injuries can cause you to have chronic pain following a whiplash injury.

Whiplash injuries usually go away in several months. However, some whiplash injuries can last more than 10 years. (L. Barnsley, S. Lord, and N. Bogduk. "Clinical Review: Whiplash Injury," *Pain* 58 [1994]: 283-307) The prevalence of whiplash injuries is higher in women as previously stated. Your health-care provider must provide you with the proper modalities and the proper individualized treatment to rehabilitate you to decrease your pain and return you to normal activities of daily living.

Treatment for Whiplash

Treatment for whiplash generally consists of heat therapy and the use of pain relievers. Be sure to properly follow your doctor's or therapist's instructions about taking any medications and performing exercises.

For Men

- Try to rest your neck for two to three days.
- If possible, use a heating pad for 15 minutes a day, 4 to 5 times per day. Be sure not to use the heating pad while you are sleeping.

- Rest your neck for two to three days if possible to keep from doing excessive bending and turning. This will help your muscles heal and keep them from further stress.
- Take any prescription medications prescribed by your doctor.
- Perform neck exercises as described in Chapter 10. Use these exercises to strengthen your neck muscles and improve your pain symptoms.
- See a chiropractor to help relieve the pain in your neck.

For Women

- Try to rest your neck for two to three days.
- If possible, use a heating pad for 15 minutes a day, 4 to 5 times per day. Be sure not to use the heating pad while you are sleeping.
- Rest your neck for two to three days if possible to keep from doing excessive bending and turning. This will help your muscles heal and keep them from further stress.
- Take any prescription medications prescribed by your doctor.
- Perform neck exercises as described in Chapter 10. Use these exercises to strengthen your neck muscles and improve your pain symptoms.
- See a chiropractor to help relieve the pain in your neck.

Chapter 15
Understanding Headaches

Have you ever had a headache? A headache is pain felt within the skull, in the forehead, in the temples, or at the base of the skull. Most headaches are caused by emotional stress or fatigue, but some headaches are a symptom of a disease within the brain. Of the many pains that you can feel throughout your body, pain in the head region is usually the most distressing. Pain in your head can arise in your head or can be referred from your neck, too.

This chapter will teach you about common types of headaches, how your doctor will diagnose your headache, what some common sources of headaches are, and current research findings about treatment for headaches. Different types of headaches such as migraines, tension headaches, cluster headaches, head trauma headaches, and temporal arteritis headaches will be discussed. You will also learn about how hormones, especially those in women, affect the onset, intensity and duration of headaches.

Common Types of Headaches

Pain in your head can be divided into two divisions: Some pain receptors exist outside your skull, and other pain receptors exist within your skull. Structures outside of your skull that can cause pain in your head include the skin and scalp over the head, muscles around your head and neck, and the outer wrapper of the bone of your skull called the *periosteum.* Your sinuses can also cause you to have head pain. Within your skull, you have a lining that can become inflamed and irritated and cause pain. Your veins can cause pain as well if they become engorged. You must tell your doctor where the location of your pain is. This will help your doctor determine the source of your headache.

Your doctor will complete a detailed neurological examination to determine what type of headache you have. The purpose of a neurological examination is to exclude any disease or tumor that could be causing your headache. If you have a history of rheumatoid arthritis, make sure that your doctor knows that you have this disorder. Headaches can arise from instability of the first bone in your neck, called the *C1 vertebral body.* Because tight muscles can also cause headaches, your doctor will check the muscles in your neck. Your doctor will then press on the arteries in your temples. If you have tenderness around the arteries in your temples, you have an inflammation of the temporal arteries. Your doctor will have you lie flat on the examining table. Your doctor will ask whether you have a change in your headache after your head is lifted. If your headache is originating from your neck, there may be some relief by lifting your head relative to your neck.

If you go to your doctor when you are having a headache, your doctor will observe you. Your doctor will record whether you look pale, have a drawn face, and whether you have dark circles around your eyes. Doctors look for tearing and redness of the eyes. Your doctor will examine your pupils to see whether they are extremely small and will look at your upper eyelids for any drooping. As mentioned, your doctor will observe your behavior during your headache. Those with migraine headaches usually want to be left alone and usually seek a quiet, dark place. Those with cluster headaches find no relief in any position; they try many positions while attempting to eliminate their headaches and usually end up pacing the floor.

Your doctor will also take your temperature. If your temperature is elevated, you may have an infection in your throat, sinuses, or even in your brain. You may be asked to fill out a psychological assessment; your doctor uses this to determine whether you suffer from any emotional disorders. Remember that emotional disorders can cause headaches. In addition, a skull x-ray may be taken. Skull x-rays can prove useful for the diagnosis of a fracture, cancers, bone destruction, or some shift of the structures of the brain. If you have pain in your neck, your doctor may order x-rays of your neck, with your neck bent forward and then bent backward. This test can determine whether you have any instability of the bones in your neck. Blood flow studies may be done to determine whether you have any compromise in the blood flow going to your brain. A decrease in blood flow can cause significant headaches.

Sometimes a CT scan is necessary to determine whether you have swelling in your brain or a brain abscess. (H.N. Raskin. *Headache.* New York: Churchill Livingstone, 1988) (M.G. Bousser, et al.

"Migraine and Pregnancy," *Neurology* 40, [1993]: 437-441) An *electroencephalogram* (EEG) study is sometimes needed to determine whether you have a seizure disorder or a sleep problem. If you have had trauma to your head, your doctor may want a CT scan, which will show whether you have bleeding within your head. An MRI scan of your brain can be done to see whether you have loss of myelin, which is a substance in your brain. With loss of myelin, you may develop neurological symptoms that include memory loss and difficulty concentrating. Occasionally a spinal tap is done. This can investigate whether you have an infection. At the time that the spinal tap is done, a pressure monitor can be used to see whether you have increased pressure in your central nervous system.

Remember that your history is important. Your doctor needs to know if you have had a headache with loss of consciousness. Loss of consciousness could indicate seizures or a hemorrhage into your brain. If you have had no previous history of headaches, your doctor will need to run tests to see whether you have a bleed in your brain from a weakness in the arteries in your brain. A weakness in the blood vessel is called an aneurysm. If you have headaches accompanied by neurological abnormalities during and after your headache, your doctor will want to make sure that you don't have a bleed within your brain.

Tumors can cause headaches with neurological abnormalities such as forgetfulness and dizziness. If you have a headache that first begins after age 50, your pain may be coming from degeneration of the discs in your neck. (H.N. Raskin. *Headache*. New York: Churchill Livingstone, 1988) (M.G. Bousser, et al. "Migraine and Pregnancy," Neurology 40, [1993]: 437-441)

Hormonal changes that occur with the decreased function of your thyroid gland can cause headaches as well. (H.N. Raskin. *Headache*. New York: Churchill Livingstone, 1988)

Remember that depression can also cause headaches. If someone has told you that your personality changes when you have a headache, your doctor will want to determine whether you have a tumor or even an infection of your brain. A headache that occurs when you have an increase in your blood pressure can indicate various medical diseases that may be causing a headache. Be aware that headaches can come from the soft tissues in your neck. An x-ray of your neck will not reveal soft tissue problems. An MRI can usually reveal problems in structures that could cause you to have a headache.

Migraine Headaches

Be aware that headaches are the most common pain syndrome in middle-aged adults. (H.N. Raskin. *Headache*. New York: Churchill Livingstone, 1988) (M.G. Bousser, et al. "Migraine and Pregnancy," Neurology 40, [1993]: 437-441) It is the most frequent symptom seen by neurologists. Be aware that there are different types of headaches. Headaches are classified so as to help doctors plan treatment strategies.

A common type of headache is the classic migraine headache. By definition a migraine headache is a headache that returns and varies widely in its intensity and frequency of the attacks and the duration. Usually the headaches occur on one side and are associated with nausea, vomiting, and a loss of appetite. Sometimes you may have visual problems associated with this headache. You can have a headache with sensations that forewarn you of an attack of an impending headache. You may have a sensation of flickering lights or blurred vision or weakness in your arms or legs. These sensations are called an aura. Some migraines occur without an aura. If you have migraines with an aura, usually you have visual disturbances. This type of visual disturbance is seen in 90 percent of patients who have migraine headaches with an aura. Migraine headaches can be triggered if you have abnormal response to stress.

Different Causes of Migraines

More than 50 years ago, doctors thought that the source of migraine pain was related to decreased blood flow to the brain, which in turn decreased the oxygen in the brain, causing headaches. However, more recent studies have demonstrated that the migraine headaches occur in brain cells. (H.N. Raskin. *Headache*. New York: Churchill Livingstone, 1988) (M.G. Bousser, et al. "Migraine and Pregnancy," Neurology 40, [1993]: 437-441)

Sometimes the blood flow in the brain can decrease and the thickness of the blood can increase. These events can release chemicals in your brain that activate the pain impulses in your brain. When you have one of these headaches, you may experience mood disturbances as well as pain. You may have nausea and vomiting, too.

Migraine headaches usually begin when you are a teenager. However, some migraine headaches can begin at age 40. (H.N. Raskin. *Headache*. New York: Churchill Livingstone, 1988) (M.G. Bousser, et al. "Migraine and Pregnancy," Neurology 40, [1993]: 437-441)

Before you suffer a migraine headache, you may have changes in your vision or speech and balance. You may notice zigzag lines in front of your eyes or small specks in one eye. You may notice different lines that come and go in front of your eyes. You may have numbness in your hands. When the headache occurs following these visual disturbances, your headache is usually on one side of your head. If you are seeing lines only in front of your left eye, usually your headache will be on the right side of your brain.

Sometimes you can have headaches that occur several times a week followed by a long period of having no headaches. Sometimes your migraine headaches can be incapacitating. Movements such as bending over, coughing, or sneezing can worsen your headache. You will want to lie down. Following your headache, it can take approximately 24 hours for you to feel normal again.

If you have a history of migraine headaches, be aware that some stressful situations such as weddings, funerals, or speaking in front of people can trigger your migraine headaches. Remember that there can be a family history of migraine headaches. Seventy percent of people inherit the tendency to have migraine headaches. If you have migraine headaches, you usually have less than two attacks per month. However, 10 percent of patients have attacks every week.

Another type of migraine headache can occur that does not have changes in sensation that can forewarn you of an impending headache. This type of headache is called a migraine headache without an aura. Sometimes these headaches occur on both sides of the head.

Prevention and Treatment of Migraines

Before your doctor prescribes medicines for your migraine, your doctor must tailor your medications and take into account your disability, your medical history, and your psychological profile. Treatment of your migraines can be divided into acute treatment of the attack as well as treatment to prevent the onset of headaches.

Whenever possible, the factors that cause your headaches should be avoided. Stay away from foods that could trigger your migraine headache. Cheese, chocolate, red wine, and some Chinese foods that contain the additive MSG are commonly considered migraine headache triggers.

If you have an onset of a headache, a mild attack can be treated with aspirin. Nonsteroidal anti-inflammatory drugs can also be used to treat your headache. Ibuprofen is commonly used to treat headaches and can be purchased without a prescription. The new nonsteroidal anti-inflammatory drugs called COX-2 inhibitors (for example, Vioxx and Celebrex) can also be effective for the treatment of headaches. If you have nausea and vomiting associated with your migraine headache, you may need to take a nonsteroidal anti-inflammatory drug by the rectal route. New drugs called triptans have been developed and can decrease your headache within a significant time after its onset. Sumatriptan was the first triptan drug to be used for the treatment of migraine headaches. Triptans are much better tolerated than the older caffeine-ergotamine medications. Be aware that the triptans are expensive. When you first suspect that you are having a migraine, take your triptan immediately.

Sometimes stronger drugs are needed for the treatment of migraine headache symptoms. Codeine and Darvocet are sometimes needed. Stronger drugs such as Percocet have been prescribed for the treatment of migraine headaches.

Stress and Migraines

If you have frequent migraine attacks and if these attacks are disabling, consider prophylactic treatment. Because migraine headaches can be activated by stress, it is important that you tell your doctor what situations trigger your headaches. You may have to make life adjustments. If you are having too much stress at work, you may need to consider changing your job. Medications can be helpful in preventing your headaches, but you should not become dependent on these drugs to solve any emotional problems that you may have. Avoid an overly busy schedule. Have one hour per day of free time to relax from a busy workday. Attempt to take one afternoon off per week and even one day off from work per month. When you have this time free, do whatever you feel like doing.

If anxiety causes you to have migraine headaches, consider relaxation techniques such as yoga or hypnotherapy. If you have significant psychological problems, consider a consultation with a psychologist. Sometimes breathing into a plastic bag for 10 minutes can prevent the onset of a headache. You may benefit from the administration of nitroglycerin placed under your tongue, which can decrease the onset of migraine headaches. Remember, however, that nitroglycerin can cause headaches if the dose taken is too high. Aspirin can prevent the onset of headaches. Benadryl has been used to prevent the onset of migraine headaches as well. Antihypertensive medications such as Nadolol and Verapamil have been used to prevent the onset of migraine headaches. Amitriptyline, an antidepressant, also has been demonstrated to prevent the onset of migraine headache.

Migraines in Women

Migraine headaches appear to be hormonally related. They are more common in women until age 60 when the incidence is about equal. (H.N. Raskin. *Headache.* New York: Churchill Livingstone, 1988)

Migraine headaches commonly occur with the onset of menses in women. These headaches may also occur in the first trimester of pregnancy. The headaches can disappear following a complete hysterectomy. After the onset of menopause, your migraine headaches may disappear or at least decrease in intensity and frequency. However, if you receive hormone therapy at the time of menopause, this can prolong your headache symptoms. Sometimes your migraine headaches can worsen when you begin using oral contraceptives. Concern exists about the use of oral contraceptives by those who suffer migraine headaches, because they run a higher risk of stroke. The risk of a stroke is further increased if you smoke.

Tension Headaches

Another type of headache that you could experience is called a tension-type headache. This is also called a muscle contraction headache or a psychogenic headache. The term "tension type" is used to imply that muscle tension plays a role in the onset of the headache. If you have chronic tension-type headaches, you may have headaches 15 days a month. For your doctor to make a diagnosis of your tension-type headache, you should have at least 10 previous headache episodes. The headaches should last from 30 minutes to 7 days. You will usually have a headache on both sides of your head. Your headaches should not be aggravated by walking or routine physical activity. If you have a tension-type headache, you should not experience nausea or vomiting. You should not have visual disturbances that are associated with migraine headaches.

Be aware that some individuals have chronic daily tension-type headaches. Migraine headaches and tension-type headaches are experienced more in women than men. Studies have been done which indicated that tight muscles around the scalp and neck can cause tension-type headaches. Studies used to objectively identify muscle tension have been done and have validated muscle tension as a cause of tension-type headaches. Remember that if you have significant stress in your life that the muscles in your neck and scalp can have sustained contractions. When you have prolonged muscle contractions of your scalp and neck, the muscles have less blood flow and, therefore, less oxygen going to your muscles. This decrease in blood flow can result in the formation of lactic acid in your muscles, which can cause you to have significant pain.

Muscle tension-type headaches can start at any age. Tension-type headaches can begin in childhood if a child is physically and emotionally abused. When you have a tension-type headache, you will feel a tight band and pressure around your head in the form of a tight cap. Your neck muscles will feel as if they are in a knot. The location of your head is usually all around your head on both sides. Try to avoid stress to prevent this type of headache from occurring. Usually a tension-type headache is seen in tense or anxious people. A family history of tension-type headaches is not as common as with migraine headaches.

Treatment for this type of headache is the avoidance of stress. Biofeedback as administered by a psychologist can decrease your muscle tension and, therefore, decrease your headaches. If you have tension-type headaches, you must learn to relax. Aspirin and acetaminophen can be of some help. Heat can also cause your muscles to relax.

If depression perpetuates your headaches, you can take antidepressants at bedtime. Sometimes muscle relaxants can be used to decrease your pain. Anti-anxiety drugs such as Valium have sometimes been used preventatively to decrease the chance of one of these headaches developing. When your headache occurs, one of the nonsteroidal anti-inflammatory drugs may be helpful in decreasing your headache. (H.N. Raskin. *Headache.* New York: Churchill Livingstone, 1988)

Cluster Headaches

Another type of headache that you should be aware of is called a cluster headache. For your doctor to make a diagnosis of cluster headache, you should have had at least five attacks before seeing your doctor. Usually the headache is on one side of your head and can be above your eye or in your temple. Usually the headache lasts 15 minutes to 3 hours if untreated. Usually you will have tearing of your eye as well as nasal congestion on the side of your cluster headache. You may have forehead sweating. Your pupil may be extremely small and your upper eyelid may droop.

You may have clustering of headaches for several weeks and then no headaches for two weeks. You may go for a year without having a headache. A cluster headache is different from a migraine headache. Usually there is no nausea and vomiting associated with a cluster headache. Usually if you have a cluster headache, you are agitated and have to pace the floor. This is different from your migraine headache, which causes you to lie down and rest during the attack. Cluster headaches can occur while you are asleep or at rest during the evening. The overall incidence of cluster headaches is extremely rare. Less than 10 percent of the population suffers from cluster headaches. You may have your first attack between the ages of 20 and 40 years. Cluster headaches are associated with cigarette smoking and trauma to your head. Also, if anyone in your family has a history of cluster headaches, you may be prone to these headaches.

The exact cause of these cluster headaches is unknown. The cluster headache occurs more frequently in men than in women. There is a 5:1 man-to-woman ratio of cluster headaches. If you suffer from a cluster headache, your doctor will want to make sure that you do not have a pituitary tumor. A pituitary tumor is an abnormal growth in your pituitary gland in your brain. (H.N. Raskin. *Headache.* New York: Churchill Livingstone, 1988)

Not only can it cause you to have a headache but sometimes it can decrease your vision. An MRI can help detect this tumor. If it is malignant not only may you need surgery but irradiation as well as drug therapy.

To treat a cluster headache attack, some doctors suggest inhalation of 100 percent oxygen using a face mask. Usually your headache will settle in 15 minutes. If this does not work, an injection of sumatriptan (Imitrex) may decrease your pain. Some studies have even recommended the use of local anesthetics on a cotton swab placed in the nose.

Steroids in high doses can sometimes be used to decrease the onset of cluster headaches. Medrol can be given in various doses and schedules as directed by your treating physician. This drug must be discontinued slowly after treatment for five to seven days. It may take up to three weeks to taper the drug. Nonsteroidal anti-inflammatory drugs may be effective to decrease the headaches. Sometimes sufferers need to see a neurosurgeon in consultation to see whether there is a surgical procedure that can be done to decrease the headache.

Head Trauma Headaches

If you have had a history of trauma to your head, you may develop headaches associated with your head trauma. These headaches continue for more than eight weeks after trauma to your head. Your headache is often severe and is throbbing. You may have nausea and vomiting associated with this headache. You may be drowsy or you may become irritable. Your memory may be temporarily impaired.

A headache following trauma can be made worse with physical exercise. A post-traumatic headache differs from migraine symptoms in that a chronic post-traumatic headache is usually generalized and permanent. However, it can be made worse by physical or mental strain. Usually this type of headache subsides in 8 to 10 weeks. You may develop a post-traumatic headache with only a minor injury to your head. In fact, the more severe the injury, the less chance you have of developing one of these headaches. (H.N. Raskin. *Headache*. New York: Churchill Livingstone, 1988)

Post-traumatic headache is reported more often in women than men. The incidence of a post-traumatic headache can be 40 percent following a head injury.

Treatment of this headache is with anti-inflammatory drugs or mild pain relievers such as Darvon. Your doctor must help you deal with any loss of memory. If you have had mood changes, your doctor may have you see a psychologist to help you through this post-traumatic psychological period.

You may have chronic headaches associated with trauma to the head if the injury occurred when you were older than 40. (H.N. Raskin. *Headache*. New York: Churchill Livingstone, 1988) If you have a low educational level as well as a low intelligence, your headache could be chronic. Furthermore, a history of previous head trauma or a history of alcohol abuse can predispose you to have post-traumatic headaches for a long time.

Temporal Arteritis Headaches

If you are over 60 years old, you could develop a headache associated with temporal arteritis. This usually occurs after you have had a fever. You have a burning pain caused by inflammation of your temporal artery on the side of your head. It is usually accompanied by a throbbing headache around your temple. You may have a burning pain around your scalp. Temporal arteritis headaches are worsened by jaw movement such as chewing. This type of headache can be accompanied by loss of vision, which is a medical emergency. The diagnosis sometimes has to be made with a biopsy of the arterial tissue. Steroids are usually the treatment of choice for this pain.

Sources of Headache Pain

Do you know what structure in your brain cause headaches? Pain in your head can come from direct pressure on structures such as muscles or blood vessels. Traction on your muscles and nerves can cause you pain. If your blood vessels become engorged and if the diameter of your vessels become enlarged, the enlarged vessel can compress your nerves in your brain and cause you pain. A prolonged muscle contraction in your neck can cause pain as well. On occasion, more than one mechanism can cause you to have a headache. If you have a migraine and tense your muscles, you can have two causes for your headaches.

Keep a diary of your headaches. Your history of your headaches is a most important part of your doctor's workup. Your doctor needs to know about your general medical health. The progression of your headaches over days to months to years is important. A history of any headaches in your family is important as well. You must know that migraine headaches tend to run in families. Muscle contraction headaches and brain tumors also run in families. You need to keep a daily diary. You should write down what factors cause your pain and how long your headaches last and what medications you took either before, during, or after your headaches have resolved. Your doctor will examine your diary to look for a consistent pattern in the occurrence of your headaches.

Psychological distress can trigger headaches. Sometimes major social trauma or anxiety triggers headaches. Physical trauma can also be a cause of chronic headaches. If you are a woman, your doctor will want to know the effects of your menstrual periods and pregnancy on your headaches. Menstrual periods and pregnancies change hormones in the bloodstream, and this change can trigger headaches.

Current Headache Research Findings

There are clear sexual differences in the incidence of headaches, with women being more likely than men to experience headaches. Women are two to three times more likely to suffer migraine headaches than men. Women experience more disabling daily muscle tension-type headaches. Be aware that there are no gender differences in children prior to puberty. This suggests that reproductive hormones have an effect on the onset of headaches. However, men have more cluster headaches than women in a prevalence ratio of 5:1. It is estimated that more than 50 percent of women suffering from migraine headaches miss approximately one week of work per year, whereas approximately 40 percent of men miss one week of work per year.

You need to remember that gender-specific medicine is a relatively new aspect of medicine. You must remember that you and your doctor should work as a team to control your headaches. Also remember that your treatment needs to be individualized. If you have any questions regarding your medications and the effects of your gender on these medications, ask your doctor and/or pharmacist. If they do not have an immediate answer for you, they will be able to provide you with the answer that you seek after they research the medical literature.

Gender and Headaches

Women who suffer from headaches are more likely than men to seek treatment for their headaches. (H.N. Raskin. *Headache.* New York: Churchill Livingstone, 1988) Women are more likely to receive a headache diagnosis than men. Further study reveals that women are more likely than men to receive prescription medications for their headaches. Women receive more prescriptions than men for all migraine headaches except for the nonsteroidal anti-inflammatory drug category.

Women are more likely to relate that weather changes, perfumes, and cigarette smoke can trigger their migraine headaches. The sex hormones estradiol and progestin are believed to cause the increased incidence of headaches in women. (R.B. Fillingham. *Sex, Gender, and Pain.* n.p.: IASP Press, 2000) A significant fall of estrogen in the bloodstream that occurs just before the onset of menstruation can cause migraines in some women. However, exactly how estrogen triggers migraine headaches remains to be further.

Recent studies report that migraine headaches with an aura are occur more frequently in women, whereas migraine headaches without an aura occur more frequently in men. (H.N. Raskin. *Headache.* New York: Churchill Livingstone, 1988) (M.G. Bousser, et al. "Migraine and Pregnancy," Neurology 40, [1993]: 437-441)

Cluster headaches and post-traumatic headaches occur more frequently in men. (H.N. Raskin. *Headache.* New York: Churchill Livingstone, 1988) (M.G. Bousser, et al. "Migraine and Pregnancy,"

Neurology 40, [1993]: 437-441) Chronic muscle tension headaches are more prevalent in women. Headaches arising from degeneration of the neck or muscle spasms of the neck are more common in women. (R.B. Fillingham. *Sex, Gender, and Pain.* n.p.: IASP Press, 2000) Some people who have been administered a spinal anesthetic develop a headache. The spinal headaches are more common in women. The reason for this finding is unknown.

Sex Hormones and Headaches

Sex hormones do affect pain, including headaches. If you are a woman and if your progesterone increases, your migraine headaches could go away. This is the reason why women have fewer migraine headaches during pregnancy. (H.N. Raskin. *Headache.* New York: Churchill Livingstone, 1988) (M.G. Bousser, et al. "Migraine and Pregnancy," Neurology 40, [1993]: 437-441) However, some individuals can still have migraines as pregnancy progresses—this should not be confused with a sign of preeclampsia.

As progesterone increases during the menstrual cycle, headaches may be fewer. Animal studies have concluded that pain in general, including headaches, is reduced during milk production. (R.B. Fillingham. *Sex, Gender, and Pain.* n.p.: IASP Press, 2000) On the other hand, if your estrogen decreases, you may have joint pain. The joint pain increases after menopause.

In men, when testosterone increases, cluster headaches become frequent. Cluster headaches are noted at the time of puberty. With the increase in progesterone, estrogen, and testosterone, there is an increase in migraine as well as tension headaches. Be aware that women produce testosterone as well as men. (R.B. Fillingham. *Sex, Gender, and Pain.* n.p.: IASP Press, 2000) When progesterone, estrogen, and testosterone increase, pain in general increases in both men and women.

The effects of sex steroids on chronic pain continue to be studied. As you can see now, the sex steroids can exert sex-specific effects on nerves throughout your central nervous system. In other words, sex steroids act not only on your reproductive organs but also on non-sex-related organs such as your spinal cord and brain as well as nerves in your arms and legs. These hormones can directly affect the chemicals in your body that affect pain impulse transmission. Your sex hormones can cause your nerves on occasion to release *substance P,* which is a pain transmitter. However, your sex hormones can also decrease some of the pain producing chemicals.

Headaches and the Menstrual Cycle

During the menstrual cycle, a woman retains more fluid. This retention of fluid increases the water content of the woman's bloodstream and dilutes the effects of any medications. Trials are being done to examine the effects of various analgesic medications during the menstrual cycle. What you need to realize is that the dose of the medication that you need may be less if you are a woman during your menstrual cycle. It is, therefore, believed that the mass of drug that needs to be administered at different times during a woman's menstrual cycle may vary. If this variation of fluid and drug responses is evident, your dose of drug will need to be changed periodically. The problem is that your doctor and/or your pharmacist may not be aware of the fact that your drug dose requirements can change during your menstrual cycle. It can also decrease following menopause. For this reason, if your medication prescribed for your headaches seems to stop working during your menstrual cycle, ask your doctor whether you should alter your dose.

Opioids as Headache Pain Relievers

Studies are currently being done to examine the effects of different types of opioids on the treatment of severe migraine headaches. One of the opioids that can be used for the management of severe migraine headaches is butorphanol (Stadol). This drug is administered nasally. Some doctors advocate the use of this drug for the treatment of headaches. This drug is believed to work better in women than in men. Women show a greater analgesic response to kappa-stimulating opioids. (R.B. Fillingham. *Sex, Gender, and Pain*. n.p.: IASP Press, 2000) The other types of opioids are mu-stimulating opioids and include morphine and demerol. These mu-stimulating opioids have been shown to work better in men than in women. For this reason, studies are being done and more studies need to be done that can evaluate the effects of these drugs for the treatment of severe headaches.

As we mentioned in our chapter on narcotic medications, different types of narcotic receptors exist in your brain and spinal cord. If you turn on one of these receptors your pain impulses going to your brain are decreased. Mu receptors bind morphine, oxycodone, and hydrocodone while kappa receptors bind Stadol or Talwin. Other receptors exist but are not currently stimulated by specific drugs that are readily available.

Treatment for Headache

Before your doctor prescribes medicines for your migraine, your doctor must tailor your medications and take into account your disability, your medical history, and your psychological profile. Treatment of your migraines can be divided into acute treatment of the attack and treatment to prevent the onset of headaches.

For Men

- Pay attention to what triggers your headaches. If you notice that certain foods or scents cause your headache to begin, avoid those things.
- Inhale 100 percent oxygen by mask.
- Tricyclic antidepressants, such as amitryptyline, are commonly used for preventing headaches.
- Physical therapy can help if you have frequent tension headaches.
- Massage therapy can help relax tense muscles and relieve headaches.
- Behavioral therapy can be used by those who have headaches that are made worse by stress, anxiety, depression, or other psychological factors.

For Women

- Pay attention to what triggers your headaches. If you notice that certain foods or scents cause your headache to begin, avoid those things.
- Inhale 100 percent oxygen by mask.
- Tricyclic antidepressants, such as amitryptyline, are commonly used for preventing headaches.
- Physical therapy can help if you have frequent tension headaches.
- Massage therapy can help relax tense muscles and relieve headaches.
- Behavioral therapy can be used by those who have headaches that are made worse by stress, anxiety, depression, or other psychological factors.

- Women may benefit from aromatherapy to relieve their headaches.
- Because of sex differences with respect to the effect of estrogen as well as progesterone on the absorption, metabolism, and elimination of medications, drug dosing may fluctuate in the female patient depending on whether or not the female is pre- or postmenopausal. The physiological changes that occur during the menstrual cycle can affect the response of a drug in the female body. You must discuss the effects of your drug with your doctor because the effect of your drug may decrease during menses.

Chapter 16
Understanding Arthritis

Arthritis is the painful inflammation of the joints in your body. Approximately one out of seven people has some form of arthritis, and there are many different types you can have. And if you know someone who has arthritis, you know that arthritis can be devastating. More than 35 million people in the United States suffer from this disease, and every year treatment costs the United States billions of dollars. (J.D. Loeser. *Bonica's Management of Pain*. n.p.: Lippincott Williams and Wilkins, 2001)

This chapter concisely describes the more painful arthritic conditions encountered by health-care givers: osteoarthritis, rheumatoid arthritis, ankylosing spondylitis, and gouty arthritis.

Attack of the Joint Tissue

Inflammation that occurs in your joints can cause you to have pain as well as swelling of your joints. For you to understand why you develop pain in arthritis, you must have some knowledge of joint anatomy. Joints in your arms and legs permit movement of your arms and legs. The bones of your joints are held together by a capsule that consists of a dense strong tissue; further, your joints are held by ligaments, which connect bones to each other. Your joint is supported by muscles or tendons that lie over your joints. (Tendons connect muscles to bones.) On the inside of your joint, the surface of your joint is covered with a tissue called a synovium. This tissue has special cells that exist within the lining of your synovial tissue. Some of these cells help to form some of the components that make the fluid in your synovial tissue thick. This thick fluid is like motor oil. A thick fluid will provide your joints with better lubricating properties than a watery fluid. The fluid that exists in your synovium lubricates the surfaces of the bones and cartilage that make up your joint. Cartilage is a tough, slippery layer of tissue that covers the surfaces where bones contact each other in joints.

Synovial tissues contains many blood vessels. Your synovium also contains sympathetic fibers. This anatomical feature can be important if one develops an entity called reflex sympathetic dystrophy. There is also a joint in your body where your back bone meets your hip bone. This is called your sacroiliac joint. This joint is only slightly movable. Even though this joint does not move freely, it can cause you significant pain. Other sites or cells exist in your joint that secretes chemicals that rebuild and degrade your joint. This process of rebuilding and degrading your joint keeps your joint anatomy in balance. If your joint becomes degraded, it will degenerate and you will develop arthritis in the degenerating joint.

Diagnosing Arthritis with Your Doctor

Each year approximately 10 percent of people in the United States have to seek a health-care provider's attention because of pain in their joints that affects their activities of daily living. (W.N. Nom [Editor]. *Environmental and Occupational Medicine.* Atlanta: Lippincott Williams and Wilkins Publishers, 1998) Most of us do not seek the services of a health-care provider until our activity is decreased. For example, if you are unable to go to work, your supervisor may require you to go to a doctor. In the United States, people suffering from significant arthritis miss, on average per person, 10 days of work per year.

Data has been published reporting that approximately 25 percent of people with arthritis were unable to carry out their normal activities of daily living. (J.D. Loeser. *Bonica's Management of Pain*. n.p.: Lippincott Williams and Wilkins, 2001) This means that they had difficulty shopping, driving, and dressing. If you suffer from arthritis, your pain may came and go. More than 50 percent of people with arthritis report that they have pain that is constant.

Start Keeping a Diary

When you go to your health-care provider, they will obtain a detailed medical history from you. You must keep a diary of the following information:

- The pattern of your pain. Your health-care provider will want to know whether your pain is localized to one joint or many of your joints. Does the pain affect the joints in your hands or feet as well as your ankles, shoulders, and hips? Or is it your neck, back, or sacroiliac joints (where the hip meets the lower portion of your back)?

- The intensity your pain is and how long it lasts.
- Whether your pain is sharp or dull.
- Whether your pain is made worse or better with physical activity as well as changes in the weather. For example, note any morning stiffness and how long it lasts.

If you have arthritis, you may realize that you have stiffness of your joints in the morning but that the stiffness progressively decreases as you become more active.

If you have the rapid onset of joint pain that involves one joint such as the joint in your great toe, this usually signifies a gouty arthritis, known more simply as gout.

You may know a young man who complains of pain in his buttocks and the back of his thigh along with morning stiffness. These symptoms can be associated with an arthritic condition called ankylosing spondylitis.

If you have any nodules under your skin, you may have rheumatoid arthritis. You should be able to feel these nodules over your elbows. If you have a relative who has a history of rheumatoid arthritis, you run the risk of developing this type of arthritis. If you have had weight loss as well as chronic fatigue, you must include this in your pain diary. Weight loss and fatigue can be associated with rheumatoid arthritis.

Diagnostic Tests

Your health-care provider will examine your joints for normal range of motion. (J.D. Loeser. *Bonica's Management of Pain*. n.p.: Lippincott Williams and Wilkins, 2001) If you have pain on passive range of motion of your joints (movements done by your health-care provider without any effort on your part), this usually indicates that you have inflammation of your joints.

Your joints will be examined for warmth as well as tenderness, and your muscles will be evaluated for strength as well as size. If you have significant pain, sometimes you will not use certain muscles in your arms or legs. This can cause your muscles to shrink in size and cause you to have weakness. Your shoulders will be examined for tenderness as well as range of motion. Your wrist joints, finger joints, elbow joints, hip joints, knee joints, and the joints in your feet will be examined.

If you suffer from one of the arthritic diseases, you may notice on occasion that your joints are swollen and red. When you go to your doctor, they may not be swollen and red at that time. This is why it is important for you to keep a pain diary.

If you are seeing a doctor for pain in your joints, your doctor may want to get some laboratory tests. Your doctor may use a needle and syringe to extract fluid from your joints. Your doctor will look at the fluid to see whether it is clear. Normal joint fluid should be clear and straw colored. If you have osteoarthritis, the fluid can be straw colored. Other types of arthritis that you may have include rheumatoid arthritis or gout. Your fluid may be yellow. Your doctor will examine your fluids for cells. Your doctor will also obtain blood from you. Your blood will be examined for any elevation in your white cells (a sign of inflammation) and a test for rheumatoid arthritis can be done at the same time.

These tests are important for your doctor to make a proper diagnosis of what type of joint inflammation that you have. Your doctor may also order x-rays or even a CT scan or MRI of your painful area. Furthermore, it is not unusual for your doctor to eventually order a bone scan if your pain persists in spite of conservative treatment. A bone scan consists of injecting a very small and harmless dose of radioactive dye into your vein. After this has been done, a special camera takes a picture. If you have arthritis, there will be an increased uptake of the radioactive material into your painful joint, showing that the joint is inflamed. Inflammation is the responses of your body's tissues to irritation or injury. Your affected tissue can become warm, swollen, and/or red. The severity of inflammation depends on the cause and the area affected.

Osteoarthritis

Osteoarthritis is the most common arthritic disease. (J.D. Loeser. *Bonica's Management of Pain*. n.p.: Lippincott Williams and Wilkins, 2001) It is also called degenerative joint disease. Most of us will eventually develop osteoarthritis as we experience wear and tear on the joints in our body. Osteoarthritis occurs in the joints of your body when your cartilage is worn down and damaged by overuse, sometimes allowing the rigid and brittle bone ends to come into direct contact with each other. Your bones that compose your joint can then break down and develop irregular growths called osteophytes that can interfere with the proper movement of the joint and cause pain. Your joints provide you with range of motion and do support your body as well. To have normal and painless range of motion, your joints must have cartilage in between your bones.

Cartilage is a tissue that coats the ends of your bones. The synovium surrounds your bones as well as the cartilage. Your cartilage does not have its own blood supply. This synovium is, therefore, filled with a liquid, and the synovial fluid supplies sugar and other nutrients as well as oxygen to your cartilage. When you are young, your cartilage contains approximately 85 percent water and it decreases to 70 percent as you age. Molecules called proteoglycans are in your synovial joint. These proteoglycans attach to the structure of a significant amount of water. Your cartilage is also composed of collagen. Collagen gives your joint support as well as flexibility.

When the cartilage in your joint deteriorates, you have the beginnings of osteoarthritis in your joints. Osteoarthritis does not cause you to have immediate pain in your joints. Your pain appears gradually. In the early phases of this disease, your cartilage swells. The cartilage will lose water. As the cartilage loses its hydration, cracks appear in the cartilage. Your synovium can become inflamed and swollen. If the disease progresses more tissue is lost and your cartilage loses its elasticity. Over time the cartilage in your joint can be completely destroyed. This will leave the ends of your bones without a protective cartilage. As a result, the two bones that form the joint can rub against each other, causing you to have significant pain.

Osteoarthritis does not spread throughout your entire body and cause problems outside of your joints as may happen in other arthritic diseases such as rheumatoid arthritis. It is confined to your joints. Other arthritic diseases such as rheumatoid arthritis can affect your lungs and heart. Pain in a joint in your arm or leg or your back or neck is usually your major symptom if you suffer from osteoarthritis. Pain is the reason why you will seek medical care. Pain is also the major reason why you may suffer functional loss of your arms or legs. Osteoarthritis can cause not only pain in your arms and legs, but also in your spine.

Osteoarthritis can affect the elastic cartilage in your discs between your bones. These discs between your bones in your back act as cushions between the bones. You also have joints where each in your back stacks on top of one another. These bones stack on top of each other and fit like Lego blocks. These joints can degenerate, which will cause you to become stiff and will decrease your range of motion. In addition to pain and decreased range of motion, you may have muscle spasms. If the holes where the nerves from your spinal cord come out of your vertebral bodies, the hole can decrease in size and compress the nerves going to your extremities. This can cause you pain, weakness, and numbness. Osteoarthritis of your spine can occur in your neck, lower back, or even your mid-back.

Degenerative arthritis can become evident in your hips. Pain usually develops in your hips slowly. The pain in your hips can be referred to your buttocks or to your groin. If you have osteoarthritis that affects your hips, you will probably walk with a limp. As you walk with a limp, the excessive stress on your knees, ankles, and back can cause you pain as well.

Osteoarthritis can also become evident in your knees. Your knee may become warm as well as swollen. You may have decreased range of motion in your knees over time. This decreased range of knee motion can make it painful for you to walk through a shopping center or go up and down steps.

Osteoarthritis can also affect the joints in your hands. You may notice a bony growth around the joints in your fingers. Osteoarthritis can cause painful range of motion around your fingers.

In all of these boney structures affected by osteoarthritis, be aware that osteophytes can form in your joints. The osteophytes that form at the margins of your joints can be a source of pain.

Your joint pain originates from nerves that transmit pain impulses located in the tendons, ligaments, periosteum of your bones, and the synovium of your joints. You also need to be aware that the periostium, which wraps your bone, contains many free nerve endings that can cause you to have significant pain if one bone of your joint rubs on the other bone of your joint. Various chemicals in your nerve endings in your joint can be released. One chemical, *substance P,* is frequently released in joints. Capsaicin cream that depletes substance P from the nerve endings can be used to manage your joint pain.

Your joint pain associated with osteoarthritis usually begins gradually and progresses slowly over years. Originally you may have the condition but not experience any pain. With the passage of time, symptoms may begin. You will become stiff and the stiffness will probably cause you to decrease your activity. You will notice an increase in your pain when it rains or when the weather becomes cold. Your pain may become severe to the point that it keeps you up at night. Osteoarthritis usually occurs in older people. Approximately 85 percent of people over 65 develop osteoarthritis. However, only half of these people experience any symptoms.

Caucasians have a higher incidence of osteoarthritis than other ethnic groups. Osteoarthritis is not common in people younger than the age of 45. (J.D. Loeser. *Bonica's Management of Pain*. n.p.: Lippincott Williams and Wilkins, 2001) Before age 45, this disease occurs more frequently in men. After age 55, osteoarthritis is seen more often in women. Osteoarthritis involving the knee is more prevalent in women than in men, perhaps a result of wearing high-heeled shoes.

Obesity puts an increased pressure and stress on your joints in your legs. Obesity is an abnormal increase in your body fat resulting in excessive weight. There must be a 20 percent weight gain greater than the ideal for your height and body build. If you are obese, you have an increased chance of developing osteoarthritis. Any excess weight that you carry may cause deterioration of the joints in your hips, knees, and ankles.

If someone in your family has a history of osteoarthritis, there is a chance that you could develop this disease as well. When you develop osteoarthritis and if your pain steadily increases, you may want to avoid using the affected joints. Disuse of a joint can cause your muscles to decrease in size. This decrease in size can cause you to become weak.

If you have morning stiffness and pain in your joints, you are more likely to report your pain to a health-care provider. You should know that women tend to report joint pain more often than men. Age does not affect the incidence of pain reporting. If you have weakness in your thigh muscles, called the quadriceps, you may be prone to develop osteoarthritis of your knees. Any type of chronic pain syndrome can cause you to suffer from depression. If you are depressed, tell your doctor so that your doctor can prescribe antidepressant medications for you.

Osteoarthritis can occur after trauma to a joint. Repetitive motions required in your job can also cause the onset of osteoarthritis. The management of your osteoarthritic pain first involves correction of any abnormal biomechanics. One way of changing an abnormal biomechanical factor is weight reduction. Obesity increases the incidence of osteoarthritis of the knees more in women than men. A cane or shoes that fit right and provide a cushion can decrease symptoms associated with osteoarthritis.

Because weak thigh muscles can be a cause of osteoarthritis, you will probably need a physical therapy evaluation to show you how you can strengthen your muscles. You will be prescribed strengthening exercises for these muscles. Therapy in aquatic environments such as a swimming pool can provide you with minimal-impact aerobics. It is important to retain joint range of motion when you have osteoarthritis. Water aerobic programs are well-suited to osteoarthritic joint rehabilitation.

Nonsteroidal anti-inflammatory medications are commonly used to treat osteoarthritis (for example, Celebrex, Mobic, and Day Pro). Be aware that nonsteroidal anti-inflammatory drugs may cause gastrointestinal complications. The new selective COX-2 inhibitors can decrease your chance of developing gastrointestinal pathology. Steroids injections into your joints can also decrease the inflammation of your joints, which will decrease your pain. Your doctor can also inject hyaluronic acid into your joints for pain modification. Glucosamine, which is available without a prescription, has been demonstrated to decrease pain associated with osteoarthritis. If you persist with chronic pain and disability, consultation with a surgeon may be indicated to see whether you quality for and would benefit from a total joint replacement.

Rheumatoid Arthritis

Another form of arthritis is rheumatic arthritis. Rheumatic arthritis is characterized by redness, warmth, swelling, and painful joints. If you have rheumatoid arthritis, you will have decreased range of motion of some of your joints in your body. You may also complain of stiffness. This disease attacks the synovial linings of your joints as well as the tendons around your joints. If you develop rheumatoid arthritis, you may suffer generalized weakness and weight loss.

The exact cause of rheumatoid arthritis is unknown, but approximately 43 million people in the United States suffer from rheumatoid arthritis. Rheumatoid arthritis affects men and women, all races, and all ages. (J.D. Loeser. *Bonica's Management of Pain*. n.p.: Lippincott Williams and Wilkins, 2001)

However, rheumatoid arthritis is three times more common in women than in men. Family history plays an important role in the development of rheumatoid arthritis. Rheumatoid arthritis may result from an abnormality in the immune system. Your antibodies may attack your joints to cause significant degeneration within your joints. It can usually have a slow onset. However, be aware that it can have an acute onset as well. The onset of rheumatoid arthritis occurs more often in the winter. If you are between the ages of 30 and 50, your chance of developing rheumatoid arthritis are increased.

You probably have rheumatoid arthritis if you have four of the following seven criteria:

1. Morning stiffness around your joints
2. Arthritis of three or more joints
3. Arthritis of your hands
4. Arthritis that occurs on both sides of your body
5. Nodules over your bony joints
6. An elevated rheumatoid factor in your bloodstream
7. X-ray changes of your joints

The treatment of rheumatoid arthritis is to relieve your pain and decrease your joint inflammation. In addition, your health-care provider will want to maintain as much range of motion around your joints as possible. Splinting, range-of-motion exercises, and strengthening exercises can be extremely beneficial to you. Occasionally, you may need a brace on one of your extremities.

Usually nonsteroidal anti-inflammatory drugs are prescribed for the management of your arthritic pain. As mentioned with regard to osteoarthritis, the COX-2 inhibitors are safer for your gastrointestinal system than the older nonsteroidal anti-inflammatory drugs. Some doctors prescribe medications such as gold compounds, antimalarials, and sulfasalazine. However, each of these drugs has the potential to cause serious side effects. Steroids may also be necessary to decrease the inflammation of your joints. Steroids typically decrease pain and swelling.

Fish oil may have some anti-inflammatory effects against rheumatoid arthritis. The most common side effect you may experience with fish oil supplementation is mild stomach upset. Be aware that fish oils can decrease your blood's ability to clot. If you are taking blood-thinning drugs, you should not take fish oils, because it will give you an increased risk of bleeding.

If these methods do not relieve your pain, you may be a candidate for immunosuppressive therapy. Immunosuppressive therapy is the administration of a drug which eliminates or lessens an immune response. Methotrexate is used frequently for the treatment of your rheumatoid arthritis. Methotrexate can cause liver pathology. Surgery is the last resort for the treatment of rheumatoid arthritis and consists of total joint replacement. If your pain becomes intolerable and if you have significant limitations in joint function, surgery can provide you with relief. Joint replacements are now available for hips, knees, shoulders, elbows, and ankles.

Be aware that sex hormones may play a role in the development of rheumatoid arthritis. (R.B. Fillingham. *Sex, Gender, and Pain*. n.p.: IASP Press, 2000) Sex hormones can block some of the mechanisms involved in the development of rheumatoid arthritis. If you are a premenopausal woman, you could develop rheumatoid arthritis if you have low levels of DHEA as well as testosterone. Postmenopausal women have high levels of both testosterone and DHEA. Both of these chemicals are called androgens. Apparently androgens are of some benefit to you in preventing progression of this disease. On the other hand, men who have rheumatoid arthritis usually have low testosterone levels. Some medical scientists think that testosterone may decrease the incidence of rheumatoid arthritis. In addition, a history of smoking is associated with an increased risk for the development of rheumatoid arthritis in men but not in women.

Ankylosing Spondylitis

Ankylosing spondylitis is a disease that predominantly affects men. (J.D. Loeser. *Bonica's Management of Pain*. n.p.: Lippincott Williams and Wilkins, 2001) Pain usually begins in the back and sacroiliac joint (the joint where the back and hip bones meet) early in life. An x-ray of the spine of a male with ankylosing spondylitis appears as bamboo and is called a bamboo spine. This pattern is also seen on MRI imaging studies. Ankylosing spondylitis usually affects men before the age of 40. If you have ankylosing spondylitis, you may develop arthritis of your spine as well as the large joints in your body. Ankylosing spondylitis is present in 8 percent of Caucasians and 3 percent of African American men. (Bonica J. The Management of Pain, 1990, Lea and Febiger) A marker in the bloodstream called HLA-B27 is present in 90 percent of patients who have ankylosing spondylitis. Ankylosing spondylitis has been observed in rats when the HLA-B27 gene is expressed.

Usually ankylosing spondylitis will become manifest in a male around age 20. This arthritic disease does occur in women, but the symptoms are more prominent in men. If you do suffer from ankylosing spondylitis, your primary symptoms may be symptoms in your hip joints. You may have progressive decrease of your back range of motion. You may have some pain in the joints of your arms and legs as well. X-rays have shown arthritis in sacroiliac joints. Over time, your spine will continue to stiffen. The onset of ankylosing spondylitis is gradual. If your disease progresses, your symptoms will go upward toward your neck. You have a normal curve in your lower back that will become straight. You may have difficulty expanding your chest to take a breath. If your ankylosing spondylitis advances, your entire spine may become fused, which restricts your motion around your spine in all directions.

The earliest x-ray changes usually occur in your sacroiliac joints. Erosion of these joints becomes evident. The outer ring of your discs in your spine become calcified. Furthermore, calcification of the vertical ligaments that run in front and back of your vertebral bones occurs. When this happens, if you have an x-ray of your spine, it will appear as a bamboo stick. Remember that rheumatoid arthritis affects mostly small joints. Ankylosing spondylitis affects large joints. Osteoarthritis does not usually affect your sacroiliac joints.

If you have ankylosing spondylitis, physical therapy and nonsteroidal anti-inflammatory drugs are important for the treatment of the pain associated with this disease. No treatment is currently available that will eradicate ankylosing splondylitis. Occasionally stronger analgesics such as opioids are needed to control your pain. Sulfasalazine is sometimes useful for pain in arthritis in your arms and legs. The problem with ankylosing spondylitis is that you can have pain that is severe over decades of your life. The severity of the pain associated with this disease varies greatly. Approximately 10 percent of patients have disability so severe that they are unable to return to work after 10 years.

Gouty Arthritis

You or someone you know may suffer from gouty arthritis, or gout. Gout is one of the most painful arthritic diseases. Gout results from crystals of uric acid that are deposited into joint spaces between your bones. These uric acid crystals deposited into your joints cause inflammation with swelling, redness, and warmth around your joint. Sufferers develop stiffness in their joints, too. Gouty arthritis is noted in 5 percent of all cases of arthritis. We all have the formation of uric acid in our bodies. Uric acid is formed from the breakdown of chemicals called purines that are found in many foods. You should avoid foods that will elevate your uric acid blood level. If you have an onset of gout, avoid meat and seafood. Do not eat gravies. Avoid yeast products, including beer and other alcoholic beverages. You must also avoid oatmeal, asparagus, cauliflower, and mushrooms.

In most people, uric acid is dissolved in the bloodstream and excreted through the kidneys. If your kidneys do not eliminate enough uric acid from your bloodstream, the uric acid will increase in your bloodstream. If you eat a lot of liver, beans, or peas, you may increase the uric acid in your bloodstream. If the uric acid forms crystals and deposits these crystals into your joints, gout will develop. In many people, the uric acid deposits affect the joints in their great toes. The big toe is affected in approximately 75 percent of people suffering gout. The ankles, heels, knees, wrists, and fingers may also be affected by gouty arthritis.

If you have a family history of gouty arthritis, you run the risk of developing this disease. Gout is more common in men than in women and is more common in adults than in children. Obesity increases the risk of developing gout. An excess consumption of alcohol also interferes with the excretion of uric acid from your body. The increased uric acid that occurs can form crystals and deposit these crystals into your joints. Adult men between the ages of 40 and 50 are most likely to develop gout. It is occasionally seen in women. It rarely occurs before menopause. For some reason, people who have had organ transplants are more susceptible to gout.

A diagnosis of gout can be made by withdrawing fluid from your painful joints and analyzing the fluid for uric acid. When your gout attack is severe, you may be totally incapacitated. If your gout is not treated, you may develop severe pathology of your affected joints. African American men have a higher incidence of gout than Caucasian men. The prevalence for men is approximately 14 cases per 1,000 men, whereas the prevalence in women is approximately 6 cases per 1,000 women. Estrogen hormones noted in women can help the body eliminate uric acid. For this reason, gout is rarely seen in premenopausal women.

When a gout attack occurs, the maximum pain associated with the gout usually occurs in approximately the first 10 hours. In general, attacks resolve in less than 14 days. Uric acid crystals can not only be deposited in your joints, they can also form in your soft tissues. A collection of uric acid crystals in your tissues can form a lump (called a tophi), often noted on the outer edges of your forearms. Be aware that if you have gout, you have an increased risk of developing kidney stones. These stones are usually composed of uric acid. If you have gout, you also have a higher risk of developing a kidney disease.

We all have uric acid in our bloodstreams. Gout develops when there is an excessive amount of uric acid. Uric acid crystals are usually formed when your uric acid level exceeds 6.8 mg/dL. Sometimes overproduction of uric acid is related to a genetic disorder. Excessive exercise can also increase uric acid, as can obesity. Starvation or dehydration can increase uric acid, too. Thyroid disease can also increase uric acid. Diuretics (medications that make you urinate, such as furosemide [Lasix] and hydrochlorthiazide [or HCTZ], a common blood pressure medicine) and cyclosporine A (an immunosuppressive medicine) can increase the uric acid concentration in the bloodstream.

Your doctor will probably obtain a blood sample from you to measure the uric acid in your bloodstream. However, this is a misused test for the diagnosis of gout. Approximately 5 percent of the population has an elevated serum uric acid level. Only approximately 10 percent of these individuals develop gout. Therefore, an elevated uric acid level in your bloodstream does not mean that you have or will develop gouty arthritis. The diagnosis of gout is made by finding uric acid crystals in the fluid of your joints.

If you develop an acute attack of gout, you need in most instances to be treated for your pain. Your doctor may give you nonsteroidal anti-inflammatory medications, steroids, or colchicine. The use of COX-2 inhibitors is under investigation. Remember other nonsteroidal anti-inflammatory drugs could cause you to develop ulcers. Steroids can be used to treat gout and can be given orally or by injection into your muscle. The steroid can be given for approximately two weeks. Sometimes your doctor will inject your painful joint with a steroid.

Colchicine is the medication that has been used extensively over the past two decades for the treatment of gout. It is most effective during the first 24 hours of an acute attack. Colchicine can cause you to have vomiting and nausea. If you have liver problems, you should not take colchicine.

Allopurinol is another drug that can decrease your uric acid levels. Allopurinol is usually used in people who produce excessive uric acid. Allopurinol should not be used during an acute gouty arthritis episode because Allopurinol can prolong the attack. Probenecid is used by some rheumatologists because it has fewer side effects than Allopurinol.

If you have developed tophi (nodules under your skin) that are painful, you may need to have these uric acid crystals removed surgically. (J.D. Loeser. *Bonica's Management of Pain*. n.p.: Lippincott Williams and Wilkins, 2001)

If you have had significant destruction of one of your joints, an orthopedic surgeon may need to surgically correct any malformation that may be related to uric acid deposition in your joints and the resultant joint destruction.

Treatment for Arthritis

After determining what type of arthritis you have, your doctor will prescribe a treatment plan for you to follow. It will most likely include medications, therapy, and exercise.

You should now be aware that any of the types of arthritis described in this chapter can be potentially disabling. Current research involves the study of new and safer medications for the treatment of all types of arthritis.

For Men

- Anti-inflammatory medications such as Vioxx, ibuprofen, and acetaminophen will help reduce the swelling and pain sensations you are experiencing.
- Physical therapy can help relieve the pain associated with your arthritis.
- Massage therapy can relax your muscles and often relieve swelling in your muscles and help your arthritis pain.
- Acupuncture can stimulate nerve fibers and help decrease your pain.

For Women

- Anti-inflammatory medications such as Vioxx, ibuprofen, and acetaminophen will help reduce the swelling and pain sensations you are experiencing.
- Physical therapy can help relieve the pain associated with your arthritis.
- Massage therapy can relax your muscles and often relieve swelling in your muscles and help your arthritis pain.
- Acupuncture can stimulate nerve fibers and help decrease your pain.
- Because of sex differences with respect to the effect of estrogen as well as progesterone on the absorption, metabolism and elimination of medications, drug dosing may fluctuate in the female patient depending on whether or not the female is pre- or post-menopausal. The physiological changes that occur during the menstrual cycle can affect the response of a drug in the female body. You must discuss the effects of your drug with your doctor because the effect of your drug may decrease during menses.

Chapter 17

Understanding Peripheral Neuropathies: Pain in Your Arms, Legs, Hands, and Feet

You probably know someone who has a carpal tunnel syndrome. This syndrome is the result of a *neuropathy*. For you to understand a neuropathy associated with a carpal tunnel syndrome, you should have some overall knowledge of what constitutes a neuropathy in general. A neuropathy by definition is any disease of your peripheral nerves. These are the nerves that exist outside of your brain and spinal cord.

A disease of these nerves can cause a weakness as well as numbness in the area where the nerve travels. If only one nerve is affected by a disease state, it is called a *mononeuropathy*. Your symptoms will depend upon the distribution of that nerve in your tissue. A *polyneuropathy* involves many nerves. With a polyneuropathy, your symptoms are more exaggerated as compared to a mononeuropathy. A polyneuropathy can involve more than one extremity and is usually related to a metabolic disease. A momoneuropathy is usually related to a nerve compression. This chapter examines both types of neuropathy.

The figure that follows shows what a peripheral nerve looks like. It includes the synapse, dendrites, nerve cell body, axon and axonal processes, which all play a role in how your body senses pain.

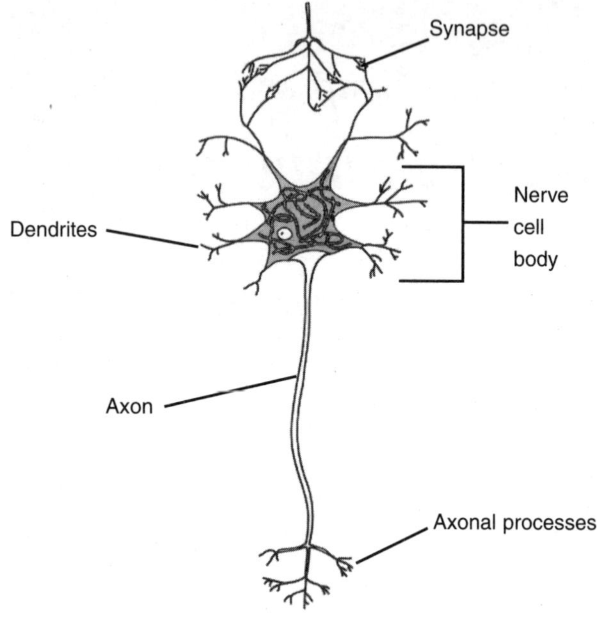

A peripheral nerve.

What Is a Neuropathy?

Basically the symptoms of your neuropathy can be divided into two groups, one of which occurs where your symptoms are spontaneous and another which involves maneuvers that can cause you to experience pain. Examples of the latter group are scratching your skin, putting pressure over the diseased nerves, or related to changes in temperature (usually cold).

Usually with the onset of your neuropathy you will feel a burning or stinging pain in the area of the affected nerve. Like neuralgias, you can also have shocklike stabbing pain. Neuralgia is "nerve pain" by definition. Sometimes the pain can radiate through your entire arm or leg. Sometimes a slight touch of the skin over your diseased nerve can cause incapacitating pain.

Your symptoms are usually individualized, which means that your symptoms may differ from other people's symptoms with the same nerve pathology. For example, if the nerve in your wrist, the median nerve, is compressed by tissue, you can develop a carpal tunnel syndrome. You may have numbness in the area of your wrist, whereas another person may complain of pain or numbness that radiates into his or her fingers. As a result, the treatment that works best for you may not work for other people with the same neuropathy.

Basically any neuropathy may cause a burning, gnawing pain. You can have some decreased sensation about the painful nerve. (T.N. Herington and L.H. Morse. *Occupational Injuries: Evaluation, Management, and Prevention.* St. Louis: Mosby, 1995) Extreme pain from just a light touch can occur in tissues over the nerve. You can have increased sweating, cold sensations, or skin discoloration in the extremity associated with your neuropathy. The onset of your pain following an injury to your nerve can either be of an immediate onset or a delayed gradual onset. Your pain intensity can be affected by both emotion and fatigue. Not all neuropathies cause pain. Some neuropathies cause only numbness.

If you go to your doctor with a neuropathy, take a detailed history of the onset of your pain and a detailed pain diary, which includes the frequency of your pain and the severity of your pain. You must also inform your health-care provider as to what methods of treatment worsen your pain and what methods improve your pain. Next your doctor will do a detailed neurological examination. You may have tests done by placing a needle into your nerves, called a nerve conduction velocity test, and an electromyography (EMG). (T.N. Herington and L.H. Morse. *Occupational Injuries: Evaluation, Management, and Prevention.* St. Louis: Mosby, 1995) Nerve conduction testing examines your nerve while the EMG examines any effects on your muscles with respect to muscle pathology. The needles used for these tests are attached to an oscilloscope and can measure the speed of the transmission of impulses in your nerves or muscles. These tests are extremely helpful to your doctor in diagnosing your pain syndrome.

Frequently a nerve biopsy is needed as well for your doctor to diagnose neuropathy. Mononeuropathies occur more often in diabetic patients than in the normal population. Diabetes can affect the muscles around your eye. A diabetic mononeuropathy can affect the nerves in your arms as well as your legs. A nerve lesion is a traumatic event to a nerve such as compression which can cause a neuropathy. If you have a peripheral nerve lesion, you will probably experience pain. The pain usually comes and goes.

You will usually have some degree of inflammation of the nerve that is affected by your neuropathy. The origin of your pain may be related to decreased blood flow to your nerve causing a decrease in the oxygenation of your nerve resulting in significant pain. Entrapment neuropathies such as the carpal tunnel syndrome are characterized by abnormal sensations in the area of the nerve as well as pain. Usually if your nerve is compressed, your blood supply to your nerve is also compromised. Entrapment neuropathies occur when a nerve is compressed. For example, tissue at your wrist can compress a nerve going to your hand and fingers which can result in weakness and pain in your hand. The basic pathology of an entrapment neuropathy is that the compression over your nerve can destroy your larger fibers that have a fatty wrapper around them called myelin. As these nerves are destroyed, it leaves only your C-fibers in the affected nerve. With the preservation of your C-fibers, you will have pain as well as tenderness at the location of your nerve entrapment.

You can have a neuropathy that is not painful but it can cause you to have abnormal feelings in the tissue around your injured nerve. You have probably heard of a Morton's neuralgia. This can cause a severe entrapment of the small nerves that are around the bones that make up the foot. If you destroy your large nerve fibers, you will have mainly the smaller C-fibers left in the diseased nerve. These C-fibers will cause you to have significant burning pain.

The exact causes of many neuropathies remain unknown, here are a few examples that are known:

- If you suffer from rheumatoid arthritis, you may suffer from a neuropathy related to your rheumatoid arthritis. A degeneration that can occur in your joints can also occur in your nerves. Some neuropathies cause you to have a loss of sensation instead of causing you to feel pain. An example of a neuropathy with a loss of sensation is called congenital analgesia with anhydrous. This means that you have some degree of numbness of an extremity but that the extremity never sweats.
- The drug Isonizid used for the treatment of tuberculosis can cause you to have pain in your nerves. You may develop a painful neuropathy related to chronic renal failure (kidney failure). This is one of the side effects of this drug. You feel some numbness but also some tingling and later significant pain that is both burning and aching. Muscles in your calves can also become painful. If you have this neuropathy, you may have difficulty walking. You may be awakened at night by the onset of spontaneous pain. On examination you will have a decreased sensation in your legs.

- Other types of drugs can also cause you to have a neuropathy. For example, arsenic has been implicated as a cause of neuropathy. In addition, people who suffer with the HIV or AIDS can have extremely debilitating neuropathies associated with their disease.
- Cancers can cause you to have a neuropathy. Your malignancy can cause you to have a progressive sensory neuropathy that usually is not painful. You may develop weakness or numbness in one or several of your nerves. If your cancer invades one of your nerves, you may develop pain that mimics reflex sympathetic dystrophy (RSD). RSD symptoms cause burning pain and swelling of your hand or foot.
- A neuropathy as a child can cause permanent anesthesia to an arm or leg. For example, if you have numbness in an area of your hand and you place your hand on a hot stove, you run the risk of a heat injury to your hand. If you have a loss of sensation in the area of one of your nerves, the tissue that does not feel sensation can be prone to future injury.
- If your thyroid glands do not produce enough thyroid hormone, you may develop pain related to a hypothyroid neuropathy. You may have pain or decreased or abnormal sensations in both your hands and feet.
- Compression of the nerves in your arms or legs for whatever reason can cause you to have pressure damage to these nerves. The neuropathy caused by this compression is called a *compression neuropathy*. Pressure over your nerve or nerves can come from a brace or cast or can come from tumors or muscle or connective tissue thickening. Compression of your nerves can occur at different points throughout your body. If you have neuropathies associated with disease states, your nerves can be more susceptible to injury with compression. You can have numbness as well as the pain in your extremities and can also have abnormal sensations. Nerve conduction studies are helpful in diagnosing neuropathies. Nerve conduction studies are done by inserting a needle into your tissue and studying the conduction of the nerve impulses. Electromyography (EMG) can also be used to evaluate a compression neuropathy. This task can determine if the neuropathy has affected your muscles.

- A *myeloma* can cause you to have pain in the distribution of one or more of your nerves. A myeloma is a malignant disease that affects your bone marrow.

The sections that follow detail some of the more common neuropathies.

Carpal Tunnel Syndrome

Carpal tunnel syndrome starts gradually with aching in your wrist that can extend to your forearm. You will develop pins and needles in your hand and fingers. This sensation can occur while you are driving, holding a phone, or reading this book. You may develop weakness in your hands and drop objects. Diagnosis of your carpal tunnel syndrome can be done by arthroscopy, which consists of putting a scope into your carpal tunnel. An MRI of your wrist and hand can be beneficial as well. You may ask whether laboratory tests can help diagnose carpal tunnel syndrome. At present, however, there are no tests that can be done to definitively diagnose this condition.

Do you think that the carpal tunnel syndrome is a condition of the new information technology age? Carpal tunnel syndrome is not new. (P.M. King. *Sourcebook of Occupational Rehabilitation*. New York: Plenum Press, 1998) It existed prior to the invention of computers. There is evidence of people suffering from carpal tunnel syndrome in the beginning of the twentieth century. The carpal tunnel is a narrow passage in your wrist about the diameter of your thumb. The purpose of this tunnel is to protect your median nerve as well as the tendons that go to your fingers. The problem is that excessive pressure on this nerve will cause you to have numbness and pain and can lead to hand weakness. With proper treatment, most people who develop carpal tunnel syndrome can have normal restoration of their hand function.

You may have heard that computer use predisposes you for carpal tunnel syndrome. An article published in the *Journal of the American Medical Association* (JAMA) in 2003 concluded that computer use is not a severe occupational hazard for developing symptoms of carpal tunnel syndrome. The real cause of your hand pain sometimes is misdiagnosed.

Repetitive-motion injuries are being reported at an increasing rate. This is reported from newsrooms to meat-packing plants to occupations where employees have to do repetitive motion daily. If you are taking birth control pills or have a sudden weight gain, which causes fluid retention, you may develop carpal tunnel syndrome.

Compression of the median nerve in the carpal tunnel is a common compression neuropathy. This entity affects women more than men. The average age of the onset of this ailment is between 40 and 60 years of age.

Your carpal tunnel is the space between your bones in your hand at your wrist and the connective tissue over your tendons. The carpal tunnel contains the tendons that flex your wrist (bend it downward) and your median nerve. A carpal tunnel syndrome can cause you to have pins and needles sensations and numbness in most of your hand except for the little finger. You can also have weakness of your thumb. This entity is caused by pressure on your median nerve as it passes through the carpal tunnel at your wrist. This condition can be caused by any continuous repetitive movement of your hand, such as typing or working with a computer. If you are obese, pregnant, have a decrease in your thyroid function, or have Raynaud's disease or diabetes or renal failure, you are at a higher risk of developing a carpal tunnel syndrome than the population in general.

If you have this syndrome, you will probably have abnormal sensations as well as pain in your affected hand while you sleep. The pins and needles sensations are usually on the palm side of your hand. You can also have wrist and forearm pain. The feeling of pins and needles as well as pain can be caused by repeated wrist and finger flexion. Remember that flexion is a downward position of your fingers as well as your hand. You may develop hand weakness. The symptoms begin in your dominant hand (the one that you use to write, to brush your teeth, comb your hair, etc.). However, your other hand can also be affected as well.

If you have carpal tunnel syndrome, your doctor will note that you have decreased sensation on the palm part of your thumb over to your ring finger. You can have shrinkage of the fleshy part of your hand at the base of your thumb. If your doctor taps over the middle of your wrist on your palm side, you may have the production of pins and needles that go from your wrist to your fingers. This is called Tinel's sign.

The Phalen test is another test to diagnose carpal tunnel syndrome. A blood pressure cuff is applied to your arm. If you have carpal tunnel syndrome, you will develop pins and needles in your hand when the blood pressure cuff is inflated.

Your doctor should examine underlying medical etioloies of carpal tunnel syndrome before determining that the carpal tunnel syndrome is related to your work activity. If you think that your work activity is causing your carpal tunnel syndrome, check with your state workmen's compensation board to see whether you are a candidate for workmen's compensation benefits. The eligibility for these benefits differ from state to state.

Repetitive motion has been downplayed as a cause of carpal tunnel syndrome. (T.N. Herington and L.H. Morse. *Occupational Injuries: Evaluation, Management, and Prevention*. St. Louis: Mosby, 1995) However, some jurisdictions allow repetitive motion as a cause of carpal tunnel syndrome. Fluid retention during menses or pregnancy is a cause of carpal tunnel syndrome.

Possible Treatment Options

It is important for you to know that carpal tunnel syndrome can be idiopathic. This means that the cause of your carpal tunnel syndrome is unknown. If you have carpal tunnel syndrome, you run a 1 percent chance that you will develop permanent injury. When you are initially seen by your health-care provider, you probably will be treated with immobilization of your wrist with a splint. This will prevent pressure on your nerve. If this method fails, you will be given an anti-inflammatory drug or an injection of Cortisone into your carpal tunnel to decrease the swelling in your tendons and ligaments within the tunnel. If this method fails, you will be a candidate for surgery.

Surgery to release the tissue that is compressing your median nerve has been shown to be effective for the treatment of carpal tunnel syndrome. There have even been cases of gout or arthritis causing carpal tunnel syndrome that have been successfully treated by surgery. You may ask whether you should have a surgical versus nonsurgical treatment for your carpal tunnel syndrome. A follow-up study of one year after surgery revealed excellent results with open carpal tunnel surgery. Surgical treatment appears to have better results than splinting.

You need to know that there could be some postoperative complications associated with carpal tunnel surgery. This can include increased pain in your scar, probably related to where the nerves in your skin come together during the healing process. You can also have recurrent symptoms of your pain and weakness of your grip. The exact causes of these problems remain unclear. This can happen whether or not your surgery is done through an open incision or by an endoscopic approach. During endoscopy your surgeon places a scope into your carpal tunnel space to be able to operate without having to make an incision. You may also develop reflex sympathetic dystrophy (RSD) for an unknown reason following carpal tunnel surgery.

Carpal tunnel syndrome is treated frequently in a primary care environment. Workplace task modification and wrist splints can defer a referral for surgical decompression. Nerve and tendon exercises can be of benefit. Steroid injections into the mouth of the carpal tunnel can be helpful in some patients, especially in women. If your doctor accidentally injects your median nerve, however, this can cause you disabling chronic pain.

If you have had surgery on your carpal tunnel syndrome and it recurs, there is a procedure using a polyester urethane patch for the prevention of recurrence of your carpal tunnel syndrome. The patch is currently being studied as a potential option if you have to have surgery again for a recurrence of your carpal tunnel syndrome. Research is being conducted on means of treating recurrent carpel tunnel and preventing RDS after surgery.

Treatment Realities

Only a small percentage of patients with carpel tunnel syndrome actually require surgery. (T.N. Herington and L.H. Morse. *Occupational Injuries: Evaluation, Management, and Prevention*. St. Louis: Mosby, 1995) Your chances of recovering completely following treatment are excellent. You should avoid re-injury by changing the way that you do repetitive movements. Research continues that is aimed at the prevention and rehabilitation of carpal tunnel syndrome. The incidence of an occupational carpal tunnel syndrome is usually a combination of genetics, your physiology, and your lifestyle factors in addition to general biomechanics. Therefore, no general rule of thumb applies to occupations in general.

You can find many different home remedies for the treatment of carpal tunnel syndrome. Before implementing these remedies and before avoiding conventional treatment, discuss alternative remedies with your doctor. Remember that the symptoms of carpal tunnel syndrome can progress. You do not want your nerve compressed for a significant period of time, because permanent injury could occur.

Carpal tunnel syndrome treatment can be expensive. The treatment can cost a company $37,000 on an average in lost work time, medical treatment, and rehabilitation for each employee who develops carpal tunnel syndrome. Because of the increased cost related to the potential workplace pain, the federal government has proposed standards that require employers to provide workspaces and equipment to support overall physical makeups to prevent from having any work-related injury. The Occupational Health and Safety Administration (OSHA) is continually doing research to see what can be done to prevent injuries in the workplace, including carpal tunnel syndrome.

Also be aware that your carpal tunnel syndrome can be due to a congenital predisposition. This means that your carpal tunnel is smaller than in other people. This can cause you to develop carpal tunnel syndrome, especially if you are doing repetitive-motion work or using vibrating hand tools. A smaller carpal tunnel noted in women may be the reason why they are three times more likely than men to develop carpal tunnel syndrome.

Preventing Carpal Tunnel Syndrome

You are probably now asking how you can prevent carpal tunnel syndrome. At work you should do on-the-job conditioning, which means performing stretching exercises and wearing splints to keep your wrists straight. Take frequent breaks. Use correct posture and wrist position. You can wear fingerless gloves to keep your hands warm and flexible. Your workstation, including tools and tool handles, as well as tasks can be designed to enable you to maintain a natural position during your job. If possible, jobs should be rotated with your fellow workers. However, even if all of these things are done, remember that workplace changes may not prevent the occurrence of your carpal tunnel syndrome.

Diabetic Neuropathy

Another type of neuropathy to be aware of, one which is fairly common, is a diabetic neuropathy. Diabetes can be associated with a polyneuropathy, which means that many nerves are involved in the disease process. If you develop polyneuropathy, it occurs usually on both sides of your body and usually in both lower extremities from the knees down to your feet. Numbness and abnormal sensations are the most frequent complaints associated with this neuropathy. You can have complaints of burning pain ranging from mild to severe in both legs. On occasion you may have symptoms of pains that are described as sharp, bolting, shocklike pain. Because diabetes can cause you to have a decrease in blood flow to your feet, make sure that you wear proper fitting shoes. Poor fitting shoes can cause ulcers on the bottom of your feet.

Sometimes both of your upper extremities can be involved with your diabetic neuropathy. The nerves in your extremities that have a myelin sheath around them will lose the sheath if you develop a diabetic neuropathy. If you have a diabetic neuropathy, you can have both pain as well as a decrease in sensation in your legs. It is interesting to note that if you have a painless diabetic neuropathy that you usually do not have reflexes in your lower extremities at your knees and ankles when your doctor taps you with a reflex hammer. However, if you have a painful diabetic neuropathy, usually your deep tendon reflexes are normal at your knee and ankle.

If you are diabetic and have an elevated blood sugar, for some reason this increased blood sugar can lower your pain threshold. This means that you will be more responsive to a certain pain stimulus than if you did not have a diabetic neuropathy. For example, if you do not have a diabetic neuropathy and prick yourself with a safety pin, your pain will be gone within a reasonable time. However, if you have a diabetic neuropathy, a simple pin prick can cause you to have significant pain because your pain threshold has been decreased. Furthermore, if you have a diabetic neuropathy with an increase in your blood sugar, your tolerance to pain will be decreased. It has furthermore been published in animal studies that an elevated blood sugar will reduce the analgesic effects of morphine in the animal model. In other words, glucose can affect your morphine pain receptors. If you have a diabetic neuropathy, you can have a decrease in tissue blood flow in your legs.

Your sympathetic nervous system can also be altered if you suffer from a diabetic neuropathy. In many instances, your sympathetic stimulation can be decreased. You can have a high blood flow in both extremities. However, this blood flow can be decreased by an increase in the activity of your sympathetic nervous system. Blood flow to certain areas of your body can be decreased by sympathetic stimulation of your sympathetic nervous system if you have a painful neuropathy. This reduction in blood flow usually results in an improvement of your pain if your pain was caused by swelling of your tissue related to an increased blood flow to your tissue. Blood flow effect in a non-painful diabetic neuropathy has just the opposite effect.

Be aware that diabetes can cause multiple nerve disorders in the nerves outside of your brain and spinal cord. However, some of the nerves coming off of your brain can transmit pain fibers and your diabetes can also adversely affect these nerves. Not only can you develop pain in your legs, you can also develop weakness in your legs as a result of your diabetic neuropathy.

Diabetic neuropathy can be potentially very disabling. You may start with a mild numbness or tingling in your legs or feet, and this will progress to a burning sensation in your feet. You may not have pain initially when the disease occurs. It may take months or years to develop your pain. Eventually the skin over your feet and ankles will become hypersensitive to touch. On the other hand, you can have loss of sensitivity of your feet. This is the reason why if you have a diabetic neuropathy that you can sustain a significant injury to your foot. Furthermore, diabetes decreases your body's ability to heal itself. For example, if you do have ulcers of your foot and so forth, you can have an impaired healing process of your involved nerves.

On occasion some individuals with a diabetic neuropathy can have constant pain. The type of diabetic neuropathy is the diabetic amyotrophy. This entity occurs on one side of your body. It occurs most often in the nerves that go to your muscles. The nerves that go to your muscles are called motor nerves. The diabetic amyotrophy is a motor neuropathy. The diabetic amyotrophy neuropathy, as well as other diabetic neuropathies, can be seen if you have poor control over your diabetes. Diabetic neuropathies are found in middle-aged as well as elderly patients who suffer with diabetes. Careful attention to control over blood sugar in the long term is the best way to prevent diabetic neuropathy.

The treatment of painful diabetic neuropathy has included anticonvulsive medications such as Tegretol. Neurontin has become more popular over the past several years. Tricyclic antidepressant drugs such as Elavil can help to relieve your pain. A drug that has been used successfully for the treatment of a painful diabetic neuropathy is mexiletine. This drug is essentially a medication that is used if you have abnormal heartbeats. This drug has been shown to be effective for the treatment of your diabetic neuropathy. You can anticipate a positive reaction to oral mexiletine if you are given intravenous Lidocaine. Lidocaine is not only a numbing medicine but it is also a drug used for irregular rhythms of your heart. If you have significant pain relief with the administration of mexiletine administered intravenously the chances are that you will have excellent relief with the oral mexiletine. The problem with mexiletene is that you can get side effects such as nausea and vomiting. Tremors, dizziness, and blurred vision can also occur. If you have any heart problems that you know of, you must tell your doctor before starting mexiletine.

Another medication that can help you control your painful diabetic neuropathy is a topical capsaicin cream. Almost 75 percent of patients with diabetic neuropathy who used this cream reported significant pain relief. The problem with this cream is that you can have side effects that include a burning sensation at the sight of the cream on application. If you take a warm bath or shower, the pain about your skin can be magnified.

Alcoholic Neuropathy

Do you know someone who consumes a significant amount of alcohol? Alcoholic neuropathy is fairly common in the United States. Approximately 20 percent of chronic alcoholics develop peripheral neuropathy related to their alcoholism. (J.D. Loeser. *Bonica's Management of Pain*. n.p.: Lippincott Williams and Wilkins, 2001) The neuropathy affects not only sensation but can affect strength in your lower extremities. Alcoholics who develop this neuropathy complain of burning feet. As the neuropathy becomes more severe, the alcoholic will develop weakness in both legs. Occasionally the arms can be affected as well. One important treatment for this neuropathy is to stop drinking. When alcohol consumption has been abolished, the neuropathy can recover, but the recovery is slow. The alcoholic neuropathy is believed to be due to a deficiency of thiamine as well as other B vitamins. Alcoholics usually have an inadequate food intake. The alcohol can affect the absorption of vitamins through their gastrointestinal systems.

Alcoholics have a greater need for thiamine but are not obtaining the thiamine in their diet. (J.D. Loeser. *Bonica's Management of Pain*. n.p.: Lippincott Williams and Wilkins, 2001) It is furthermore known that alcohol itself can exert a direct toxic effect on nerves in the arms and legs. Besides stopping alcohol consumption, alcoholics should take nutritional supplements containing both thiamine and a vitamin B complex. Tegretol or Neurontin or a tricyclic antidepressant such as Elavil can also be used for the treatment of this disease.

Uremic Neuropathy

If you or someone you know has kidney failure, a severe neuropathy can occur that is called a uremic neuropathy. This type of neuropathy is associated with chronic renal failure. Uremia is the presence of an excessive amount of urea as well as other nitrogen waste compounds that are in your bloodstream. Normally these waste products are excreted by your kidneys into your urine. However, if you have kidney failure, your urea is not eliminated from your bloodstream. This will cause your urea to accumulate in your blood. This will cause you to have drowsiness as well as nausea and vomiting and can progress to death.

If you have uremia, you have a 50 percent chance that you can develop a uremic neuropathy. (J.D. Loeser. *Bonica's Management of Pain*. n.p.: Lippincott Williams and Wilkins, 2001) This disease is becoming less prevalent because of the treatment of kidney failure with hemodialysis as well as kidney transplants. This disease progresses slowly. At first it affects your sensory nerves. It can progress to cause weakness in the muscles about your feet. You can have cramps in your calves. With dialysis, this disease will stabilize. It can even improve with dialysis. If this disorder worsens during dialysis, the frequency and duration of your dialysis will be increased until your symptoms improve. After renal transplant, you can expect to have a significant improvement in your renal neuropathy.

Nutritional Neuropathy

As previously mentioned, thiamine deficiency as seen in alcoholics can cause neuropathies. This is another class of neuropathy called nutritional neuropathy. This class of neuropathy is seen not only in alcoholics but in individuals who are on restrictive diets.

Thiamine deficiency can lead to heart failure. With this nutritional neuropathy, you may have hand, feet, and calf pain. You can have extreme pain just from light touch. You may have some numbness and weakness in your extremities. The administration of thiamine can reduce your symptoms. Severe nutritional deficiency can cause you to develop significant pain related to your nutritional neuropathy. If you don't get enough thiamine, you can develop beriberi. This is a result of a deficiency of vitamin B1 (thiamine).

Beriberi is another nutritional neuropathy that is widespread in rice-eating countries. It is noted in individuals who eat polished rice from which the thiamine-rich seed coat is removed. Two types of beriberi exist. One form is called wet beriberi. In this type of beriberi, there is an accumulation of tissue fluid in your body. With dry beriberi, there are signs of starvation. If you starve yourself, you will become too thin. The nervous system can degenerate if you are not obtaining a proper amount of thiamine. Also, nutritional deficiencies in a woman at the time of conception can cause abnormalities in a fetus, which can cause significant harm.

Pellegra is another neuropathy caused by nutritional deficiency. It is characterized by weakness, tingling, and even pain. This neuropathy is caused by niacin deficiency. Niacin is also a B vitamin. Pellegra is a result of a poor diet that does not have enough niacin or doesn't have sufficient tryptophane. Tryptophane is an amino acid from which niacin can be synthesized in your body. Pellegra is more common in corn-eating communities.

Chemical Neuropathy

Chemicals can also cause you to develop a neuropathy. (T.N. Herington and L.H. Morse. *Occupational Injuries: Evaluation, Management, and Prevention*. St. Louis: Mosby, 1995) Cisplatin is an agent used in chemotherapy to treat tumors. This chemical can cause you to develop a painful peripheral neuropathy as well. The neuropathy associated with this drug can cause you to have severe pain in your extremities. However, this neuropathy is reversible at the end of your chemotherapy. Arsenic is another chemical associated with a painful neuropathy. It can also cause you to have renal failure. Arsenic can be toxic to your heart and can cause your heart to stop. It takes one to two weeks for you to develop a neuropathy associated with arsenic ingestion. You will have burning pain as well as tingling and numbness in your extremities associated with this neuropathy. If you have a severe neuropathy from arsenic poisoning, you may not have a good prognosis on your recovery.

Thallium is an insecticide as well as a rodentcide (kills rats and mice). It can also be used to image your heart by your cardiologist when examining you for heart disease. If you suffer from thallium poisoning, you will now develop the pain in your gut including nausea and vomiting. Your symptoms can progress through a stoppage of your heart. You can develop a psychosis as well as confusion, which can lead to a coma. You can develop a neuropathy within 48 hours of adjusting to this chemical. You can develop pain in both your arms and legs. In severe cases, the nerves coming off of your brain can be affected as well. This chemical can affect your nerves that are involved in your breathing. If you recover from this poisoning, your recovery may never be complete. One of the hallmarks of this disease is loss of hair.

Treatment for Peripheral Neuropathies

Each type of neuropathy requires a different type of treatment. Specific treatments are outlined in each section that describes the different neuropathies.

For Men

- For carpal tunnel syndrome, workplace task modification and wrist splints are helpful.
- For carpal tunnel syndrome, perform nerve and tendon exercises.
- Steroid injections into the mouth of the carpal tunnel can help relieve pain.
- Diabetic neuropathy pain control includes anticonvulsive medications such as Tegretol and Neurontin.
- Tricyclic antidepressant drugs such as Elavil are helpful in controlling diabetic neuropathy pain.

For Women

- For carpal tunnel syndrome, workplace task modification and wrist splints are helpful.
- For carpal tunnel syndrome, perform nerve and tendon exercises.
- Steroid injections into the mouth of the carpal tunnel can help relieve pain.
- Diabetic neuropathy pain control includes anticonvulsive medications such as Tegretol and Neurontin.
- Tricyclic antidepressant drugs such as Elavil are helpful in controlling diabetic neuropathy pain.

Chapter 18
Understanding Osteoporosis

Osteoporosis is the most common type of bone disease that is related to the breakdown of substances that exist in your bones. If you suffer from osteoporosis, you will have a progressive reduction in your bone minerals as well as the structural components of your bones, but the normal composition of bone is preserved.

Osteoporosis affects 20 million Americans and results in more than 1.3 million bone fractures in the United States every year. In a lifetime, women lose more than half of their spongy bone, which comprises the center of bones, and approximately 30 percent of the nonspongy (compact) bone, which composes the outer aspect of bones. (T.E. Andreolli, et al. *Cecil Essentials of Medicine*. n.p.: W.B. Saunders, 2000)

Osteoporosis can be a significant bone disease because it is potentially disabling. Approximately 30 percent of all postmenopausal Caucasian women will suffer from fractures related to osteoporosis. More than one third of all women and one sixth of all men over 65 years of age will sustain a hip fracture. (T.E. Andreolli, et al. *Cecil Essentials of Medicine*. n.p.: W.B. Saunders, 2000)

This is a frightening statistic because hip fracture complications can be fatal. It is estimated that the annual cost of health care for those with osteoporosis in lost national productivity as well as medical costs exceeds $10 billion in the United States alone.

This chapter reveals the seriousness of osteoporosis and the possible devastation if left untreated. Remember that osteoporosis is a silent disease that can often be prevented. If you suspect that you may be a candidate for this disease, discuss your concerns with your doctor.

What Is Osteoporosis?

During your lifetime, bone is constantly being made and is constantly being lost. In normal circumstances, the production and reduction of your bone is balanced. Osteoporosis can result if you do not make enough bone or if you have an accelerated decrease in your bone minerals and the matrix structure (the components of your bone which make your bones hard) of your bone or both.

Bone Density

Your bone density increases significantly during puberty. This increase in bone density is the result of your response to sex steroids. Sex steroids increase your bone density. When you are a young adult, your bone density is twice what it is when you were a child. If you have had a delay in the onset of puberty, you may have a decrease in your bone density. (T.E. Andreolli, et al. *Cecil Essentials of Medicine*. n.p.: W.B. Saunders, 2000)

Factors that can affect your bone mass include exercise or lack of exercise, calcium intake, growth hormones, sex hormones, genetics, race, and gender. If you have a relative who has a history of osteoporosis, tell your primary-care doctor. Genetics play an important role in the development of osteoporosis. Studies have demonstrated that bone density is lower in the daughters of women who have osteoporosis than in those women who do not have osteoporosis.

Bone density tests in identical twins have been done indicating that genetics is an important factor in the development of osteoporosis. (W.H. Kirkaldy-Willis, et al. *Managing Low Back Pain*. New York: Churchill Livingstone, 1992) These studies have suggested that most of the genetic differences in bone density are the result of a gene that is linked to your vitamin D receptor gene. Further study has revealed that variations of the vitamin D receptor gene result in differences in bone density changes of 10 percent to 12 percent in osteoporosis-prone individuals. Further study is being done on the effect of the vitamin D receptor gene and the severity of osteoporosis in both men and women.

Men in general have been shown to have higher bone densities than women. Furthermore, African American men have higher bone density than Caucasian men. (T.E. Andreolli, et al. *Cecil Essentials of Medicine*. n.p.: W.B. Saunders, 2000) The same is true with African American and Caucasian women. Even though osteoporosis is a disease that mostly affects women, osteoporosis can be seen in a small percentage of men.

If you are a woman and if you have had a delay in the onset of your menstrual periods by several years, you may be susceptible to osteoporosis. A woman's first menstruation occurs when her reproductive organs become active and can take place at any time between the ages of 10 and 18. Studies have revealed that calcium supplementation can enhance prepuberty bone accumulation. An increase in physical activity can also increase bone density around the time of puberty. (T.E. Andreolli, et al. *Cecil Essentials of Medicine*. n.p.: W.B. Saunders, 2000)

Your bone density will continue to increase throughout your life until you reach an age where your bone density becomes stable. When you approach 40, your bone density can begin to decline. Bone density decreases are noted in women before menopause. In men, a decrease in their bone density occurs somewhere between 20 to 40 years of age. In women, after menopause has occurred, the rate of bone loss accelerates. During the first 10 years of menopause, the women's spongy bone is lost faster than the outer bone.

Bone Fractures

Osteoporosis is usually without symptoms until a fracture occurs. (W.H. Kirkaldy-Willis, et al. *Managing Low Back Pain*. New York: Churchill Livingstone, 1992) Usually the fracture is in one of the bones of the back. However, your wrists, hips, ribs, pelvic bone, and your leg bones can sustain fractures. The bones in your spine can have a loss of height, which is called a compression fracture.

If you have osteoporosis, you can sustain a fracture in one of the bones in your back with minimal stress. It usually takes significant stress to fracture a normal bone. Even bending over to pick up an object off the floor can cause a compression fracture. You will most likely notice the immediate onset of pain in your mid- or lower back at the time of the compression fracture. Usually your pain decreases over several weeks. If you have multiple fractures in your back, your pain may become chronic. Usually your back pain is worse with standing vertically. The increased weight on the bones in your back will cause you to have pain. Lying down will decrease your spine pain. (W.H. Kirkaldy-Willis, et al. *Managing Low Back Pain*. New York: Churchill Livingstone, 1992)

You will also lose height as the bones in your back compress. If you fall, you may sustain a hip fracture. Hip fractures are dangerous for elderly patients. Usually a hip fracture will cause you to need hospitalization. On occasion your total hip has to be replaced surgically. If you are elderly, you may need nursing home care following a hip replacement. Medical complications, such as pulmonary embolus, that can be associated with hip surgery in elderly patients can be fatal.

Causes of Osteoporosis

If you have osteoporosis, your bones become more porous. This means that the bones in your body develop holes, which in turn weaken the structure of your bones. All of your bones can be affected, and each of your bones can be at an increased risk for a fracture. If you have a low calcium intake and are not physically active, you are also at risk of developing osteoporosis.

There is a type of osteoporosis that is called idiopathic osteoporosis. The cause of this type of osteoporosis is unknown, but it does affect middle-aged men and premenopausal women. Did you know that being weightless in space can contribute to the onset of osteoporosis? Individuals who suffer from anorexia nervosa also develop osteoporosis.

There are other causes of osteoporosis besides the ones just mentioned. Hyperthyroidism and hyperparathyroidism in addition to your body's overproduction of cortisone (a steroid) are causes of osteoporosis. As previously mentioned, if you have a decrease in your growth hormone, you are prone to develop osteoporosis.

It is important for your body to absorb calcium through your gastrointestinal system. If you have a history of a gastrectomy (removal of a portion of your stomach), cirrhosis of the liver, or any other gastrointestinal malabsorption syndrome, you are more prone to develop osteoporosis. If you have a history of multiple myeloma or leukemia, you may develop osteoporosis. The exact cause of this finding is presently unknown.

If you have been immobilized for any reason, you may develop osteoporosis. If you are unable to walk or exercise for whatever reason due to your immobilization, you may develop osteoporosis. Alcohol can contribute to your development of osteoporosis. Chemotherapy can also cause osteoporosis. Steroid use has been implicated in the development of osteoporosis.

Other diseases have a link to osteoporosis. An autoimmune disease is a disorder in which your body attacks its own tissue. Your joints can become damaged by your own antibodies. Systemic lupus erythematous is an autoimmune disease commonly known as lupus. If you have lupus, you will become fatigued and have painful joints in addition to developing skin rashes. Ninety percent of individuals diagnosed with lupus are women. (W.H. Kirkaldy-Willis, et al. *Managing Low Back Pain.* New York: Churchill Livingstone, 1992) If you have lupus, you are at an increased risk for developing osteoporosis. Steroids are prescribed for the treatment of lupus. However, remember that steroids can trigger osteoporosis. The fatigue caused by lupus results in a decrease in exercise and activity. These factors increase your risk of developing osteoporosis. Furthermore, the disease itself can decrease your bone mass.

Individuals who are HIV positive can also develop osteoporosis. The reason for the increase in osteoporosis in patients with HIV infection is not known. It is possible that the virus may infect the cells that produce bone.

In addition to Caucasian women being more prone to developing osteoporosis, Asian American women are also at a high risk for developing osteoporosis. African American and Hispanic women are at a lower risk for developing osteoporosis. The reason for the effect of race on the development of osteoporosis remains to be seen.

Testing and Diagnosing for Osteoporosis

A diagnosis of osteoporosis can be made by a plain x-ray. If you have a vertebral bone compression in your mid-back, for example, there will usually be a decrease in the height of your affected (compressed) bone that can be seen on x-ray. Sometimes a bone scan is needed to diagnosis osteoporosis. If you have a bone scan, a doctor will inject a radioactive material into your vein. You will have a picture of your body taken by a special camera. Compression fractures, which were not diagnosed by other means, can be detected on a bone scan.

Osteoporosis can also be diagnosed by measuring your bone mineral density. Your bone density value will be compared to a normal value that is noted for young adults of your same sex. A bone density test can predict the probability of you developing a fracture related to your bone density value.

Quantitative computed tomography can also be used and is effective for diagnosing osteoporosis because it will not only measure your bone mineral density, this test can also measure the density of your spongy bone within your back and hip bones. However, this test is expensive and will expose you to radiation. Different types of tests are being used and being developed to diagnosis osteoporosis. Bone scanning can be useful for the diagnosis of compression fractures. If you have a decreased bone density, your doctor should attempt to determine the cause of your osteoporosis.

Sometimes your doctor needs to obtain blood from you for further testing. Your doctor may take some blood from you to be sent to a lab to measure the calcium, organic phosphate, and alkaline phosphatase in your bloodstream. These minerals are usually normal if you have osteoporosis. However, your alkaline phosphate may be higher if you have a fracture.

Hormones Associated with Osteoporosis

Not all fractures associated with osteoporosis are painful. You may have a fracture and not know it. Your doctor will probably measure the level of your parathyroid hormone in your blood if you develop nonpainful bone fractures, which are not associated with bone trauma such as a fall. This is important because an elevation of parathyroid hormone can decrease your bone mass. Because a decrease in testosterone may be associated with osteoporosis in men, male patients should have their testosterone blood levels measured when they have their yearly physical examinations.

Preventing Osteoporosis

Bone density testing is important early in the development of osteoporosis because there is no cure for osteoporosis. In other words, there is no way to reverse osteoporosis after it has become established. However, early treatment can prevent the progression of osteoporosis.

If it has been determined that alcohol is a cause of your osteoporosis, you must stop consuming alcohol. If your thyroid levels are elevated, this disease should be treated early to decrease the progression of your osteoporosis. Physical therapy and mild aerobic exercise may be important in slowing down the early development of osteoporosis. If you have a compression fracture of one of your bones in your spine, a back brace can provide you with pain relief. Your physical therapist may want to strengthen your stomach muscles as well as the muscles in your back.

Talking About Osteoporosis with Your Doctor

Not only should you be educated in the diagnosis and treatment of osteoporosis, your doctor may also need education in the diagnosis and treatment of this disease. A study published in an orthopedic surgeon journal reported that orthopedic surgeons are frequently the first health-care providers to evaluate patients with fractures. (T.E. Andreolli, et al. *Cecil Essentials of Medicine*. n.p.: W.B. Saunders, 2000)

This study reported that orthopedic surgeons, however, have been slow to develop an awareness for identifying individuals who have osteoporosis who could benefit from drug therapies. Only 50 percent of patients who have a history of a hip fracture were referred for bone density testing.

Furthermore, a Canadian survey done in 1998 revealed that orthopedic surgeons had little interest in evaluating and treating osteoporosis in patients who had fractures. Doctors need to realize that a patient who sustained a hip fracture is identified as an individual who has a high probability of developing osteoporosis. This individual is at a high risk for having a future bone fracture. If you have had a hip fracture, you are a probable candidate for bone density testing. Communication between a patient's orthopedic surgeon and primary-care doctor is essential. This communication could facilitate the diagnosis of decreased bone density in individuals who have suffered hip fractures.

Compression Fractures

Cortical bone is a compact form of bone that makes up the outer shell of your bones. It consists of a hard, solid mass made up of bony tissue that is arranged in concentric layers. This is similar to the layers noted in a tree. Your compact bone will surround your spongy bone. Bone is composed of collagen fibers that contain bone salts, which are mainly calcium carbonate salts as well as calcium phosphate salts. As previously stated, during the first 5 to 10 years of menopause, women can lose 10 to 15 percent of their compact bone and 25 percent of your spongy bone. It is important for you to know that this bone loss can be prevented by estrogen-replacement therapy. However, estrogen therapy can be associated with an increased risk of a stroke and heart disease.

The amount of bone loss varies among women, which has led medical investigators to derive a classification of osteoporosis. If your osteoporosis is more severe than is expected for your age, you have type I postmenopausal osteoporosis. If you have type I osteoporosis, you are at a higher risk to have compression or crush fractures of the bones in your spine. You may also be prone to a fracture at the bone above your wrist on the side of your thumb. This type of fracture is called a Colles fracture. If your bones are weak and fragile, you can easily sustain a bone fracture. These types of fractures are related to bone density loss. If you have a decrease in your estrogen, you may have the production of chemicals that may decrease your bone mass.

An initially rapid rate of bone loss in the postmenopausal period is followed by a slower loss of bone throughout the rest of life. Your loss of bone mass does result from normal aging and occurs in both men and women. This type of bone loss is called type II osteoporosis. Fractures can occur in type II osteoporosis as well as in type I osteoporosis. Fractures can occur in your hip, pelvis, wrist, the bones in your legs, and the bones in your back.

Sometimes type II osteoporosis is associated with a defect in the absorption of calcium through the gastrointestinal system.

As you age, your calcium absorption through your stomach and intestine can decrease. A decreased absorption of this important substance will decrease the amount of calcium in your bloodstream.

Hormones and Bone Density

In your body you have various chemicals stimulated by growth factor. Growth factor tells your body to make new cells and to maintain the cells that are already present in your body. These chemicals sit on the outer surface of your cells. Growth factor is needed in wound healing if you have had an injury to one of your tissues (bone, muscle, nerve). Estrogen, a female sex hormone, increases the production of this growth factor. Be aware that growth factor stimulates bone formation. (R.B. Fillingham. *Sex, Gender, and Pain*. n.p.: IASP Press, 2000) If you have a decrease in estrogen, you can diminish your formation of bone. As a result, a decrease in estrogen will decrease your ability to form bone.

In your body you have two parathyroid glands. These glands are around your thyroid gland at the base of your neck above your breastbone (your sternum). Your parathyroid glands stimulate the production of parathyroid hormone, which is produced if you have a decrease in calcium in your bloodstream. Parathyroid glands produce parathyroid hormone. This hormone produced by your parathyroid gland is released into your bloodstream. The parathyroid hormone controls the distribution of both calcium and phosphate throughout your body.

A high level of parathyroid hormone will cause transfer of calcium from your bones to your bloodstream. If your parathyroid hormone level decreases in your bloodstream, it will lower your blood calcium level. If you have a decrease in your estrogen hormone, you will have a decrease in your blood calcium levels as well. If your estrogen goes down, your bone sensitivity to the transfer of calcium from your bones to your bloodstream is increased. Therefore, you will lose your bone density as your blood level of estrogen decreases. If your calcium in your bloodstream increases, you will decrease your parathyroid hormone secretion. Estrogen deficiency can decrease your bone matrix formation in your body. You should now be aware that sex hormones play an important role in the maintenance of your bone structure. You should now realize that when your sex hormones decrease as you age, this decreased hormone level could adversely affect your skeletal system.

Osteoporosis in Men

Osteoporosis occurs more often in women than in men. However, it is also seen in men. It is estimated that more than 2 million men in the United States suffer from osteoporosis. Approximately 20 percent of all hip fractures in the United States occur in men. Compression fractures in the bones of the spine can occur in men as well. Bone fractures related to osteoporosis accounted for $2.7 billion, which is one fifth of the total cost of osteoporotic fractures, in the United States in 1994. This observation demonstrated that osteoporosis is not solely a "woman's disease." Osteoporosis develops less often in men than in women because men have more bone mass and larger skeletons. Therefore, the bone loss in men starts later and progresses more slowly.

The development of osteoporosis in men has been recently recognized as an important public health issue. Men suffering from osteoporosis are a long-neglected group of individuals. The National Institutes of Health are currently studying osteoporosis in men. The results of this study should help doctors understand how to prevent and treat osteoporosis in men. Remember that when bone is lost, it cannot be replaced. Middle-aged and elderly men should have their testosterone levels measured periodically. As previously stated, a reduced level of testosterone in men can cause osteoporosis. Thirty percent of men with osteoporotic fractures of the bones in their spine have low testosterone levels. Testosterone therapy may slow the development of osteoporosis in men. The research has shown that a decrease in estrogen in men can be a cause of osteoporosis. (T.E. Andreolli, et al. *Cecil Essentials of Medicine*. n.p.: W.B. Saunders, 2000) Be aware of the fact that men also have estrogen secreted in their bodies.

Prevention of Osteoporosis

The prevention and treatment of osteoporosis includes synthetic estrogen or progesterone therapy if you are postmenopausal. However, you must take calcium in addition to the hormone therapy. A synthetic estrogen called raloxifene has been approved for the treatment of osteoporosis. This drug will increase your bone density. It has fewer side effects than other types of estrogen drugs.

Postmenopausal women who exercise for 60 minutes 3 times a week and take calcium supplements can stop bone loss. It is recommended that individuals over 50 use calcium supplements. If you do not want to use a calcium supplement, calcium-rich foods such as milk, yogurt, and cooked dry beans will provide you with calcium. Furthermore, some cheeses can increase the calcium in your bloodstream. Most individuals have trouble getting enough calcium in their diet and end up needing calcium supplements.

Remember that vitamin D is also an important vitamin that is necessary for strong bones. (B. Riggs and L. Melton. "The Prevention and Treatment of Osteoporosis," *New England Journal of Medicine* 327 [1992]: 620-627)

If you are not out in the sun, you should drink vitamin D-fortified milk or eat vitamin D-fortified foods. Remember that vitamin D is important because it helps your body to absorb calcium. Vitamin D can help you increase your calcium absorption through your gastrointestinal tract by up to 65 percent.

Be aware that drugs used to treat asthma can increase your risk of fractures if you are prone to osteoporosis. Inhaled steroids can be used for the treatment of asthma. This drug increases your risk of sustaining a bone fracture. Steroids are used not only for the treatment of asthma but also for the treatment of rheumatoid arthritis and some bowel disease. (B. Riggs and L. Melton. "The Prevention and Treatment of Osteoporosis," *New England Journal of Medicine* 327 [1992]: 620-627)

If you are taking steroids for longer than three months, you may need to discuss this with your doctor and you and your doctor should consider a prescription for Fosamax, which is used to treat osteoporosis.

Smoking also increases bone loss. Hip and spinal bone fractures are higher in men and women who smoke. Research is being done to determine how nicotine damages bone. Preliminary investigations reveal that nicotine can inhibit absorption of calcium that is needed for bone health. Just like women, men need to take calcium. Men can inherit osteoporosis from their fathers. Caucasian men are at a higher risk of developing osteoporosis than other races. Osteoporosis in men can be diagnosis by a bone mass measurement. This is a special type of x-ray that emits a trace amount of radiation. Middle-aged men who have complaints of back or hip pain may be candidates for a bone mass measurement as well as a measurement of the testosterone in their bloodstream.

Research has demonstrated that there is gender bias with respect to men who have suffered hip fractures. Doctors in the past have felt osteoporosis was a woman's disease. We now realize that osteoporosis affects both women and men. Medications to prevent bone loss are for the most part ignored for middle-aged and older men who have sustained hip fractures. Hip fracture complications are a cause of death in approximately 17 percent of women and 6 percent of men in the United States. By the age of 70, bone loss is equal in both men and women. As previously stated, the absorption of calcium from your gastrointestinal system decreases with age. (T.E. Andreolli, et al. *Cecil Essentials of Medicine*. n.p.: W.B. Saunders, 2000) (B. Riggs and L. Melton. "The Prevention and Treatment of Osteoporosis," *New England Journal of Medicine* 327 [1992]: 620-627)

The United States recommended dietary allowance of calcium is up to 1,000 milligrams per day. Calcium can slow your osteoporosis but cannot completely stop it. An increase in calcium in your bloodstream may not protect you from compression fractures of the bones in your spine. Calcium therapy can help you if you are a woman and postmenopausal. Some endocrinologists have recommended that if you are postmenopausal that you should consume 1,500 milligrams per day of calcium.

As stated earlier in this chapter, sex steroids are important for the maintenance of proper bone density. Oral estrogen as well as estrogen in the form of a patch worn on the skin can prevent bone loss if you are estrogen deficient. Bone loss is rapid in the first years of menopause, so estrogen therapy is of great benefit if it is administered before you begin to lose a significant amount of bone mass. Studies have demonstrated that estrogen therapy decreases the risk of bone fractures in postmenopausal women. It is recommended that if you are taking estrogen supplements that you also take calcium supplements.

Estrogen supplements are not without side effects. If estrogen is not administered along with progestin, you run the risk of cancer. Estrogen replacement can be related to breast cancer as well as heart disease. These studies with respect to cancer are controversial, however. Other studies have noted that estrogen therapy can decrease the chance of you having a heart attack by up to 50 percent.

However, routine use of estrogens is not recommended by most physicians because of potential side effects. Consult your doctor about the risks and benefits of estrogen therapy and make your own decision before using estrogen therapy.

Calcitonin is another drug that you could take to prevent bone loss in your vertebral bodies throughout your spine. Calcitonin is most effective in early and late menopause. (T.E. Andreolli, et al. *Cecil Essentials of Medicine*. n.p.: W.B. Saunders, 2000) (B. Riggs and L. Melton. "The Prevention and Treatment of Osteoporosis," *New England Journal of Medicine* 327 [1992]: 620-627) Calcitonin is available for intranasal use. Calcitonin has been shown to produce pain-relieving effects. Calcitonin is most useful if you have a history of osteoporosis and have chronic pain due to fractures related to your osteoporosis.

Elderly individuals appear to be prone to vitamin D deficiency. Decreased vitamin D and decreased calcium in elderly patients' bloodstreams can lead to accelerated bone loss. It has been shown that vitamin D plus calcium can reduce the incidence of fractures in elderly women.

Current Research on Osteoporosis

Studies have been done that suggest eating foods rich in soy protein helps protect older women from bone loss. However, a new study reveals that this is not true for young women. Women in their 20s who ate diets that were high in soy protein did not demonstrate any improvement in their bone density. Some compounds found in soy are chemically similar to human estrogens. Some studies suggest that eating a soy diet can slow bone loss in postmenopausal women. A new form of vitamin D supplements can help women regain some bone mass loss due to osteoporosis. This new vitamin D supplement is more potent than previous vitamin D supplements. This new compound is called 2MD. It promotes the growth of cells that are responsible for making bone. Current studies that are being done in animals are prominent. This new form of vitamin D may become an important alternative to hormone therapy. However, 2MD has not been tested in humans.

Falls can cause significant injury to your hips or the bones in your legs if you have osteoporosis. A recent study has demonstrated that vibrating shoe insoles can help elderly individuals improve their balance and prevent falls because the soles increase awareness as to where the feet are positioned. The rationale for this device is that the nervous system in elderly individuals, both women and men, decreases touch and position sense. Touch and position sense are needed to maintain balance. (B. Riggs and L. Melton. "The Prevention and Treatment of Osteoporosis," *New England Journal of Medicine* 327 [1992]: 620-627)

It is thought that if you can stimulate the nervous system in the soles of the feet, improvement will be seen in the balance and posture control of elderly individuals. Improvement in the balance of elderly individuals is extremely important because bone fractures can be potentially lethal for them.

Recent research has revealed that one in five elderly individuals who have suffered a hip or wrist fracture because of osteoporosis received the treatment that they need to prevent future fractures of their bones. (T.E. Andreolli, et al. *Cecil Essentials of Medicine*. n.p.: W.B. Saunders, 2000)

Only 22 percent of elderly women and elderly men received a prescription drug for one of the drugs used to treat osteoporosis. It is important that elderly individuals who have sustained a fracture receive osteoporosis treatment medications because they are five times more likely to suffer another fracture. By using osteoporosis drugs, they can reduce the risk of a future fracture by as much as 60 percent. (B. Riggs and L. Melton. "The Prevention and Treatment of Osteoporosis," *New England Journal of Medicine* 327 [1992]: 620-627)

Be aware that more than 550,000 hip and wrist fractures occur in elderly individuals suffering from osteoporosis every year. An initial fracture in an elderly individual should signal a red flag to a doctor that this individual probably has osteoporosis and needs prescription medications.

An experimental drug is currently under development for the treatment of osteoporosis. This drug is to be used in women suffering from osteoporosis. An injection of this drug is administered every three months. This new drug that is being tested in preliminary studies has been shown to prevent osteoporosis in women who are susceptible to osteoporosis.

A new test is becoming available that can diagnosis osteoporosis by taking a sample of your saliva. This test hopefully will be available within five years. Studies are currently being done on sheep.

If you have had a fracture of one of the bones in your spine, treatment that puts bone cement into your bone can be used to treat any compression fracture that you may have. Be aware that leakage of this bone cement, called polymethylmethacrylate, can be associated with an embolus to your lungs, heart and lung failure, and death.

The techniques that use this cement are called vertebroplasty and kyphoplasty. Value and safety of these procedures continues to be studied. Vertebroplasty involves the injection of the bone cement into your vertebral bones. Kyphyplasty introduces a surgical instrument into one of the bones in your spine with intent to elevate the compressed bone. When this instrument is withdrawn, the space left is filled with bone cement. Each of these procedures remains to be studied.

A study is currently being done examining the use of fluorides to possibly strengthen bone. A small dose of sodium fluoride can increase your spinal bone density. As a result, you can have a reduced incidence of vertebral body fractures. A study continues demonstrating that parathyroid hormone can prevent bone loss in young women who are estrogen deficient.

Be aware that a new drug recently developed for the treatment of osteoporosis, Forteo, has been shown to cause bone cancer in laboratory rats. No cancers were seen in humans to date. If you do have a prescription filled for this medication, your pharmacist will give you an FDA information sheet. This way the FDA can track any complications associated with this drug.

Treatment for Osteoporosis

If you have decreased bone density, you must take the medicines prescribed for you. Studies have shown that compliance is sometimes as low as 66 percent. This means that only 66 percent of individuals in a study actually took the medications prescribed for them. Women who did not take their osteoporosis medications developed significant further decrease in their bone densities. On the other hand, a study of postmenopausal women who had a history of a fractures related to osteoporosis did not receive drug treatment for the osteoporosis within a year following their fracture. Improved adherence to osteoporosis treatment can be done if women are educated regarding their bone densities and the effects of drugs on their bone density.

Bisphosphonates are an important class of drug for osteoporosis. These drugs can increase the minerals in the bones in your back. Furthermore, the chance of you having a vertebral fracture is decreased if you are in late menopause. These drugs can also prevent bone loss in early menopause. Examples of these drugs include etidronate and alendronate. Further research is being done with respect to these drugs in the prevention of bone fractures. However, these drugs will not reverse osteoporosis.

There are other drugs available for women who have osteoporosis. Fosamax and Actonel are two of the drugs commonly used to decrease the progression of osteoporosis. This new drug is called ibandronate. This drug can cause generalized body aches.

Some researchers thought that two drugs would be better for replacing bone loss than one drug. Fosamax was combined with parathyroid hormone but was not any better than either drug alone in building stronger bones. Fosamax is a bisphosphonate, as previously mentioned. Fosamax slows the cycle of bone breakdown. If the rate of bone breakdown is decreased, there is a reduced chance of you having a fracture.

During the acute stage of fractures, attention is directed toward relieving your pain with pain pills, including narcotics and muscle relaxants for spasm that occurs related to the fracture. Heat, massage, and rest can also be of benefit to you. Physical therapy in many instances can help you with your pain. If you have a fracture of one of the vertebral bodies in your spine, a corset or a back brace can decrease your pain. Exercise can be useful if it strengthens your abdominal and back muscles.

For Men

- Prevention is the best treatment.
- A calcium supplement that contains vitamin D, such as OsCal-D, will strengthen your bones and help prevent osteoporosis.
- Prescription medications such as Fosamax will keep you from losing more bone mass.
- Perform weight-bearing exercises to help maintain and build your bone mass.
- Be sure to follow all of your doctor's recommendations for exercises and medications.

For Women

- Prevention is the best treatment.
- A calcium supplement that contains vitamin D, such as OsCal-D, will strengthen your bones and help prevent osteoporosis.
- Prescription medications such as Fosamax will keep you from losing more bone mass.
- Perform weight-bearing exercises to help maintain and build your bone mass.
- Be sure to follow all of your doctor's recommendations for exercises and medications.

Chapter 19

Understanding Irritable Bowel Syndrome and Other Stomach-Related Pains

Pain in your abdomen can be disabling and can be severe. Abdominal pain in general occurs more often in women than in men. However, this incidence of abdominal pain decreases with age. A study is currently being done to attempt to find out what physiological or psychlogical change associated with aging may protect you against continuation of your abdominal pain. Stress, diet, and the work environment are currently being investigated as causes of abdominal pain in general. Your gastrointestinal pain will decline after age 40. The pattern of declining abdominal pain is consistent in both sexes. However, overall, the incidence of abdominal pain is higher in women than in men from childhood years to old age. These findings of various abdominal pains include pain in your upper, mid, or lower abdomen.

Cramping and intermittent pain is easily caused by disorders of your bowel, gallbladder, ureter, or fallopian tubes. This chapter includes information about an irritable bowel syndrome that can be associated with bloating.

Irritable Bowel Syndrome

A common syndrome in adults is the irritable bowel syndrome (IBS), which is frequently diagnosed in the general population. Approximately 30 percent of patients seen by gastroenterologists suffer from IBS. It is more common in women and may even be seen in adolescents. (R.B. Fillingham. *Sex, Gender, and Pain.* n.p.: IASP Press, 2000) (P. Wall and R. Melzack. *Textbook of Pain.* New York: Churchill Livingstone, 1999)

If you have IBS, this disease can impair your quality of life. This disease has begun to become more closely studied and the pharmaceutical industry has begun marketing new drugs to decrease the symptoms of IBS.

The exact cause of IBS remains to be discovered. IBS has become a defined clinical entity. IBS can be caused by physiological, psychological, and behavioral factors. Sometimes you may have severe symptoms without any physical findings. A diagnosis of IBS is determined by your symptoms. If you have IBS, you will frequently report pain or discomfort in your stomach area.

This pain is not confined to one area of your gut but it is global over your stomach. Usually this abdominal pain is relieved followed a bowel movement. You may suffer diarrhea alternating with constipation. You can suffer bloating or the feeling of incomplete evacuation of your stool. Some investigators believe that your colon is the cause of IBS. You can have symptoms daily or you may have symptoms once a week or once a month. If you have IBS, you may also have heartburn and nausea. If you have IBS, you can suffer from *fibromyalgia* or other muscle pains. (R.B. Fillingham. *Sex, Gender, and Pain*. n.p.: IASP Press, 2000) (P. Wall and R. Melzack. *Textbook of Pain*. New York: Churchill Livingstone, 1999) You can have headaches or bladder symptoms. In addition to other body disturbances, you may also suffer from chronic fatigue and significant depression.

IBS can involve the *central nervous system* (your brain and spinal cord) as well. If you suffer from psychological distress, you can have a negative effect on your central nervous system that may send signals to your *peripheral nervous system* and cause you to have hypersensitivity with respect to your gastrointestinal (mouth to rectum) system. IBS can coexist with ulcerative colitis or *Crohn's disease*. If you suffer from IBS, the underlying causes may be psychological.

Pain associated with IBS can be a result of depression or other illness. If you have psychosocial factors, these factors can influence the frequency of your symptoms as well as the severity of your symptoms. If you suffer from IBS, you may have a history of physical, sexual, or emotional abuse. (R.B. Fillingham. *Sex, Gender, and Pain*. n.p.: IASP Press, 2000) (P. Wall and R. Melzack. *Textbook of Pain*. New York: Churchill Livingstone, 1999) Usually extensive diagnostic tests are not utilized for your doctor to diagnose your IBS because there are no definitive tests for this disease.

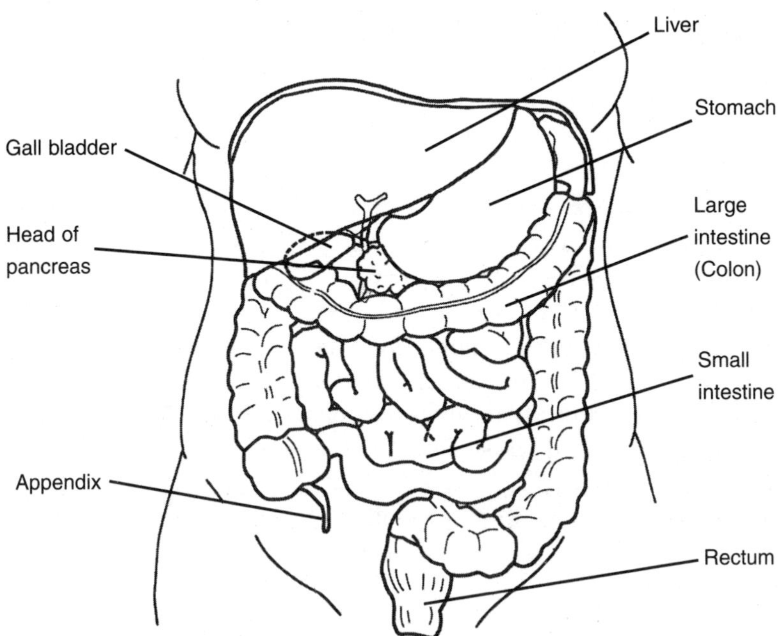

Organs in the gastrointestinal tract.

Diagnosing Irritable Bowel Syndrome

A diagnostic criteria for the diagnosis of IBS is hard to establish because of the variety of physical complaints associated with IBS. In other words, the pattern of the pain as well as the location and severity differs among patients. To be diagnosed with IBS, you need to have abdominal pain first of all. Your pain must be relieved with a bowel movement. The onset of your pain must be associated with a change in the frequency of your stool habits. The onset of your pain must be associated with a change in the appearance of your stool. You may possibly have IBS if you have an abnormal stool (in which it differs in appearance from usual stool appearance) one out of every four defecations.

Be aware that just because you have continuation of your symptoms, this does not justify expensive diagnostic testing. You do not have a severe life-threatening medical disease if you have IBS. Your doctor will reassure you that you do not have a dangerous disease. If you do notice blood in your stool, notify your doctor so that your doctor can determine whether or not you need further diagnostic tests. If you develop weight loss, symptoms that are worse at night, blood in your stools or have a family history of colon cancer, follow up with your doctor.

Symptoms of Irritable Bowel Syndrome

If you have feelings of having to strain or have a feeling of incomplete evacuation of your stool in one out of four defecations, you may possibly have IBS. If you have bloating or abdominal distention in one out of four days or passage of mucus in one out of four defecations, there is a high probability that you have IBS. You should have symptoms for at least 12 weeks or more over the previous 12 months. Your symptoms do not have to be consecutive. Approximately 70 percent of individuals with IBS have only mild symptoms. On the other hand, 25 percent of patients have symptoms that can interfere with work, school, or social functions. (R.B. Fillingham. *Sex, Gender, and Pain.* n.p.: IASP Press, 2000) (P. Wall and R. Melzack. *Textbook of Pain.* New York: Churchill Livingstone, 1999) Approximately 5 percent of individuals have severe symptoms that severely limit their activities of daily living and their quality of life. If you have mild or moderate symptoms, these symptoms can be managed by your primary care doctor. You may only need a dietary or lifestyle change.

Be aware that upper abdominal pain not associated with ulcers can be present in 50 percent of the IBS population and nausea and vomiting can also be present in 50 percent of the IBS population. Increased urination among women is also associated with IBS. Women who have IBS can also have chronic pelvic pain and other gynecological symptoms. If you have a history of physical or sexual abuse or have suffered the loss of a parent or other important person during childhood, you are more prone to develop IBS. You can have sexual dysfunction if you have IBS. Decreased sexual drive has been seen in both men and women who suffer from IBS. If you are a female, you may suffer significant stomach pains premenstrually. Stomach pain as well as pelvic cramping were noted to be higher in individuals with IBS during menses.

Psychological Testing and Treatment

At one time, doctors thought that IBS was a *psychosomatic* (mental) entity. If you suffer from IBS, you are not "crazy." It is now known that nerves in your gastrointestinal system can become oversensitive, causing them to overreact to both gas as well as food passing by these nerves. The stimulation of your nerves in your gastrointestinal tract will cause you to have pain as well as cramping. Current studies reveal that symptoms associated with IBS are not imagined but are real and have a neurological basis.

If you have moderate symptoms, you may require psychological treatment and occasionally pharmacologic management. If you have severe and constant symptoms, you may require antidepressants as well as psychological testing and treatment and you may need to be referred to a gastroenterologist. As previously stated, your doctor may want to test for parasites in your blood. A general consensus among treating doctors in general is that you do not need extensive testing when you initially present to your doctor. You will be re-evaluated over time and any additional diagnostic tests will be done depending on your clinical status and your response to treatment.

In 1999, it was published that more than 50 percent of patients with IBS who were seen in a gastroenterologist clinic had psychiatric problems. (R.B. Fillingham. *Sex, Gender, and Pain.* n.p.: IASP Press, 2000) (P. Wall and R. Melzack. *Textbook of Pain.* New York: Churchill Livingstone, 1999) The possibility of developing IBS is extremely high in individuals who suffer panic disorders. If you have depression, you are also prone to IBS. Greater sympathetic nervous system responses to abdominal pain have been reported in men when compared to women. Studies have demonstrated that men have heightened sympathetic nervous system activation. In other words, women have lower sympathetic nervous system activation when compared to men.

Treating Irritable Bowel Syndrome

In 1917, a German scientist determined that in the wall of the gut was a self-contained nervous system that could function on its own without impulses from either the brain or the spinal cord. In other words, your gut has a brain of its own. Small nerves are in the lining of your esophagus, stomach, small intestine, and your colon. Because of new findings associated with IBS, a pharmaceutical company has developed a drug called Lotronex. This new drug can help manage your symptoms associated with IBS. Be aware, however, that your gastrointestinal system is closely connected to your brain.

Your brain can affect the nerves in your stomach, on the other hand. For example, if you are anxious or have to give a speech in front of a large crowd, you may develop "butterflies" in your stomach. In other words, you feel the effect of your stress within your gastrointestinal system. If you are facing a stressful situation, your brain can influence specialized cells in your gastrointestinal system called mast cells to release histamine. Histamine makes the nerves in your gastrointestinal system to contract the smooth muscle in your gut. This will cause you to have cramps. It can also cause you to have diarrhea. Be aware that medications that affect your brain can also affect your gut.

Prozac can work on serotonin in your brain and spinal cord but also cause you to have abdominal cramping and diarrhea. Anti-anxiety drugs are currently being studied to determine whether they can decrease your symptoms associated with your IBS. Imitrex, which is used to treat migraine headaches, is being studied for the treatment of your IBS symptoms. Lotronex is an anxiety type of drug. This drug is becoming increasingly popular for the treatment of IBS.

IBS has become the most diagnosed but the least understood medical ailment. The new drug Lotronex is used to treat abdominal pain and discomfort as well as any diarrhea. Be aware that more individuals suffer from IBS than asthma or diabetes. Lotronex is the first drug approved by the FDA to be used for IBS treatment. At one time, you did not hear much information about IBS in the lay press. The reason for this was that subjects about the bowels and defecation were considered taboo by the press. Now you may note that there are television advertisements touting the use of medications for the treatment of IBS. It is important for you to be able to talk to your doctor openly about your IBS. You must talk openly and not suffer any embarrassment when you talk to your health-care provider about your symptoms. As people age, the incidences of women suffering from IBS outnumber men by three to one. (R.B. Fillingham. *Sex, Gender, and Pain.* n.p.: IASP Press, 2000) (P. Wall and R. Melzack. *Textbook of Pain.* New York: Churchill Livingstone, 1999)

A new drug now available is called Zelnorm. It is a drug that is in a class of medications called gastrointestinal serotonin agonists. This drug is used for the treatment of constipation, bloating, and abdominal pain. It is anticipated that this new drug will improve your quality of life if you suffer from IBS. In the United Kingdom, another drug called renzapride is being studied for the treatment of IBS. Preliminary studies that are being done with respect to this drug for the treatment of IBS symptoms are extremely promising. It is unknown whether and when the Canadian and the United Kingdom drugs for IBS treatment will be available in the United States. Research continues into the development of new drugs for the treatment of IBS because this disease costs the health-care system approximately $30 billion per year.

Sometimes anti-anxiety drugs can be used for the treatment of your IBS. Anti-anxiety drugs can be effective if you get abdominal cramps when you become stressed. In addition to the utilization of drugs for the treatment of your IBS, also consider meditation, exercise, yoga, and getting enough sleep. All of these methods can decrease your stress, which ultimately could decrease your symptoms associates with IBS. Another method that you may want to consider for the treatment of your IBS is hypnosis. Hypnosis has been shown to be effective for the treatment of symptoms associated with IBS.

Sex steroids may work to modulate abdominal pain associated with IBS. They can have direct effects on your gastrointestinal motility and inhibit the emptying of your stomach. Studies have shown that pre-menopausal and postmenopausal women who are taking hormones had slower stomach-emptying times with solids when compared with men and when compared with postmenopausal women who were not taking hormones. Testosterone has no influence on the gastric emptying in men. However, estrogen and progesterone will slow down the gastric emptying time in men. A study has demonstrated that a male's complaint of discomfort with distention of a balloon in the male's rectum was higher if the male had a low testosterone level. (R.B. Fillingham. *Sex, Gender, and Pain.* n.p.: IASP Press, 2000)

When considering your treatment for your IBS, your doctor will assure you that your symptoms are not from a serious illness. Your doctor will recommend a change in your diet with an emphasis on a high-fiber diet and low fat. You will be prescribed medications for constipation, diarrhea, and pain. You may require antidepressant medication as well as psychological intervention. Because of the differences in gender with the prevalence of IBS, pharmaceutical companies are now looking at gender as they search for new IBS gender-specific medications. One drug company has asked for approval to study the drug for the treatment of IBS in women only. Early studies have revealed that Alosetron may demonstrate gender specificity for the treatment of IBS in women.

Reducing the Effects of Irritable Bowel Syndrome

If you have severe IBS, you may have had stomach and bowel problems all of your life. If you have IBS, you will be fearful that your symptoms can occur at any moment. Therefore, you will always attempt to know where the closest restroom is. As a result, this can influence your social interaction. Traveling can become a problem for you. In addition to the medication mentioned, dietary fiber and biofeedback as well as occasional antidepressants can alleviate your symptoms.

If you suffer from IBS, you may want to minimize your fat intake. Many foods inhibit your intestinal gas transit. By decreasing the passage of gas through your gastrointestinal system, bloating and the expansion of your bowel can cause you to have pain. Fructose is another food substance that can worsen your IBS symptoms. Fructose is found in honey, fruit, and in some soft drinks. Fructose can cause you to have bloating, cramps, and diarrhea. Bacteria in your colon may use fructose as their food source. In the process of utilizing fructose, hydrogen gas is liberated in your colon from the breakdown of sugars.

Inflammatory Bowel Disease

Inflammatory (as opposed to irritable) bowel disease is another entity that can also cause you to have significant pain. Both IBS and inflammatory bowel diseases have similar symptoms. Your IBS is characterized by pathology within your intestine. Both IBS as well as inflammatory bowel disease can be affected by stress. They both can be affected by your central nervous system as well as your immune system within your gastrointestinal system. Antibiotics and anti-inflammatory agents are used in inflammatory bowel syndromes. There has been some suggestion that these pharmacologic methods can be useful also in IBS.

Inflammatory bowel disease is believed to be a disease of your immune system. IBS can respond to diet. However, the inflammatory bowel disease rarely responds to changes in diet. Inflammatory bowel disease includes ulcerative colitis and Crohn's disease. Ulcerative colitis is a chronic disease and a recurrent disease. It involves inflammation of the lining of the colon and can also involve your rectum. Crohn's disease can involve any part of your gastrointestinal tract, including your mouth all the way to your anus. The cause of Crohn's disease and ulcerative colitis are unknown.

Inflammatory bowel disease is more common in Caucasians and more common in Jewish men and women. The incidence is almost equal in men and women. (R.B. Fillingham. *Sex, Gender, and Pain.* n.p.: IASP Press, 2000) (P. Wall and R. Melzack. *Textbook of Pain.* New York: Churchill Livingstone, 1999) The incidence of ulcerative colitis and Crohn's disease is similar. Usually inflammatory bowel disease begins in early adult life. However, there are cases reported in the elderly. Genetic factors can make you prone to inflammatory bowel disease. If you have a disorder of your immune system, you are again prone to develop irritable bowel disease. It is possible that your immune system may attack the lining of your gastrointestinal system. Emotional stress can worsen your symptoms of inflammatory bowel disease.

Crohn's Disease

Crohn's disease usually involves the lower ileum (the lowest part of the small intestine). Your rectum can be involved. Approximately one third of Crohn's disease patients have their pathology in the colon, whereas one third of patients have their pathology in the ileum and one third have their pathology in both the ilem and colon. The inflammation of your gastrointestinal system can go from the inside of your bowel to the outside. The inner lining of your gastrointestinal system can develop ulcers. An ulcer is a break in the lining of the wall of your gut. This break in your gut lining can fail to heal and can be accompanied by inflammation. A fistula from the inside of your bowel to the outside can develop. A fistula is an abnormal communication between a hollow organ and the exterior.

With Crohn's disease, you can have fever, diarrhea, pain, and tenderness in the right lower part of your abdomen. You can also develop an abscess around your anus. (P. Wall and R. Melzack. *Textbook of Pain*. New York: Churchill Livingstone, 1999) The inner aspect of your intestine or colon can decrease in diameter, which is called a stricture. If you have Crohn's disease, you can have an increased incidence of gallstones. The bile salts are not absorbed properly through your ileum. You can also develop kidney stones. You can have a history of frequent liquid bowel movements. Because of absorption problems of nutrients, you may have a poor nutritional status. You can feel fatigued and suffer from a loss of energy. If your bowel becomes swollen, you can feel the inflamed bowel, which feels like a mass. This thickened loop of inflamed bowel can be tender to deep palpation. If you develop a tract from the inside of your bowel to the outside, this fistula can cause you to develop an abscess behind the lining of your bowel. You will have fever, chills, and tenderness to deep palpation about your abdomen. Your health-care provider will obtain a complete blood count from you.

A chronic inflammation of your gastrointestinal system can cause you to have anemia. You may suffer from iron deficiency or a vitamin

B12 deficiency. Your gastrointestinal system may not be able to absorb protein. Your doctor may want to obtain a stool sample from you and have it examined for parasites. Your doctor will want to do an x-ray series involving your upper gastrointestinal system. A barium enema and a colonoscopy may be necessary as well.

A barium enema is an enema with opaque contrast liquid that outlines your intestines on x-ray images. This test helps your doctor look for abnormalities in your bowel. To examine your lower bowel, your doctor may also use air with the barium to distend your bowel. Through the colonoscope (a flexible fiberoptic instrument), your doctor can obtain biopsies of your colon and ilium. White blood cells protect your body against foreign substances. If your white cells are elevated and your abdomen is tender, this will necessitate a CT of your abdomen (because you might have a serious infection). You will be given antibiotics as well as nutritional supplements. Occasionally surgery is required to drain the abscess.

If your gastrointestinal system develops an obstruction somewhere in your system, your food cannot pass through this obstruction. You will be treated with fluids through your veins, and a tube will be placed through your nose to suction out substances that are unable to pass through your bowel. Steroids can be necessary to treat the inflammation caused by Crohn's disease. Be aware that chronic cramping, abdominal pain, and diarrhea are noted in both IBS and Crohn's disease.

The problem with Crohn's disease is that it is a lifelong illness. You must eat a well-balanced diet. If you have Crohn's disease, you may have intolerance to milk products. You may need B12 shots monthly. Steroids are usually indicated as part of your treatment. Your diarrhea will be treated pharmacologically. Your doctor will treat your pain with the appropriate pain medication. Antibiotics can be used for your treatment. Sulfasalazine is effective in reducing the symptoms of your disease. Drugs that can affect your immune system such as azathioprine and mercaptopurine are also useful in the treatment of your disease if it is unresponsive to the other methods that we mentioned. If you smoke, stop smoking; smoking can cause you to have a recurrence of Crohn's symptoms. If conservative treatments fail, you may require surgery.

As previously stated, there is no cure for the disease. However with proper medical and surgical treatment, you should be able to cope with this disease as well as its complications and lead a productive life. Ulcerative colitis is another form of inflammatory bowel disease. Ulcerative colitis involves the inner lining of your colon. You remember that Crohn's disease can go through the entire lining of your gastrointestinal system. You will have bloody diarrhea if you have ulcerative colitis. You will have pain in your abdomen. You will develop anemia, and the protein in your bloodstream, albumin, will be decreased. A scope in your colon is the key to the diagnosis of your disease.

Other Sources of Intestinal Pain

Be aware that other structures in your abdomen can cause you to have abdominal pain. If you have a problem in one of the major arteries, for instance, you can have abdominal pain. It is difficult for your health-care provider to diagnose and treat your pain without a detailed history of your symptoms as well as with an examination. For this reason, you must keep an accurate pain diary. You may need x-rays or an MRI. Your examination by your doctor will be important. Your kidneys and ureters (as well as your ovaries and uterus if you are a female) can cause you to have abdominal pain on occasion.

Endometriosis is a common and painful disorder in women where tissue that normally lines the inside of the uterus becomes implanted on tissue outside the uterus. This can cause women to have pain in their abdomen. However, organs that are part of your gastrointestinal system are usually the cause of your abdominal pain. If you have pain in your upper abdomen on the right side, you may have an inflamed gallbladder or an ulcer. Hepatitis can cause you to have pain. Pancreatitis, a painful inflammation of the pancreas, can cause pain in your mid abdomen that radiates to your back. Renal stones and kidney stones on occasion can cause abdominal pain in addition to pain in your flanks.

Interstitial cystitis is an inflammatory disease of your bladder that can cause you to have lower abdominal pain. If your abdominal pain is associated with your menstrual cycle, keep a diary of how the pain is affected. Ovarian cysts can cause you to have pain in your lower abdomen. Abdominal pain is the pain that you feel in your abdominal area which is between your chest and groin. Another term for abdomen is your stomach or "belly." Always be aware that pain in your abdomen can originate from your chest or your pelvis (the area below your abdomen).

There are many organs in your body. You can have pain in any one of these organs. For example, you can have pain in your stomach, your large and small intestines, your liver, gallbladder, and pancreas, for instance. Your aorta, which is a major blood vessel that comes off of your heart, runs down through your abdomen. If you have an aneurysm, which is a defect in the wall of this great vessel, you can have pain in your abdomen. An aneurysm needs to be evaluated by your doctor. An aneurysm is a weakness in the wall of your aorta. This weak area could rupture, which could be fatal.

Your appendix, if it is inflamed, can cause you to have abdominal pain as well. Your appendix is part of your gastrointestinal system. A viral infection in your intestine or gas can cause you to have significant abdominal pain. As you probably know, this pain can be severe. This should alert you that the severity of the pain does not correlate with the severity of the disease. In other words, you can have cancer of your colon and have only mild pain. Causes of abdominal pain include gas, constipation, milk intolerance, stomach flu, an irritable bowel syndrome, indigestion, esophageal reflux, ulcers, gallstones, and diverticular disease.

If you have an obstruction of your bowel, you can have significant disabling pain. A food allergy can cause you to have gastrointestinal pain. Kidney stones and urinary tract infections can also cause you to have pain. If you have a sickle cell crisis, you can also experience abdominal pain. Crohn's disease and ulcerative colitis are two types of inflammatory bowel disease that can cause you to suffer significant pain. If one of your inflamed organs ruptures, you will have excruciating pain and your stomach will be as hard as a board. You will probably have a fever associated with this pain. These symptoms are usually seen in peritonitis. Peritonitis is an inflammation of the membrane which lines your abdominal cavity.

If you have abdominal pain that occurs during your period, your pain may be from menstrual cramps. Pneumonia can cause you to have referred abdominal pain, and even a heart attack can occasionally cause you to experience abdominal pain. Cancer of the stomach, colon, and pancreas can also cause abdominal pain. Emotional upset can also cause you to have abdominal pain.

Parasites as well as heliocobacter pylori can cause you to have abdominal pain. (T.E. Andreolli, et al. *Cecil Essentials of Medicine.* n.p.: W.B. Saunders, 1997) This bacteria is called in microbiological terms a gram-negative bacteria and can be found in the moist membrane lining of your stomach. It can cause you to develop a progressive gastritis (an inflammation of the lining of your stomach) as well as stomach cancer, heart disease, and gastric and duodendal ulcers. Your doctor will help your body eradicate this bacteria with antibiotics and other drugs.

Keep a diary of your stool frequency and note the amount of rectal bleeding, cramps, and abdominal pain that you have. If you have frequent diarrhea, the fluid volume of your body can become depleted. You may have up to 10 bloody bowel movements a day, which can cause you to develop severe anemia. If you have ulcerative colitis, you may also have ankylosing spondylitis, which is an arthritic type of disease that can affect your joints. Plain x-rays of your abdomen can be helpful for the diagnosis of ulcerative colitis. There may be increases in the diameter of your colon in certain areas of your abdomen.

Sometimes children can have abdominal pain. The ratio of girls to boys with abdominal pain is four to three. There can be a psychological origin of their abdominal pain in a significant number of these children. Chronic abdominal pain in children without obvious pathology such as a diseased appendix is psychogenic in approximately 90 percent of cases. Psycogenic means that the origin is in your mind as opposed to your body. The etiology of this abdominal pain arises from stress, anxiety, and/or depression. Sometimes this entity can be caused by inflammatory bowel disease or an ulcer.

Treatment for Irritable Bowel Syndrome and Other Stomach-Related Pains

As you can see, the diagnosis of abdominal pain can be complex. (R.B. Fillingham. *Sex, Gender, and Pain.* n.p.: IASP Press, 2000) (P. Wall and R. Melzack. *Textbook of Pain.* New York: Churchill Livingstone, 1999) Unfortunately, other things besides your gut can cause you to feel stomach pain. What can you do to help your doctor? You need to keep a diary of your pain. Tell your doctor if you have pain all over your abdomen or if it is in a specific location.

You need to keep a diary as to whether or not your pain is severe, cramping, persistent, or constant. Does your pain only awaken you at night? Have you ever had a similar pain pattern previously? How often do you have the pain? In other words, does it occur daily, weekly, or monthly? Does it occur after meals? Is the pain referred to your back, shoulder blades, or legs? Is it worse after lying down or after drinking or eating greasy foods? Is the pain worse with stress? Is your pain relieved after eating or after drinking milk? What medicines are you taking? If you are taking over-the-counter nonsteroidal anti-inflammatory drugs, you need to tell your doctor. Have you had a recent injury to your stomach? As you can see, your history is an important factor in helping your doctor diagnose what is causing your abdominal pain.

Sometimes your doctor will obtain laboratory values, including blood samples, stool samples, and a urinalysis. An x-ray of your abdomen may be necessary to diagnose the cause of your pain. A barium enema or an upper GI and small bowel series are sometimes done as well. A scope can be placed into your gastrointestinal tract to attempt to diagnose the cause of your pain as well.

Your treatment goal of any gastrointestinal disease is twofold. The first is your doctor will terminate your acute symptoms (symptoms of recent onset and not necessarily of great severity), and then your doctor will attempt to prevent a recurrence of your symptoms. If you have mild symptoms, eat a regular balanced diet but decrease your intake of caffeine and any vegetables that can produce gas. Fiber supplements decrease diarrhea. Your doctor may prescribe medications for you to take for your diarrhea. If your disease is confined to your rectum, your doctor may prescribe topical medications only. Topical steroids and steroid suppositories can also be used.

If you have mild to moderate symptoms, you will be given oral medications. Sulfasalazine can be prescribed to treat your symptoms. Mesalamine can also be used. For some reason, the use of a nicotine patch has been shown to be effective in some patients suffering from this disease. The reason for this finding remains unknown. Steroid enemas can be used to treat your symptoms. Oral steroids can be used as well. If you develop severe symptoms, you may require hospitalization. Approximately 15 percent of individuals with ulcerative colitis develop symptoms that are severe. You must stop all oral intake. You will require fluids. Stop all opioid drugs. If your disease progresses, your fluid volume can decrease, which can make you dehydrated. You may require blood transfusions if you are hemorrhaging.

If your abdomen distends and becomes increasingly tender, you run the risk of perforation of your bowel (the creation of a hole in your tissue). Your colon can become excessively dilated. This finding is in less than two percent of cases of ulcerative colitis. This expansion of your bowel can cause a decrease in the blood flow to the bowel tissue. This is called toxic megacolon. If you have this disease, you run the risk of developing colon cancer. If your symptoms remain severe, you may require surgery. Severe bleeding as well as the perforation of your bowel are indications for surgery. You may want to try to avoid surgery because of your self-image as you will probably require placement of an external pouch to evacuate your feces. However, if your colon is removed, your surgeon may be able to do a surgical procedure where you don't need an ostomy (opening into a tissue). Be aware that ulcerative colitis is a lifelong disease. In most instances, your symptoms will be controlled by medical therapy. You probably will not need surgery. You may never need hospitalization. Be aware that if you do need surgery, however, this could result in a complete cure of your disease. If you do suffer from ulcerative colitis, you have a better overall prognosis than if you suffer from Crohn's disease.

If you have pain related to your gastrointestinal system, be sure to keep a comprehensive pain diary. Notify your doctor if you have any changes in your symptoms. Be compliant in the taking of any medications prescribed to you. Do relaxation techniques. Eat proper diet as advised by your doctor. Remember that you are a member of your pain-care team.

For Men

- It is important for your and your doctor that you keep a detailed pain diary. Be sure to note what you ate and what time you ate, along with how you felt afterward.
- Eat a well-balanced diet. Exclude caffeine and gas-producing vegetables from your diet to help prevent gastrointestinal pain and diarrhea.
- Correctly take any medications for diarrhea that your doctor prescribes. This will help relieve some pain related to cramping.
- Steroids and other prescriptions from your doctor can be helpful in relieving the symptoms of stomach-related pain.
- Performing relaxation techniques can help you cope with your pain as well.

For Women

- It is important for your and your doctor that you keep a detailed pain diary. Be sure to note what you ate and what time you ate, along with how you felt afterward.
- Eat a well-balanced diet. Exclude caffeine and gas-producing vegetables from your diet to help prevent gastrointestinal pain and diarrhea.
- Correctly take any medications for diarrhea that your doctor prescribes. This will help relieve some pain related to cramping.
- Steroids and other prescriptions from your doctor can be helpful in relieving the symptoms of stomach-related pain.
- Performing relaxation techniques can help you cope with your pain as well.

Chapter 20
Understanding Fibromyalgia

"Doctor, I have pain all over my body. I'm depressed and I can't sleep at night. I feel miserable. What's wrong with me? Can you give me something for the pain?" If you have fibromyalgia, you know this scenario all too well. You know the pain can affect multiple sites throughout your body and often cause you to miss work and interrupt your daily living.

Fibromyalgia is a chronic pain syndrome that affects soft tissue, tendons, and fascia. Also referred to as fibromyositis, it affects about 5 percent of the population, 90 percent of which are women of childbearing age. (C. Germano and W. Cabot. *Nature's Pain Killers: Proven New Alternatives and Nutritional Therapies for Chronic Pain Relief.* New York: Kensington Books, 1999) (Fillingham, Roger B., et al. "Gender Differences in the Response to Noxious Stimuli," *Pain Forum* 4 [1995]: 209-221)

Chronic means that your doctor does not have an immediate fix for your pain. You must choose a physician who you feel comfortable with because you will probably see this person every month. You and your doctor must take control of your pain and not let your pain control your life. Changes in diet and exercise or lack of exercise must be addressed by you and your physician. You and your physician must function together as a team.

Fibromyalgia causes you to have muscle pain throughout the body, joint stiffness, and fatigue. You also may experience sleep disturbances and depression. It can cause many places on your body to become extremely tender. You are only diagnosed with fibromyalgia after other pain-causing conditions have been eliminated as the reason for your pain. Fibromyalgia is a condition that can be painful, but it is benign and will rarely cause you to be totally disabled. Only you can let it become disabling.

This chapter will teach you about the signs and symptoms of fibromyalgia, how it differs between men and women, and how hormones can affect your fibromyalgia pain. You also will learn about the various treatment options you have for fibromyalgia and why they work, including medication and physical therapy options. Since the entity of fibromyalgia can be complicated to deal with emotionally, psychological techniques are recommended to help you cope with your pain.

Signs, Symptoms, and Gender Differences in Fibromylagia

The reasons for diagnosing fibromyalgia vary and are based on the complaints that you have mentioned to your doctor. Right now no laboratory tests lead to a specific diagnosis of fibromyalgia, so your doctors must rely on you to explain the specific complications you are having. Your doctor will also test you by taking a small amount of blood from your vein to make sure that you do not have arthritis or another condition that could be causing your pain. You must tell your doctor if you have been bitten by tics or mosquitoes in the past six months, because West Nile virus symptoms and Lyme disease symptoms may mimic the symptoms of fibromyalgia.

The criteria for the diagnosis fibromyalgia are as follows:

- Aches, pains, and stiffness involving three or more places on your body for at least three months.
- No traumatic injury to your body.
- Knowing that you do not have a rheumatic disease, but that you do have three or more places on your body that are extremely sensitive to pain.
- Your symptoms of pain either get better or get worse when you do a lot of physical activity.
- Your pain gets worse when the weather changes.
- Your pain gets worse when you are under a lot of stress.
- You have a history of anxiety.
- You have a history of a lot of headaches.
- You have a history of irritable bowel syndrome.
- Your doctor finds tender spots on your body in at least 12 of 14 specific places.

- You have a history of being extremely sluggish and tired in the morning.
- Lab tests show that you have normal connective tissue on your muscles.

People without fibromyalgia may also have similar tender points on their body like you do. (C. Germano and W. Cabot. *Nature's Pain Killers: Proven New Alternatives and Nutritional Therapies for Chronic Pain Relief*. New York: Kensington Books, 1999) (Fillingham, Roger B., et al. "Gender Differences in the Response to Noxious Stimuli," *Pain Forum* 4 [1995]: 209-221) Their tenderness could be caused by diseases such as rheumatoid arthritis, or they may be experiencing tenderness after a traumatic event such as a whiplash injury or a lifting injury. The difference is that your tender areas will be more sensitive to pressure than the surrounding areas of muscle. In other words, there will be one small extremely tender area of the muscle that is surrounded by a nontender area of the same muscle. It is common for these tender "trigger points" on your body to be extremely sensitive. This is because the fibromyalgia causes you to have less of a pain tolerance in all the muscles throughout your body.

If you are like other people with fibromyalgia, the muscle pain that you experience is probably most common in your neck and lower back. However, it can affect any muscle part of your body. Your pain can range from sharp or cramping to a burning sensation. Your pain may be worse in one specific area, even though the pain can be felt all over your body. You also will notice that fibromyalgia pain affects tender areas on your body that are symmetrical, or located in the same places on the opposite side of your body.

Tenderness and swelling of the hands or feet is common. Other common places where you may notice tenderness include the areas under the base of the skull; above the shoulder blade, elbows, the buttocks (gluteal muscle); the front of the neck midway from the chin to the collar bone; the chest; the sides of the body over the hip regions; and the inner aspects of the knees.

It is more common for women to have fibromyalgia than men. (C. Germano and W. Cabot. Nature's Pain Killers: Proven New Alternatives and Nutritional Therapies for Chronic Pain Relief, New York: Kensington Books, 1999) (Fillingham, Roger B., et al. "Gender Differences in the Response to Noxious Stimuli," *Pain Forum* 4 [1995]:

209-221) Because of this, researchers are trying to find gender-specific causes of fibromyalgia. In general the amount of pain that women can withstand is lower than the amount of pain that men can withstand. (R.B. Fillingham. *Sex, Gender, and Pain.* n.p.: IASP Press, 2000) Some researchers think that the differences in hormones between men and women can cause the differences in the amount of pain they can each withstand. Fibromyalgia is seen mostly in women between 20 and 50 years of age. However, it can affect children and elderly people as well.

Musculoskeletal Pain and Fatigue

The exact cause of fibromyalgia remains unknown. Studies of muscle tissue in people with fibromyalgia have shown changes that are similar to muscle tissues that have not been used very much. As a fibromyalgia sufferer, you may not be getting enough deep sleep. Even in normal people, not getting enough sleep can produce symptoms of fibromyalgia. It is not known if the lack of deep sleep is a cause of the beginnings of fibromyalgia. Some doctors think the loss of this deep sleep pattern can speed up the symptoms of fibromyalgia once they show up, but they do not think this explains what causes the syndrome.

You may have either an increase or a decrease in blood flow to your muscle tissues. (C. Germano and W. Cabot. *Nature's Pain Killers: Proven New Alternatives and Nutritional Therapies for Chronic Pain Relief.* New York: Kensington Books, 1999) This may be the direct result of an abnormal nervous system. As a result of either an increased blood flow or a decreased blood flow, your blood vessels can become a filter for blood to leak into your muscle tissues. The blood or plasma that is leaking into your muscles is the reason why you may sometimes notice that individual tissues, such as your hands or feet, are swelling up on your body.

If you have a decreased flow of blood to your muscle tissues, the tissue then does not have enough oxygen (C. Germano and W. Cabot. *Nature's Pain Killers: Proven New Alternatives and Nutritional Therapies for Chronic Pain Relief.* New York: Kensington Books, 1999) This causes a type of pain called ischemic pain (meaning a decrease or loss of oxygen supply to a tissue). This is the type of pain someone having a heart attack may experience. In much the same way, your feeling of pain results when your muscle has a sudden loss of its oxygen supply.

Not having enough oxygen going to your muscle cells lowers the levels of some chemicals in your muscles, causing you to feel pain.

Your specific muscle groups that are affected by the fibromyalgia pain will usually become weaker than your other muscles. The rest of your muscle groups should continue to show their normal strength. This weakness in your muscles is what lessens your ability to function normally. On occasion, you may feel overly fatigued.

How Hormones and Other Chemicals Affect Pain

Hormones and other chemicals released by your body also affect symptoms of pain. Serotonin and norepinepherine are two chemicals in your central nervous system (brain and spinal cord) that calm down pain signals traveling to your brain. Not having enough serotonin going to your brain and spinal cord can cause you to not get enough deep sleep, which can cause symptoms of depression as well as fibromyalgia pain. (C. Germano and W. Cabot. *Nature's Pain Killers: Proven New Alternatives and Nutritional Therapies for Chronic Pain Relief*. New York: Kensington Books, 1999)

Fibromyalgia also affects your levels of norepinepherine, which is a chemical in the central nervous system that functions in response to your short-term stress (such as work-related or spousal problems). Urine studies in people diagnosed with fibromyalgia have shown above normal urinary norepinephrine levels. (R.B. Fillingham. *Sex, Gender, and Pain*. n.p.: IASP Press, 2000) These same high urinary norepinepherine levels also are seen in patients with anxiety. Just the opposite, people who don't have fibromyalgia, but who have a history of depression, do not show high urinary norepinepherine levels.

Another chemical in your body that causes pain is substance P. Substance P is found basically in all neurons of your central nervous system as well as nerves that go to your muscles. After your muscle tissues have been hurt, substance P is released. This can trigger burning pain sensations in your body. High substance P levels have been noted in the spinal fluid of people with fibromyalgia. Endorphins, substances produced by your body and deposited in the spinal cord to decrease pain transmission to your brain, are known to slow down the pain-causing effects of substance P. The low levels of endorphins in your brain and spinal cord may be another cause of pain associated with this condition.

It is well known that vigorous exercise can produce endorphins that are then released in your body. Along with decreasing the pain signals that are sent to your brain, endorphins can affect your mood.

It is thought that a lower than normal blood level of endorphins may be another cause of fibromyalgia. People with and without fibromyalgia who do physical exercise have noted a decrease in their pain following aerobic exercise. Normal people usually have an increase in endorphins in their bloodstream following exercise. However, you may show no increase in endorphin levels after you exercise.

One good finding is that a two- to three-year follow-up of people with fibromyalgia showed that those who did regular aerobic exercise did not progress to more serious conditions such as rheumatoid arthritis or hypothyroidism. Another theory of the cause of fibromyalgia is related to the increase in substance P in the spinal fluid of people with fibromyalgia. An increase in substance P in your spinal fluid can cause the nerves that go to your muscles to become excited. After these nerve endings are stimulated, your muscles will become excited and they will tense up and contract. After they have been contracted for a period of time, your muscles will not get enough blood to them. This causes your muscles to become injured. Incorrect posture can also cause your muscles unnecessary contraction. This can be an additional cause of fibromyalgia.

Your complaints may also be the same as complaints from people who have hormone deficiencies. Growth hormone helps your body to heal muscle trauma. (C. Germano and W. Cabot. *Nature's Pain Killers: Proven New Alternatives and Nutritional Therapies for Chronic Pain Relief*. New York: Kensington Books, 1999) Their production in your body depends on certain sleep patterns. If you do not get enough sleep or you are fatigued a lot, your body may not produce as many growth hormones. If your growth hormone level is decreased, your muscles will not heal as well as they should. In some studies, injections of growth hormones have decreased the symptoms of fibromyalgia, but many people are unhappy with the overall effects of the growth hormone and the extremely expensive cost of regular injections of growth hormone. You may also have symptoms similar to someone with low thyroid hormone production. This low blood level of thyroid hormone can cause you to have symptoms that include fatigue, weakness, and muscle aches. It is possible that the lower levels of serotonin in your bloodstream and central nervous system cause these symptoms.

Some doctors and researchers think that mental illness could also be a cause of fibromyalgia. Some doctors think that fibromyalgia is a made up expression from people with depression or anxiety. The thought that fibromyalgia may be the result of a bipolar disorder is also being looked into. Researchers have discovered a higher lifetime rate of anxiety and depression among people suffering from fibromyalgia. In one study, 64 percent of patients suffering from fibromyalgia had depression for at least 12 months prior to its beginning. However, in some people with chronic pain, depression and anxiety can be a result of their chronic pain symptoms. About 40 percent of people with fibromyalgia are depressed, whereas 10 percent of the healthy population suffers from depression as well. The common thinking among current researchers leans toward the assumption that depression does not cause fibromyalgia, but that it occurs after the fibromyalgia itself sets in.

Current Research Findings

Your sex hormones interact with the nerves that go out to your arms and legs as well as with the nerves going to and from your spinal cord. They can also affect the nerve pathways in your brain and spinal cord, which are involved in determining how sensitive you are to pain. The sex hormones in your spinal cord can reduce the pain signals that are ultimately going to your brain.

Related to women's hormones, researchers are now examining the effects of menstrual cycle-related hormone changes in women with fibromyalgia. One study showed that 72 percent of women with fibromyalgia said they had more pain during the premenstrual phase of their menstrual cycle. (Fillingham, Roger B., et al. "Gender Differences in the Response to Noxious Stimuli," *Pain Forum* 4 [1995]: 209-221)

This means that right before the beginning of their menstrual cycle, levels of certain hormones are changing that cause women to experience more pain.

Women with fibromyalgia have a decrease in a body chemical called nociceptin. This is similar to morphinelike chemicals that reduce pain. Women suffering from fibromyalgia have a lower blood level of nociceptin than do normal women throughout the entire menstrual cycle. This could be a cause for their increase in pain sensitivity during that time. However, women suffering from fibromyalgia do not appear to have a decrease in their symptoms following menopause when their hormone levels are decreasing.

There is increased evidence that fibromyalgia can be genetically inherited. (R.B. Fillingham. *Sex, Gender, and Pain*. n.p.: IASP Press, 2000) You may even know of a relative who has symptoms similar to yours. The exact gene that causes fibromyalgia has not been isolated, but several genes have been proposed as a possible explanation for the genetic inheritance of fibromyalgia and they are being studied. Research into the causes of fibromyalgia must continue. Continued research may ultimately lead to the answer of why men and women respond to pain differently. You must tell your doctor if other family members suffer with fibromyalgia. This information may help your doctor make the diagnosis of fibromyalgia. You must give your doctor as much information as possible regarding your health as well as the health of your family members.

Treatment of Fibromyalgia

There is no agreement among doctors from different specialties as to the best treatment of fibromyalgia. Different doctors will advise you of different treatments for your fibromyalgia. Anesthesiologists will inject your muscles with a steroid mixed with a numbing medicine. Physical medicine and rehabilitation specialists will prescribe heat, cold, and other physical modalities for the treatment of your pain. Internists will prescribe various pills to control your pain. Whatever method your doctor chooses for you, it should definitely include educating you about the condition and the reassurance that it is not imaginary or life threatening.

Your understanding of fibromyalgia will diminish some of the fears associated with this disorder that you may have and help you to understand why certain methods of treatment have been prescribed by your doctor. This will help you to become more involved in your own treatment. It is important that you see only one doctor for your treatment of fibromyalgia. This will ensure that your condition is closely and consistently monitored. If you have any concerns about your treatment, tell your doctor.

Always stay away from things that cause you to become stressed or depressed. Stress and depression cause the hormones and other chemicals in your body to become unbalanced and could lead to more symptoms of pain. If you live in a cold environment, it is important that you keep warm to keep your blood flowing properly. Otherwise, your muscles will not get enough oxygen, causing you more muscle injury and pain.

It is a good idea for you to keep a daily diary of your activities and pain levels. When you visit your doctor, be sure to take your diary with you so your doctor can see your daily activities such as exercise, sleep, and eating habits. Also be sure to write down any medications you have taken and what their effects were. This will help your doctor determine what areas you need help in the most, and can help the doctor prescribe an effective treatment to relieve your pain symptoms. Let your pain-management doctor know if your primary-care doctor diagnosed any new disorder or prescribed any new drug since your last visit with your pain doctor.

It is important that you do exercise or any type of low-impact aerobic activity. Aerobic exercise is extremely helpful in decreasing your pain and improving your sleep pattern. Swimming and water aerobics are excellent ways for you to accomplish this goal. They are some of the best exercise activities for patients with fibromyalgia. These types of nonimpact activities will help strengthen and condition your muscles, unlike high-impact exercise that can actually do more damage to your muscles. A study published in 1996 said that following physical exercise, almost 50 percent of people had a significant decrease in their signs and symptoms of fibromyalgia. Exercise will improve your muscle range of motion.

You should also include some form of physical therapy for the treatment of your fibromyalgia. Massage and heat therapy (ice may cause decreased blood flow to muscle tissue and make symptoms worse) are both good options. Acupuncture has also been shown to be of some benefit due to its effect on the release of the body's endorphins.

Most doctors agree that medications, injections, and therapy alone will not be able to eliminate your pain, but rather it will help you to manage your pain and cope with it better. Taking steroids to treat your fibromyalgia will not improve your symptoms of pain. People with other muscle or bone conditions such as rheumatoid arthritis do respond well to steroids. However, nonsteroidal anti-inflammatory medications such as ibuprofen may relieve or at least decrease your muscle pain.

Most pain medicine physicians who treat fibromyalgia agree that you should not use morphinelike drugs. Tramadol (Ultram or Ultracet) may be extremely helpful to people suffering from fibromyalgia. It has two mechanisms of action that can effectively reduce your pain. First, Tramadol exerts its pain-relieving effects by stimulating receptors in your brain and spinal cord. Activation of these receptors can significantly block the amount of pain impulses that ultimately reach the pain center in your brain. Second, the added advantage of using this drug to treat your pain is that it increases the levels of serotonin and norepinephrine in your spinal cord and brain. These two substances in turn can decrease the amount of pain signals that reach your brain. This drug should not cause you to become addicted to it.

The main goal in treating your fibromyalgia is to attempt to break the pain cycle. One way of accomplishing this goal is to correct any disturbance in your sleep pattern. Amitriptyline (Elavil) can be an important drug in restoring your sleep. Numerous studies have shown that getting enough sleep can significantly reduce your pain. If you are allergic to Amitriptyline, cyclobenzaprine (Flexeril) can be used. In some people, nonsteroidal anti-inflammatory medications such as ibuprofen can be successfully used. Amantadine hydrochloride (Symmetrel) may also be used. This medication is an antiviral as well as an anti-Parkinson medication. Serotonin reuptake inhibitors (Paxil) may also have a positive effect on reducing your pain.

As stated previously, avoid any narcotic types of pain-relieving medications. These narcotic medications could cause you to feel depressed. They can also reduce your hormone production. A reduction in the levels of the hormone testosterone can occur in both men and women. In men, a large decrease of testosterone in the blood can cause depression and osteoporosis. It is also possible that you could become addicted to narcotic-type medications. In many cases, people with a lot of pain request narcotic therapy because they think it is the only thing that could possibly take care of relieving their pain. However, there is rarely a need for you to use these types of medications for the management of your fibromyalgia pain. If they are prescribed to you at all, only take them for three to five days.

Pain-relieving creams that can be applied directly to your skin are also an effective way to reduce your pain symptoms. (R. Melzack and P. Wall, *Handbook of Pain Management a Clinical Companion of Textbook of Pain*, New York: Churchill Livingstone, 2003) Capsaicin cream contains chemicals that are obtained from red peppers. These substances lessen the amount of substance P in the nerve endings around your muscle tissue. Zostrix or a similar cream may also be effective for you. This cream is expected to be more effective for managing pain than creams such as Ben-Gay that contain menthol. Be aware of the fact that capsaicin-containing creams can cause your skin to feel like it is burning. This is a normal occurrence and will lessen with repetitive applications. Ben-Gay is most useful in managing inflammatory pain such as arthritis. You may even find it helpful to have an injection of a local anesthetic and a steroid directly into your most sensitive areas of pain.

Nerve stimulation is another method of relieving pain that you may find helpful. A TENS unit (Transcutaneous Electrical Nerve Stimulator) is useful in managing fibromyalgia pain in many patients. This small battery-powered instrument has two to four patches that are placed over your painful muscle areas. Electrical impulses will stimulate the nerves around your areas of pain. This stimulation will cause the production of the pain-relieving chemical enkephalin into your spinal cord. Enkephalin will diminish the intensity of your pain signals which ultimately reach your brain.

Another useful machine that is gaining in popularity is a muscle stimulator. These devices have six to eight patches that are placed over your painful muscle areas. The muscle stimulator machine will stimulate and work your muscles until they are fatigued and weakened. It is possible for your muscles that have been weakened by the fibromyalgia to be strengthened this way.

The MEDEX system is another machine that you can use to improve your muscle strength. It is found in physical therapy departments. These machines can address many muscle groups throughout your body. There is a machine for every muscle group in your body. Beyond muscle strengthening, a computer in the machine can analyze your muscle strength and compare it to the muscle strength of normal people. It can also track your progress in strengthening your muscles. This is a way to independently evaluate your progress.

Your muscles are not the only entity that needs to be treated in order to manage your pain. You may have psychological needs related to coping with your fibromyalgia that should be addressed. (R. Melzack and P. Wall, *Handbook of Pain Management a Clinical Companion of Textbook of Pain*, New York: Churchill Livingstone, 2003) Fibromyalgia support groups exist in many communities. In these groups you will share with each other what treatments work best for you. You may discover a new treatment you would like to try, and you may even find a friend to exercise with or just talk to about your experiences with fibromyalgia. Psychological counseling can be another useful way to cope with your pain. A psychologist can help you deal with the suffering aspect of your pain. Your psychologist may also want to teach you biofeedback. This is a good way for you to learn relaxing techniques that can significantly reduce your pain. Your psychologist may want you to listen to a CD or cassette tapes at home. Aromatherapy could also be effective for helping you manage your pain. This method is more effective in women because their scent perception is better than a man's. You may also find that hypnosis can decrease your pain intensity. You may want to try self hypnosis as another modality for the management of your chronic pain.

You can see that there are many proposed causes of fibromyalgia and there are as many treatments recommend for the control of fibromyalgia pain. Empower yourself by becoming involved in your treatment. No matter what treatment method your doctor prescribes, make sure you understand why it is being suggested and that you can correctly follow the treatment guidelines. Always be honest with your doctor and let him or her know how you feel during your treatment. With good communication, you and your doctor together can find the causes of your pain and learn how to manage them effectively with the treatment modality or modalities that works best for you.

For Men

The symptoms of fibromyalgia in men are generally fewer and milder than those of women. However, the conditions caused by this syndrome can be just as painful. It is important that you discuss treatment with your doctor and follow your doctor's advice carefully. It is equally as important to educate yourself on the condition and pay attention to actions that may be aggravating your symptoms.

Habits:

- Change your lifestyle habits. Keep a diary of your daily activities. Try to pinpoint actions that could be causing your fibromyalgia symptoms to worsen and eliminate them.
- Assess your posture. If you slouch while sitting or standing, learn and follow proper posture techniques. This will keep your muscles from being unnecessarily contracted, which can cause you pain.
- Get more sleep. The more sleep and rest you accumulate, the more your muscles will be allowed to rest.

- Begin an exercise program. Exercising your muscles can help reduce some of the symptoms of fibromyalgia. Water aerobics and swimming are good, nonimpact types of exercise that are beneficial. Exercising will also produce serotonin, which will in turn help you sleep better.
- If maneuvers that you do at work worsen your pain, notify your supervisor. If you continue to work with pain you could ultimately injure yourself or a co-worker. If you frequently use a computer, do not keep your neck in a bent position.

Medications:

- Take nonsteroidal anti-inflammatory medications such as ibuprofen to decrease your muscle pain.
- Applying topical pain-relieving creams such as capsaicin or Zostrix over your area of pain will help reduce your muscle pain.
- If your pain is keeping you awake at night, take a sleep-inducing medication such as Elavil to help you sleep. Getting enough sleep is important to helping your body heal.
- Tricyclic anti-depressant medications will help stabilize chemicals in your brain that respond to pain and reduce some of that pain.
- Taking pain medications such as Tramadol can provide you with some relief of your pain symptoms.

Therapy:

- Try massage or heat therapy on your affected muscles to relieve your muscle stress and fatigue and help relieve some of your pain.
- You could see your doctor for nerve stimulation by a TENS unit to help release pain-relieving chemicals that will help decrease your pain.
- Your doctor or physical therapist will be able to stimulate your muscles with a muscle stimulator machine or a MEDEX machine. Muscle stimulation can strengthen your weak and painful muscles. The machine will work your muscles for you, since you may not be able to because it is too painful. This will also help relieve some of your pain.
- If you are depressed or need psychological help to deal with your pain, psychological therapy or support groups can help you cope with the suffering aspect of your pain.

- Biofeedback with a psychologist can teach you techniques that will help you relax and deal with your pain.

For Women

Fibromyalgia occurs more often in women of childbearing age and is often more painful in women than men. Women need to work closely with their doctor to achieve the best treatment plan. Because different hormone levels are present in women's bodies in different amounts during their menstrual cycle, it is especially important to keep a daily diary and chart your pain symptoms carefully. This will help your doctor prescribe the proper medications and other treatment methods most appropriate for you.

Habits:

- Change your lifestyle habits. Keep a diary of your daily activities. Try to pinpoint actions that could be causing your fibromyalgia symptoms to worsen and eliminate them.
- Assess your posture. If you slouch while sitting or standing, learn and follow proper posture techniques. This will keep your muscles from being unnecessarily contracted, which can cause you pain.
- Get more sleep. The more sleep and rest you accumulate, the more your muscles will be allowed to rest.
- Begin an exercise program. Exercising your muscles can help reduce some of the symptoms of fibromyalgia. Water aerobics and swimming are good, nonimpact types of exercise that are beneficial. Exercising will also produce serotonin, which will in turn help you sleep better.
- If maneuvers that you do at work worsen your pain, notify your supervisor. If you continue to work with pain you could ultimately injure yourself or a co-worker. If you frequently use a computer, do not keep your neck in a bent position.

Medications:

- Take nonsteroidal anti-inflammatory medications such as ibuprofen to decrease your muscle pain.
- Applying topical pain-relieving creams such as capsaicin or Zostrix over your area of pain will help reduce your muscle pain.

- If your pain is keeping you awake at night, take a sleep-inducing medication such as Elavil to help you sleep. Getting enough sleep is important in helping your body to heal.
- Taking pain medications such as Tramadol can provide you with some relief of your pain symptoms.
- Taking serotonin reuptake inhibitors such as Paxil will help stop serotonin depletion in your brain and help your sleep patterns.
- Because of sex differences with respect to the effect of estrogen as well as progesterone on the absorption, metabolism and elimination of medications, drug dosing may fluctuate in the female patient depending on whether or not the female is pre- or post-menopausal. They physiological changes that occur during the menstrual cycle can affect the responses of a drug in the female body. You must discuss the effects of your drug with your doctor because the effect of your drug may decrease during menses.

Therapy:

- Aromatherapy can decrease your pain sensitivity and relieve some of your pain.
- Try massage or heat therapy on your affected muscles to relieve your muscle stress and fatigue and help relieve some of your pain.
- You could see your doctor for nerve stimulation by a TENS unit to help release pain-relieving chemicals that will help decrease your pain.
- Your doctor or physical therapist will be able to stimulate your muscles with a muscle stimulator machine or a MEDEX machine. Muscle stimulation can strengthen your weak and painful muscles. The machine will work your muscles for you, since you may not be able to because it is too painful. This will also help relieve some of your pain.
- If you are depressed or need psychological help to deal with your pain, psychological therapy or support groups can help you cope with the suffering aspect of your pain.
- Biofeedback with a psychologist can teach you techniques that will help you relax and deal with your pain.

Chapter 21

Understanding Myofascial Pain

Have you ever had a muscle cramp? You may have had a myofascial pain syndrome at one time if you are active playing sports or working in your garden, for example. You may have what is called a myofascial pain syndrome. A myofascial pain syndrome is a soft tissue disorder of your muscles that can cause you not only to have pain for a long time, but it can also cause you to have some disability. (D.G. Simons, et al. *Travell & Simons' Myofascial Pain and Dysfunction: The Trigger Point Manual.* Atlanta: Lippincott Williams and Wilkins, 1999)

Your overall activities of daily living, including work, can be significantly decreased. Myofascial pain is pain related to muscle injury or overuse resulting in taut bands and palpaple areas of pain which is referred to other areas of your body.

The problem with a myofascial pain syndrome is it can be present with your pain symptoms that are similar to other muscle-causing pain syndromes such as fibromyalgia. Fibromyalgia is a disorder characterized by pain in the fibrous tissue of muscle. Muscle strains and ligament sprains can cause pain in your muscles and can contribute to the onset of the myofascial pain syndrome. Be aware that your myofascial pain syndrome is a distinct entity. This chapter will show you that just as there are criteria for fibromyalgia, there are criteria for the diagnosis of your myofascial pain syndrome.

What Is Myofascial Pain?

The pain intensity of myofascial disorders can vary from painless decreases in range of motion about your arms, legs, neck, and lower back, which are common in older individuals, to pain that is agonizing and incapacitating. (D.G. Simons, et al. *Travell & Simons' Myofascial Pain and Dysfunction: The Trigger Point Manual.* Atlanta: Lippincott Williams and Wilkins, 1999)

This latter type of pain is seen if you are young and are extremely active. If you have a severe attack of myofascial pain, the pain may be so severe that it can cause you to fall to the floor. Pain related to myofascial pain syndrome can be as severe as that caused by a heart attack or by kidney stones. On the other hand, you need to realize that myofascial pain is not life threatening. However, the pain can be severe enough to cause you to lie in bed until the pain is gone. Myofascial pain can decrease your activities of daily living and if it becomes chronic, can be a major cause of time lost at work. The good news is that most myofascial pain can be relieved with an appropriate diagnosis and specific treatment tailored to your gender, age, and overall medical condition.

In 1843, painful areas around muscles called "muscle callouses" were described. The doctor who identified these tender spots reported that the areas felt like a rope cord or a wide band. In the latter 1800s, it was thought that this muscle pain was associated with rheumatism.

In 1904, fibrositis was a term used to describe inflammation of muscles. The muscles were noted to be hard to touch, and by the scientist who reported these findings thought that the pain was due to inflammation of the muscle tissue. Some health-care providers still use the different term fibromyositis.

In 1938, a doctor reported that pressing on the tender spots in a patient's muscle(s) could cause the individual to experience pain in other areas that were remote from the tender points. Before 1938, medical investigators did not realize that the pain was referred to areas distant from the tender spots. To define areas of the referred pain, the scientist injected saline or saltwater into areas that were painful (the volume of fluid induced pain).

He then observed an individual's complaints of pain and established referred pain patterns that were related to an individual's trigger points. In 1942, Dr. Travell emphasized that referred pain to areas away from the trigger point was evident if a patient had a myofascial pain syndrome. (D.G. Simons, et al. *Travell & Simons' Myofascial Pain and Dysfunction: The Trigger Point Manual.* Atlanta: Lippincott Williams and Wilkins, 1999)

It was not until 1973 that scientists took biopsies of muscle tissues from areas of myofascial trigger points. Researchers reported abnormalities in the muscle tissue. Because it is known that there is an abnormality in your muscle tissue if you have muscle pain syndrome and that palpation of these areas causes you to have referred pain, the term "myofascial trigger points" is now used to define your painful areas throughout your body.

Myofascial trigger points occur when there is trauma to your muscle or prolonged tension to your muscle from slouching over a desk or slouching over a work table. This slouching results in disruption of the muscle cell. When your muscle cell becomes disrupted, your cell releases calcium. Calcium released inside of the muscle cell stimulates another contraction of your muscle. The prolonged contraction will exceed the available oxygen, glucose, and other nutrients that are needed for the energy to allow your muscle to continue to contract. With a sustained contraction, you run out of oxygen as well as other nutrients. This allows your muscle cell to build up a substance called lactic acid.

Lactic acid is seen when your body does not have sufficient oxygen. This substance then causes your body to produce pain-causing substances such as *prostaglandins.* These pain transmitters then stimulate nerve endings around your muscle cells. These nerve endings go to other structures in your body. This is why you notice a referred pain pattern when you have a myofascial pain syndrome. You will notice nodular, ropelike bands under your painful muscles when you have myofascial pain syndrome. The lack of oxygen in your muscle tissue will cause some of your muscle cells to die. This will cause scar tissue to form around your muscles. This scar tissue gives you the nodular feeling when you press over these painful areas.

Not all pain in your muscles is from myofascial pain. Sometimes arthritis can cause muscle pain surrounding your joints. Myopathy is a disease of muscles that can occur and cause you to have muscle pain. If you have a disc herniation, you can have referred pain to your muscles as well. Rocky Mountain Spotted Fever or Lyme disease can also cause you to have muscle pain.

Diagnosing Myofascial Pain Syndrome

A myofascial trigger point in your muscle needs to be distinguished from tender areas around your ligaments as well as around your bone. The diagnosis of your myofascial pain syndrome is made by your health-care provider's history and physical examination and expertise. No laboratory tests are useful for the diagnosis of this syndrome. (D.G. Simons, et al. *Travell & Simons' Myofascial Pain and Dysfunction: The Trigger Point Manual.* Atlanta: Lippincott Williams and Wilkins, 1999)

If you have the myofascial pain syndrome, you will complain of localized muscle pain and tenderness as well as the referred pain. If you have myofascial trigger points around your head and neck, you may complain of headaches as well as problems with your vision. Remember that you can have myofascial trigger points in one muscle or many muscles.

To make a diagnosis of myofascial trigger points, you must have the presence of painful areas on examination. These painful areas must be nodular and must be reproducible. Different amounts of pressure from your examining health-care provider will give you trigger point referred pain. Your doctor will record whether you have a "jump sign." This means that when your doctor applies pressure on your trigger point, you jump away from the pressure. Your health-care provider will usually notice a twitch around the area that has had pressure applied to it. At the time of your examination, your health-care provider will notice that your pain diminishes with stretching or injection of your muscle with local anesthetics.

Your trigger points are classified as either active or latent. Your active trigger point causes you to have pain at the time of palpation. The latent trigger point on the other hand does not cause you to have pain at rest but can cause you to have restriction of movement around a certain part of your body and will cause weakness of the muscle that has the trigger point. Remember that we described a latent trigger point that can persist for years after recovery from an injury. However, this latent trigger point will predispose you to have attacks of pain with overuse of your muscle. Sometimes in cold weather, your muscle will contract and cause you to have pain. Remember, only the active trigger points cause you pain. The latent trigger points, if they do become active, cause you to suffer some degree of pain.

Normal muscles do not have trigger points that can be felt. You should feel your normal muscles. Normal muscles have no ropelike, nodular areas or tender areas to pressure and exhibit no observable twitch when the muscle is palpated by your health-care provider. Furthermore, you will not have referred pain with this applied pressure. You can have different degrees of severity of myofascial pain. Some trigger points are much more sensitive than others. An extremely sensitive trigger point can cause you to have greater referred nerve pain than a less-severe or less-intense trigger point. Myofascial pain is usually not symmetrical on either side of your body. However, medical conditions that cause muscle pain such as fibromyalgia are symmetrical.

Usually, patients come to their doctor with complaints due to the most recent active trigger point. When this trigger point has been eliminated, you may have other active or latent trigger points. These trigger points must also be inactivated. Usually the most severe trigger point is manifest. In other words, you can have three trigger points but the most severe trigger point is the one that actives the pain processing center in your brain. After this trigger point has been eliminated, the next most severe trigger point will be appreciated value. The three trigger points were always there but you concentrated on the more severe trigger point. This is why you have "movement" of your trigger points. Usually when your trigger point returns, it will return to the same areas that have been treated.

Trigger points are usually activated by overuse of your muscle. You stretch your muscle beyond its normal capability, which will cause your muscle to become injured. (D.G. Simons, et al. *Travell & Simons' Myofascial Pain and Dysfunction: The Trigger Point Manual.* Atlanta: Lippincott Williams and Wilkins, 1999) Bleeding can occur within your muscle tissue, which will cause scar formation in your muscle. Active trigger points can develop in your muscles following excessive, repetitive, or sustained motions. For example, if you work in a warehouse and load heavy boxes all day over months, you can begin to develop active trigger points.

Be aware that emotional stress can cause the formation of trigger points. Remember that stress causes your muscles to stay in a contracted state. When your muscles are contracted for a length of time as previously stated, you lose oxygen and other nutrients to your muscle tissues. This is the reason that you must attempt to relax and do the breathing exercises and range-of-motion exercises recommend in Chapter 10. You must take control of your myofascial pain. Use heat if you develop myofascial pain. The application of cold can decrease your active myofascial trigger points. However, you should not use cold packs more than two days because chilling can contract your muscles and cause your myofascial pain to become worse.

Your active trigger points can vary in pain severity from hour by hour or from day by day. The stress required to produce pain is variable. Again, if you are under much stress, it does not take much muscle stress to produce myofascial pain. The amount of stress that is needed to make your latent trigger become an active trigger point depends on your degree of conditioning of your muscles and your exercise tolerance as well. If you do not exercise and do aerobic activity and are under a lot of stress, you have susceptibility to develop active trigger points. If your muscle is stiff, avoid placing cold packs on a muscle that may already be contracted. Viral illnesses can cause muscle pain. If you have a virus, do not put cold packs on your muscles.

Your myofascial pain will outlast any precipitating traumatic event. The pain duration is longer in duration than the muscle strain duration. The problem exists that when you were injured, your muscles have developed a way of trying to prevent further pain. In doing so, these other muscles will cause your injured muscle to be protected. Eventually your active trigger points will become latent. If you rest your muscle and use a splint or an elastic bandage, your active trigger point may revert to become a latent trigger point. Occasionally you may do an activity that will activate your latent trigger point.

Many of your muscles around your active trigger point can decrease their function, causing your muscles to become weak. If enough of your muscles lose a significant portion of their function, you can develop weakness.

You should remember that your pain is frequently caused by pressure over your muscles. When you are lying in bed, you may have some pressure on your body in the area of the trigger points from your mattress. This pressure from your bed can cause you to have pain. On the other hand, be aware that sleep disturbances can cause your muscles to contract and become stiff and can worsen your myofascial pain syndrome. When this happens, consult your doctor as to whether you should be prescribed sleep aids. At times, melatonin before retiring at night can enhance your sleep.

Active Trigger Points

You should attempt to avoid allowing your painful muscles to become stiff while you are at work or doing recreational activities. To decrease the change of stiffness, you must do range of motion lightly using the muscle. For example, if you have myofascial pain in your shoulder, do range of motion around your shoulder without a weight in your hand. Your muscle stiffness can increase the painful muscle with inactivity. Therefore, when you wake up in the morning, do range-of-motion exercises. Stretch the contracted muscle. If your pain is in your arm, neck, or shoulder, be aware that this extremity can become weak. Also be aware that you could unexpectedly drop an object from your hand. If you are picking up an expensive vase, for example, use both hands.

When you have an injured muscle and if you go to pick up an object, your brain through the spinal cord has developed a protective mechanism to keep you from injuring your muscle further. This is the reason why you will occasionally drop an object. This is another reason why you will become weak if you are suffering from the myofascial pain syndrome. If your weakness persists in the extremity, concentrate on using the other extremity until the pain in your affected extremity has resolved.

If you have active trigger points when your health-care provider examines you, your health-care provider will stretch your muscles. A slight stretch of your activated trigger point may provide you with some relief. However, a further stretch can cause you to have an increase in your pain. As your muscles become further stretched, they may go into spasm. The spasm will block any further lengthening of your muscle. Your health-care provider will examine your muscle strength. If you have myofascial pain, your pain will be increased when your muscle contracted against resistance. Sometimes when you have pain in the area of your myofascial trigger points, you can develop goose flesh as well as sweating and sometimes discoloration. This is due to increased activity of nerves that go to your blood vessels and sweat glands called sympathetic nerve fibers. (D.G. Simons, et al. *Travell & Simons' Myofascial Pain and Dysfunction: The Trigger Point Manual.* Atlanta: Lippincott Williams and Wilkins, 1999)

If your health-care provider does not notice spasms of your muscle, this individual may snap your muscle to see if you truly have a myofascial trigger point. This essentially amounts to pinching and pulling your muscle up. When this happens, usually your muscle will demonstrate a visible muscle twitch. This muscle response can also be seen if you have latent trigger points.

You can have pain in the skin over the muscle. When your doctor attempts to roll your skin over your painful area, you may have significant pain. If your health-care provider is knowledgeable in the pathology of trigger points, your health-care provider will know that this is an infrequent observation but can occur. Furthermore, it does not mean that you have a psychological problem.

No blood tests show any abnormalities attributed to a myofascial pain syndrome. X-rays, MRI images, and CT scans have not demonstrated any changes that can be associated with myofascial trigger points either active or latent. There have been no reported electromyographic

(EMG) changes when you have a myofascial pain syndrome. However, the needle tip can touch a trigger point that can elicit a twitch which will be manifest on the EMG screen.

There is conflicting information on temperature changes associated with myofascial trigger points. Some investigators have noted that your temperature can be decreased over the area of the trigger point. (D.G. Simons, et al. *Travell & Simons' Myofascial Pain and Dysfunction: The Trigger Point Manual.* Atlanta: Lippincott Williams and Wilkins, 1999) However, for some reason, other investigators have noted increased temperature in the area of your trigger points. The reason for the discrepancy in these findings remains unknown at the present time.

Any serious sports injuries that you may have had years ago must be noted as well as any work-related injuries. Do you remember lifting a heavy box at work? You may have had some pain in your back following this injury. Usually this type of pain will go away. However, you may have trigger points that have been present in your body. However, if you have not stretched some of these muscles, you may not have experienced any pain since your original injury. However, if you go out and do something that you don't do daily such as twisting in a garden and moving rocks, you may use previous muscles that were injured years ago. These motions of your body can trigger the onset of a myofascial pain syndrome. Medical disease can cause you to have muscle pain. This is the reason why your health-care provider must take a detailed medical history from you.

Latent Trigger Points

The muscles of your skeleton are collectively the largest organ of your body. These muscles account for approximately 40 percent of your total body weight. You have approximately 696 muscles in your body. (D.G. Simons, et al. *Travell & Simons' Myofascial Pain and Dysfunction: The Trigger Point Manual.* Atlanta: Lippincott Williams and Wilkins, 1999) The problem is that any one of these muscles can develop pain. What is even worse is that any of these muscles can cause you to have referred pain. Your muscles receive minimal attention in medical textbooks. And as stated before your muscles are collectively the largest organ in your body; and if any part of this muscular organ can cause you to have pain, be aware that myofascial pain is a common occurrence.

As you move your muscles around daily, the muscle tissue itself is subject to wear and tear. Myofascial trigger point areas are common and can significantly increase your activity of daily living. Myofascial pain can even cause you to miss work if it is severe. The first part of this chapter mentioned that a previous injury could cause you to have current manifestations of myofascial pain. The areas of pain that are now manifest from a previous injury are called latent myofascial trigger points. Be aware that latent trigger points are more common than more recent active trigger points. A previous study examined 200 adults who had no history of pain. On examination, scientists found latent trigger points in the neck and shoulder muscles of 54 percent of women and 45 percent of men. Referred pain to other sites of the body was demonstrated in 5 percent of all the subjects collectively.

Further studies have demonstrated that the greatest number of trigger points occur between ages 31 and 50. When you are over 50, maximum activity will cause you to suffer from myofascial pain. As you continue to age and reduce your activity as a result of pain, your range of motion as a result of latent trigger points will become manifest. Many health-care providers are aware of myofascial trigger points. Chiropractors treat myofascial trigger points, as do physical therapists. Acupunturists, anesthesiologists, dentists, pediatricians, rheumatologists, and specialists in physical medicine and rehabilitation all treat myofascial pain syndrome. The manner in which each of these health-care providers treats myofascial pain will vary from each of the health-care provider specialties.

Myofascial Pain vs. Fibromyalgia

As stated previously, a myofascial pain syndrome is a distinct entity from fibromyalgia and other pain syndromes. There are different signs but the same symptoms. Myofascial pain was recognized approximately 200 years ago. In the 1800s, doctors noted that some of their patients had tender areas that they noted by pressing on the muscles around the neck, back, arms, and legs.

Following his PT boat injury in World War II, John F. Kennedy who went on to become president of the United States, was treated by Dr. Travell. John F. Kennedy had significant neck and back pain as a result of commanding a PT boat that was struck by an enemy ship. John F. Kennedy sustained muscle injuries as well as other injuries as a result of this accident. Dr. Travell noted that John F. Kennedy had areas throughout his body that when touched or when pressed upon caused him to have significant pain. (D.G. Simons, et al. *Travell & Simons' Myofascial Pain and Dysfunction: The Trigger Point Manual.*

Atlanta: Lippincott Williams and Wilkins, 1999) She first reported that he was suffering from "tender points" throughout his body. However, as time progressed, she noted that his condition was chronic. She also noted that if she pressed deeply into his muscle tissue that he would have pain that was referred to other areas about his body.

Eventually the term "tender points" was changed to "trigger points" because palpation of the muscle would elicit referred pain elsewhere in the body. (D.G. Simons, et al. *Travell & Simons' Myofascial Pain and Dysfunction: The Trigger Point Manual.* Atlanta: Lippincott Williams and Wilkins, 1999) For example, if you suffer from a myofascial pain syndrome, if your doctor presses on one of your painful areas in your shoulder for example, you may have referred pain that actually goes to your neck. Your health-care providers will frequently refer to this book to determine whether your referred pain pattern corresponds with one of these trigger points that these doctors have mapped out.

If you suffer from the myofascial pain syndrome and if you are receiving adequate treatment for this syndrome, you will know that the diagnosis of myofascial pain syndrome needs to be accurate for you to receive the appropriate treatment. For example, traction on your spine could increase your myofascial pain but improve your pain if you have a disc herniation. Your chiropractor, doctor, or physical therapist may make the diagnosis of a myofascial pain syndrome. Your may note that you have areas in your body that are nodular like a rope and painful and if you press on these nodular areas it causes you to have pain. Your diagnosis is made by your health-care provider following a detailed medical history of your pain as well as an examination of your body.

A detailed history must be obtained from you by your doctor. Because other painful syndromes such as fibromyalgia can cause muscle pain, you must keep a pain diary of how your pain occurred, where your pain is located, and how severe your pain is. You must keep your diary information as to whether your pain stays in an isolated area or whether your pain moves in areas throughout your body. If you have had a motor-vehicle injury at some time in your life, you must tell your doctor. For example, you may have had a whiplash injury 2 to 10 years ago. You may not have noticed significant muscle pain following the injury. However, with a muscle stretching, injury can become evident and can now cause you daily pain.

You must remember that in myofascial pain you will have a history of a sudden onset of pain following a stressful event to your muscles. You can have a gradual onset if you are doing chronic manual lifting. On the other hand, with fibromyalgia, the pain will be gradual and will be on both sides of your body, whereas your pain from your myofascial pain syndrome will be on one side. Remember that you will have tight ropelike bands in your muscles if you have myofascial pain but will have normal muscle tone if you have fibromyalgia.

Treatment for Myofascial Pain

Your health-care provider will determine what is the best treatment for you following a detailed history and medical examination. Different types of treatment can be used to treat your myofascial pain syndrome. As with other tissues in your body, the muscles in your injured area go through different changes. If your muscle has direct trauma to it, it can develop some scar tissue around your injured muscle. These developing scars will limit your muscle's ability to either contract further or relax. This phenomena can result in a shortened, weakened muscle. If you sustained a sprained ankle, you may have been placed in a brace. You will then have disuse of your muscles, which can cause your muscles to shrink in size, called atrophy.

If you had a fracture of one of your bones, you may have been placed in a cast by your doctor for six to eight weeks. The muscles around the injured joint under the cast will become weak. As you attempt to regain strength in the muscles, you may experience the onset of trigger points. Therefore, your therapist will need to do stretching exercises and conditioning exercises to help you regain strength and eliminate any active or latent trigger points that may be present. In addition to strengthening and stretching exercises, your therapist may want to apply moist heat over your muscle pain. On occasion your therapist may progress the heat to ultrasound, which is a deeper application of heat. On occasion a massage may help to loosen your muscles. Your therapist may want to do deep, vigorous massage to break up any scar that has developed around your muscle tissue. This form of massage is called myofascial release therapy. Whatever method is chosen, the choice of treatment is usually based on the location of your myofascial trigger point and the sensitivity of the pain over the muscle. The choice of treatment is also based on the expertise of your clinician.

A technique called spray and stretch is sometimes used to decrease myofascial pain. The spray-and-stretch technique involves stretching painful muscle while using a cold spray. This cold spray is a *vapocoolant* and decreases the pain conduction in muscles from the pain fiber nerve endings. Furthermore, this vapocoolant helps muscles to relax. This form of therapy can provide you with immediate relief of your pain. However, when you go home you will need to stretch your muscles yourself. This type of therapy is used for mildly painful myofascial pain. The vapocoolant releases a jet stream of a substance. The vapocoolant is applied in sweeps in different directions around the entire length of your muscle. It is directed toward the area of your referred pain. The stretch-and-spray technique is used until your muscle length is back to normal. Because the vapocoolant can cause your muscles to contract, your therapist or chiropractor may immediately apply moist hot packs. These hot packs will rewarm your skin and help you to relax your muscles. After your muscles have been relaxed and rewarmed, the spray and stretch can be repeated. Your therapist or chiropractor will do several cycles of stretch as well as relaxation.

If you still complain of pain and have active trigger points, you may be a candidate to have ischemic compression massage. This type of massage consists of applying a local force to tissues surrounding your trigger point and then releasing it. This maneuver will cause some inflammation around your trigger point. This inflammation will cause your blood vessels to increase in caliber and will increase blood flow to your injured muscle. By increasing your blood flow, you will have an increase in oxygen, glucose, and other nutrients necessary for normal muscle function. This type of therapy is usually used in conjunction with injections of numbing medicine into your painful areas.

Trigger point injections administered by your doctor into your muscles can relax your muscles. The volume of fluid that goes into your muscle tissue is anywhere from one to three milliliters. This volume of fluid can disrupt the scar that has formed around and within your muscles. Some doctors do not inject any local anesthetic or steroid into your muscle. They use what is called a dry-needle technique. They think that insertion of the needle into your muscle can break up some of the scar around the muscle itself. Injection therapy into your trigger points can provide you with significant relief. The procedure is usually done with you in a lying position. The procedure consists of using a small needle about the size of an acupuncture needle. Your skin is cleansed with alcohol prior to injection therapy. The small needle is injected into your trigger point. At that time, you receive a small volume of local anesthetic. Some doctors mix a local anesthetic with a steroid. The numbing medicine relaxes your muscle and decreases the pain so that your physical therapist can spray and stretch the muscle back to its original length. The steroid works to take the inflammation out of your muscle cells.

Following injection therapy, your therapist will do spray and stretch. Following the spray and stretch, hot packs will be used to heat the cold muscle from the spray technique. After this is done, your physical therapist will have you move your muscle through its complete range of motion. It is always important that you have a stretching maneuver following your trigger point. Some practitioners use saline or saltwater to inject your muscle. The purpose of the saltwater is to break up the scar around your muscle. Occasionally your doctor will inject you with a long-acting numbing medicine called bupivacaine or marcaine. Etidocaine (Duranest) can also be used and can give you pain relief for up to seven days after the procedure.

Acupuncture is another method that can be extremely valuable in the treatment of your myofascial pain syndrome. (B. Goldberg. *Alternative Medicine, The Definitive Guide*. Berkeley: Celestial Arts, 2001) Acupuncture does not use numbing medicines or steroids. Remember that you can be allergic to some numbing medicines as well as steroids. The acupuncture needle tip can break up some of the scar around your muscle tissues. Furthermore, placement of the acupuncture needle can stimulate your body's productions of endorphins and other natural chemicals that you have stored within your body to decrease your pain. Acupuncture therapy has been shown to be an extremely viable treatment of a myofascial pain syndrome.

If you continue to have significant pain associated with your myofascial pain syndrome, another method that can decrease your pain is a botulism toxin injection into your painful muscle. This botulism toxin (Botox) is a gram-negative bacteria. In small doses it can relax or even paralyze small muscle fibers. The relief of the Botox can last up to three months. The problem with the Botox injection is that some individuals develop what appears to be fever and generalized joint pain associated with the bacteria that gets into their bloodstream.

Sometimes inflammation of your muscle cells can cause you to have pain. Overexertion will lead to a certain degree of inflammation around your muscle cells. For this reason, nonsteroidal anti-inflammatory drugs can decrease your pain. You will probably only need these medications for several days to a week. Over-the-counter ibuprofen is an effective treatment for your muscle pain. Remember that nonsteroidal anti-inflammatory drugs can potentially cause you ulcers. Another drug that you may be prescribed by your doctor is a muscle relaxant. Muscle relaxants can significantly decrease your pain. However, these drugs can cause drowsiness, and some of them can cause you to become weak.

With respect to gender specificity, it appears that men suffer more from acute myofascial pain, whereas women suffer more from latent myofascial pain syndromes. Latent myofascial trigger points are more prevalent in women who are not active with respect to aerobic exercise. On the other hand, active trigger points are more prevalent in men who are doing vigorous exercises or who are doing heavy manual labor. (R. Melzack and P. Wall, *Handbook of Pain Management a Clinical Companion of Textbook of Pain*. New York: Churchill Livingstone, 2003) Future research continues with respect to the treatment of your myofascial pain syndrome.

For Men

- Use vapocoolant with a spray-and-stretch technique on your affected painful muscles to relieve the soreness and pain.
- Acupuncture could be an effective way to stimulate and release endorphins and other chemicals in your body that can reduce your pain.
- You can try compression massage directly on your painful areas to improve blood flow to your muscles and help relieve some of your pain.
- Trigger point injections can relax your muscles and therefore relieve some of your pain. Your doctor may even want to inject a steroid or local anesthetic to relieve your pain, depending on your specific symptoms.
- Botox injections can relax or paralyze small muscle fibers in your painful areas and temporarily reduce or relieve your pain.
- Take nonsteroidal anti-inflammatory medications such as ibuprofen to reduce your muscle inflammation.

For Women

- Use vapocoolant with a spray-and-stretch technique on your affected painful muscles to relieve the soreness and pain.
- Acupuncture could be an effective way to stimulate and release endorphins and other chemicals in your body that can reduce your pain.
- You can try compression massage directly on your painful areas to improve blood flow to your muscles and help relieve some of your pain.
- Trigger point injections can relax your muscles and therefore relieve some of your pain. Your doctor may even want to inject a steroid or local anesthetic to relieve your pain, depending on your specific symptoms.
- Botox injections can relax or paralyze small muscle fibers in your painful areas and temporarily reduce or relieve your pain.
- Take nonsteroidal anti-inflammatory medications such as ibuprofen to reduce your muscle inflammation.

Chapter 22
Understanding Facial Pain

Neuralgias or pathology of the nerves of the face has been recognized for centuries. These types of pain, especially trigeminal neuralgia, can be some of the most severe pain that you could ever experience. The pain associated with trigeminal neuralgia has been well defined.

Sometimes your facial pain can be idiopathic, which means that there is not a defined cause for your pain. There can be an area of maximum pain in your upper or lower lip. When this area is stimulated by washing your face, talking, or opening and closing your mouth, your pain can be severe. (J.D. Loeser. *Bonica's Management of Pain*. n.p.: Lippincott Williams and Wilkins, 2001) It may last a few seconds to several minutes. If you go untreated, the pain can progress to become severe. You may drool from your mouth. As your pain gets worse, you will be unwilling to open or close your mouth or touch the area that triggers your pain.

This chapter will teach you about some of the forms of facial pain, such as temporomandibular joint pain (TMJ), trigeminal neuralgia, and other general facial pains. You will learn how facial pain is diagnosed and treated as well.

Temporomandibular Joint Pain (TMJ)

A common type of pain syndrome is pain related to temporal mandibular joint disorders. (J.D. Loeser. *Bonica's Management of Pain*. n.p.: Lippincott Williams and Wilkins, 2001) This usually involves the joint between your lower jaw, which is called the mandible, and your temporal bone, which is called your maxilla. When these two bones meet, they form a joint.

If you have a temporal mandibular joint (TMJ) disorder, you will probably be referred to an individual who has expertise in this area. This health-care provider will examine the movements of your jaw, your muscles around your jaw, your ligaments, and the way your teeth align. If your pain appears to be related to your TMJ, your specialist will determine whether your problem is within your joint or outside of the joint. This is an important diagnosis because the treatment differs.

Problems outside of your temporal joint are usually related to the muscles that are used to chew. A thorough examination is necessary because your teeth can cause pain to be referred to your face. A third molar, for example, can refer pain to your ear. If you have a history of arthritis, you can have joint problems within your TMJ. You can have dislocations of the small discs within your TMJ. This can result in inflammation as well as dysfunction of your joint and cause persistent and chronic inflammation, which in turn will cause you to have chronic pain.

If you do suffer from TMJ, you usually have many problems, including the following:

- Misalignment of your teeth
- Emotional stress
- Poor body mechanics
- A history of generalized myofascial pain

Because many factors can cause you to have TMJ, a multidisciplinary approach to the management of your pain is usually indicated. This will include a dental specialist, a doctor, and a psychologist.

Understanding TMJ

To understand TMJ pain, you should have some knowledge of the anatomy of this joint and how it works. This joint is a true joint. It is composed of cartilage. This type of cartilage in your TMJ can regenerate. Your TMJ is involved in mouth movement. Within your TMJ, you have a disc. Your joint is stabilized by muscles around your joint. The muscles that are involved in chewing that exist around the TMJ are also responsible for TMJ functioning.

Your jaw movement is both up and down as well as some lateral movement. These movements are involved in chewing. You can develop myofascial pain in any of the muscles involved in chewing. You can develop pain of extra-articular origin. This means that your pain is outside of your TMJ joint. If one of your chewing muscles dysfunctions, you can have pain around your joint. If you have myofascial pain, you have trigger areas which are zones of hypersensitivity located within the spasmodic muscle. If you or your health-care provider provides a direct, constant pressure on the trigger area, it can cause pain that is referred to other areas about your jaw. If this happens, your pain can be treated with a trigger point injection consisting of a local anesthetic usually combined with a steroid.

The muscles that you use to chew can refer pain to your teeth and gums. Pain from some of the muscles can be referred to your upper teeth. If you have muscle pain at the angle of your lower jawbone, your pain can travel upward to the outer ring of your eye. Other muscles involved in chewing can refer pain to the sides of your head. Sometimes heat and muscle relaxants can relieve some of your pain.

TMJ from Psychological Causes

Your TMJ muscle pain can originate from psychological causes. Stress, which can cause you to grind your teeth, leading to dental irritation, can cause your muscles to become overactive. This can cause your muscles around your jaw to become spasmodic and can fatigue easily.

If you have TMJ, you will complain of pain as well as have muscle spasms and clicking of your TMJ. This will result in limited motion on attempting to open your mouth. If you are under significant emotional stress, you may clench your teeth especially at night. This can increase the pressure within your TMJ, which can cause you to have abnormal TMJ movement.

You must remember that psychological symptoms such as depression and anxiety occur more among females than males. Also remember that depression and anxiety are associated with increased pain symptoms. Psychological or emotional distress causes more pain symptom reports and also increases the severity of pain. Because females can have greater emotional distress than males, they are predisposed to increased pain associated with TMJ. You also need to be aware that female TMJ patients have a greater need for treatment of their symptoms than males. Depression has been associated with greater pain severity among females, whereas depression causes more activity impairment in males. However, levels of anxiety are associated with increased pain severity. Anxiety can cause greater pain disability in males.

Studies published as early as 1973 reported greater sensitivity to painful stimuli in individuals with TMJ when compared to the general healthy population. (J.D. Loeser. *Bonica's Management of Pain.* n.p.: Lippincott Williams and Wilkins, 2001) These findings supported the idea that changes in your central nervous system pain regulation could contribute to the onset of your TMJ pain. This report is important because a greater sensitivity to pain among females, who because of sex differences are associated with an increased risk of developing TMJ. Females have been reported to develop greater jaw pain than males after experimental jaw clenching.

Your ability to control your pain using your body's own opioid system may be gender specific. Beta endorphins in males can inhibit some types of pain that are not seen in females. (R.B. Fillingham. *Sex, Gender, and Pain*. n.p.: IASP Press, 2000) This data tells us that there are differences in pain regulatory systems in females than in males. For example, if you are female and have decreased beta endorphins, you are more prone to develop pain.

You must realize that fibromyalgia is more common in individuals with TMJ than in the general population. Almost 20 percent of TMJ patients meet the criteria for fibromyalgia. However, 75 percent of fibromyalgia patients may have TMJ. Irritable bowel syndrome occurs more commonly if you have TMJ. (J.D. Loeser. *Bonica's Management of Pain*. n.p.: Lippincott Williams and Wilkins, 2001)

Depression is more common in TMJ than in the healthy population. In 1996, and again in 1998, it was reported that TMJ may be a result of stress-related disorders that are characterized by your pain. (J.D. Loeser. *Bonica's Management of Pain*. n.p.: Lippincott Williams and Wilkins, 2001) Be aware that if you have chronic pain, you have a 60 percent chance of having a relative who suffers from chronic pain as well. Therefore if one of your parents or an older brother or sister has a history of TMJ, you may be at risk as well for developing this disorder.

TMJ from an Abnormal Mouth Bite

If you have an abnormal mouth bite, you can develop pain in your TMJ joint. When your teeth are properly aligned, especially during chewing, your muscles will be of a normal tone. If you have an abnormal bite, your muscles around your jaw can develop areas of spasm. Sometimes your muscles that are involved in chewing fail to relax. This muscle behavior causes you to have myofascial trigger points in your muscles involved with chewing. Not only will you have pain in your muscles and your TMJ, you will also eventually have TMJ dysfunction. Your dental specialist can make a special orthotic device for you that can be placed intermittently which will allow your jaw muscles to relax. This modality will ultimately decrease your myofascial trigger points.

Studies have been done to evaluate the muscles involved in TMJ pain. Most of the muscles that you use to chew can cause you to have pain around your TMJ. Furthermore, if you have TMJ, you can have ringing in your ears and hearing loss as well as pain around your ear. Heat and massage as well as analgesic medications can reduce your TMJ pain. You may want to try a soft diet for a while as well as use nonsteroidal anti-inflammatory medications. Alternating heat packs with ice packs can be of benefit as well. You should also do self-relaxation techniques.

TMJ from Your Nervous Habits

Your nervous habits can result in TMJ pain as well. Do you chew your fingernails or chew on a pencil eraser or have any other habit that keeps your jaw in a forward position for a prolonged period of time? These maneuvers can cause you to have abnormalities that exist in your muscles and can ultimately cause you to have myofascial pain. If you have an occupation in which you talk on a telephone for a significant amount of time, use a headset. There have been reports of TMJ pain related to individuals holding their telephone on their shoulder for hours at a time. These maneuvers compress some of your muscles, leading to myofascial pain and trigger points. It has been shown that women are more prone to TMJ than men.

TMJ from Worn Out Discs

The discs in your joints can displace or wear out and cause you TMJ pain. This is called intra-articular TMJ pain. If your disc is displaced forward, you may develop clicking, popping noises when you open and close your mouth. You can also have pain as well as limitation of your jaw movement. Over time you will develop wear-and-tear changes, leading to osteoarthritis of your joint. The capsule around your TMJ can become inflamed as well as deranged.

You should keep a diary as to when your jaw clicks when you open your mouth. The clicking can occur early or late depending on your jaw-opening position. If your disc is dislocated forward, a chronic problem around your joint can occur. You can injure the ligaments around your joint as well as cause further degenerative changes around your TMJ. These changes can be observed on x-ray. When you get to this point, you will have pain and limited opening of your mouth on the affected side. You will have difficulty eating some foods such as an apple. The disc in your TMJ will not return to its normal position and over time degenerative arthritis called osteoarthritis can occur. This arthritis occurs after prolonged displacement of your TMJ disc. Your pain is most severe with wide opening of your mouth.

A family history of disc displacement may have an effect on the inheritance of TMJ. There is a higher incidence of TMJ among family members of TMJ patients who have a displaced disc in the joint as compared to TMJ patients who do not have a disc displacement.

TMJ from Inhibitory System Impairment

In the central nervous system there are areas that exist in the spinal cord and the brain that inhibit painful impulses from reaching the pain center in your brain. It is possible that TMJ may be associated with impairment in your inhibitory system. (J.D. Loeser. *Bonica's Management of Pain*. n.p.: Lippincott Williams and Wilkins, 2001) This allows pain impulses from your jaw to reach your brain without being filtered or decreased in intensity. If you have a decrease in your inhibition in your spinal cord, you will have exaggerated responses to both painful stimuli and psychological stimuli. For some reason, increased pain sensitivity throughout the body is more prevalent in patients with TMJ. The enhanced pain sensitivity noted among patients with TMJ was done in a clinical laboratory setting.

TMJ Pain Related to Stress

TMJ patients in general have a lower pain threshold than normal subjects for an unknown reason. TMJ patients in general can have more physical and psychological symptoms of stress. TMJ individuals report greater stress than healthy individuals. This finding is important because stress can cause you to clench your teeth. This clenching of teeth can affect your muscles for chewing as well as your TMJ joint. Tests have been done to determine tension in your chewing muscles. This test, called an EMG, has been done in study subjects. In individuals with TMJ there is a noted increase in the muscle tone in some or all of the muscles involved with chewing.

Diagnosing and Treating TMJ

TMJ disorders occur in 12 percent of individuals in the United States. (J.D. Loeser. *Bonica's Management of Pain*. n.p.: Lippincott Williams and Wilkins, 2001) The actual cause of TMJ remains unknown. We have presented different theories of the cause of TMJ. You should note that if you have TMJ, you may have symptoms similar to other chronic pain syndromes. You may have symptoms but not have objective, physiologic findings. Maladaptive behaviors can be seen in TMJ syndromes. If you clench your teeth as a result of stress, you can develop TMJ. If you have TMJ, you may have excessive use of a health-care system. This is because if you have psychological problems, you may focus entirely on your pain. TMJ can be debilitating. There are sex differences in TMJ, with women having a higher percentage of TMJ. (J.D. Loeser. *Bonica's Management of Pain.* n.p.: Lippincott Williams and Wilkins, 2001)

If a health-care provider diagnoses you with TMJ, your diagnosis will consist of three examination categories. Muscle pain with opening of your jaw will be recorded. If you have any displacement of your jaw with range of motion around your jaw, this information will be recorded as well. Your disc function within the joint will be analyzed by your health-care provider as well. Different health-care providers use different criteria to report that you have TMJ. It is a general consensus that you must have pain in order to be diagnosed with TMJ. If you do not have pain associated with your jaw movement, you probably do not have TMJ. Pain is the most important factor for which TMJ patients seek treatment. TMJ can also be seen in children. In children, however, there are no sex differences with regard to frequency of TMJ occurrence.

Both fatigue as well as psychological distress can increase your pain. As time progresses, your pain will become constant. X-rays can identify changes in your TMJ space. Traumatic injuries can also cause you to experience TMJ pain. If you have rheumatoid arthritis, you can develop TMJ pain. Rheumatoid arthritis is usually on both sides of your body, whereas osteoarthritis is usually confined to one side. If you have rheumatoid arthritis, this disease can progress to your TMJs on both sides of your head. In addition to x-rays, you may need a magnetic resonance image (MRI). A CT scan can also be used to examine your TMJ. At the present time MRIs are the most effective tool for diagnosing TMJ problems. (J.D. Loeser. *Bonica's Management of Pain.* n.p.: Lippincott Williams and Wilkins, 2001) Your TMJ specialist can also inject dye into your joint. This injection of dye, called an arthrography, can help diagnose the disc displacement.

As your health-care provider examines you, this individual will examine your facial muscles as well as your TMJ. Remember your muscles, teeth, and TMJ all interact to help you open and close your mouth and to help you chew. Your health-care provider will measure your jaw opening. Furthermore, your health-care provider may inject a local anesthetic into the muscle that may be causing your pain. If you have significant relief, your health-care provider has a diagnosis of the origin of your pain. The injection demonstrated that your muscle was the source of your pain.

If you have a displacement of your TMJ disc, your mouth will deviate to one side as you open your mouth. If you have popping or clicking, this indicates that you have a disc pathology. An important tool for your doctor or dentist to diagnose the source of your pain is with an injection of numbing medicine. If an injection into your TMJ provides you with significant relief, your pain is intra-articular or coming from within the TMJ itself. However, if injection into your muscle provides you with pain relief, this tells your health-care provider that the pain is coming from outside your joint. Furthermore, by injecting around the nerve that goes to your TMJ, this maneuver can provide information as to whether your TMJ is the source of your chronic pain. These injections are safe.

Surgery is sometimes indicated for the management of a TMJ problem. When less-invasive procedures fail to alleviate TMJ pain, oral surgery procedures can be done. These include using a scope to reposition your discs. Your oral surgeon can also remove your discs. Implantations can be done into your TMJ. Using a scope is less invasive than opening your TMJ joint. You need to remember that the most conservative therapies are usually the best therapies.

TMJ Differences in Men and Women

TMJ prevalence peaks between the ages of 25 and 44. After age 44, the chance of you developing TMJ decreases with increasing age. For some reason, female patients who develop TMJ were more likely than males to have chronic pain. Studies have shown that sex is a definite risk for the development of TMJ. TMJ is most noted in women during their reproductive years. The reason for this finding is not known. The problem with doing gender-specific studies on TMJ patients is that only a small number of males actually seek treatment for TMJ. A study in 1994 demonstrated that women have more physical and psychological symptoms with TMJ than males. However, in the study, males had greater psychological-related symptoms.

Studies have also been done to determine whether TMJ psychosocial symptoms were different from women when compared to men.

Higher levels of stress, depression, and anxiety have been reported in the TMJ population in general when compared to healthy individuals who do not suffer from TMJ. In 1996, it was reported that if you suffer from TMJ that you have a higher rate of psychopathology than normal control individuals. You must be aware that psychopathology is strongly associated with generalized muscle pain throughout the body. The psychological disorders reported in TMJ patients are higher in females than males. In other words, females have more depression and anxiety than males. If you have a history of sexual abuse or trauma, you have a higher risk of developing TMJ.

In 1998, it was reported that close to 50 percent of TMJ patients have a history of sexual or physical abuse. (R.B. Fillingham. *Sex, Gender, and Pain.* n.p.: IASP Press, 2000) An abuse history makes you more prone for depression and anxiety. An abuse history in general is associated with increased physical as well as psychological symptoms if you suffer from chronic pain. An abuse history is related to your increased pain complaints as well as your psychological disturbances. Sexual abuse has been noted to be associated with an increased risk of generalized muscle pain in females but not in males. (J.D. Loeser. *Bonica's Management of Pain.* n.p.: Lippincott Williams and Wilkins, 2001) Be aware that females are more often the victims of sexual and physical abuse. As a result, the effect of abuse on pain response is more likely to be noted by females than by males.

The Role of Hormones in TMJ Development and Treatment

Hormones play an important part in your development of TMJ. (J.D. Loeser. *Bonica's Management of Pain.* n.p.: Lippincott Williams and Wilkins, 2001) Your ovarian hormones, if you are a female, can be related to TMJ. A study has examined women with TMJ. The prevalence of TMJ occurs in females during their reproductive years. Note that if you are a female that your ovarian hormones are at their greatest peak during your reproductive years. If you take oral contraceptives or have had estrogen hormone-replacement therapy, you are at an increased risk for developing TMJ. If you use oral contraceptives, your TMJ pain can be worse during your menstrual cycle. If you suffer from premenstrual symptoms, you are more likely to report TMJ than women who do not have any premenstrual symptoms. No one to date knows exactly how sex hormones produce TMJ effects. It is believed that your sex hormones alter pain processing in the nerves in muscles, TMJ joints, gums, and so on. It is interesting to note that estrogen receptors have been defined in the TMJ of animals. No one knows how these receptors affect TMJ. Psychosocial issues are important in the development of TMJ.

Important sex differences exist in the efficacy or treatment for TMJ. The treatment need is higher in women than men. Remember in general that women seek more health care than men. Women in general have more chronic pain severity than men. (J.D. Loeser. *Bonica's Management of Pain*. n.p.: Lippincott Williams and Wilkins, 2001) Female patients are treated more often by oral surgery than males. It is important to note that females have a greater success rate with treatment modalities of TMJ than males. The question that remains to be answered is whether various treatments are gender specific for males and females. Women are twice as likely as men to experience TMJ. It is believed that hormonal factors as well as psychological pathology and social factors contribute to sex differences in the onset of TMJ. Research continues into the effect of ovarian hormones on the cause and treatment of TMJ. Further research into TMJ in general will increase our understanding of this disorder and may lead to improved treatment of this disorder.

Trigeminal Neuralgia

Trigeminal neuralgia is also called tic douloureux. Tic douloureux is defined as a sudden stabbing pain felt in your face. It usually occurs on one side of your face. One of the nerves that supplies sensation to your face is the trigeminal nerve. This is the nerve that comes off of your brain stem. This trigeminal nerve is the cause of your trigeminal neuralgia. If the exit of the trigeminal nerve from your brain stem is depressed by a blood vessel or other tissue, this can be the cause of your pain. Compression of your trigeminal nerve with blood vessels occurs in approximately 80 percent of trigeminal neuralgia.

Sometimes an aneurysm or changes in your bone architecture about the skull can compress your nerve. Multiple sclerosis can contribute to trigeminal neuralgia as well. It is rare for trigeminal neuralgia to occur on both sides of your face but it can happen. Light touch over your face will usually trigger your pain. (J.D. Loeser. *Bonica's Management of Pain*. n.p.: Lippincott Williams and Wilkins, 2001)

The incidence of trigeminal neuralgia is twice that in women as seen in men. (J.D. Loeser. *Bonica's Management of Pain*. n.p.: Lippincott Williams and Wilkins, 2001) Usually the first occurrence will happen when you are 40, and it will usually reach a peak by age 50.

For some reason the right side of the face is affected more often than the left side. There are three branches of the trigeminal nerve. One goes to the area around the forehead and eyes. The second goes to the upper jaw. The third goes to the lower jaw. Sometimes pain will occur in the second and third branches of the trigeminal nerve. However, you must realize that the first branch can also be involved, but it is extremely rare to have this branch involved.

When you have trigeminal neuralgia, your pain will be transient. It can last from seconds to minutes. It can occur daily or sometimes once a week or once a month. Your pain will be like an electric shock. It can be of a stabbing nature as well. Between the episodes of your pain, your sensations over your face should be normal. Your trigeminal neuralgia can last for months. However, these painful episodes can subside, or they can return years later.

Your trigeminal neuralgia usually responds to anticonvulsant medications. Tegretol and Neurontin are two drugs commonly used for the treatment of trigeminal neuralgia. Baclofen and Klonopin can help you as well. Injection of numbing medicine with a steroid into areas around your face that trigger your pain can relieve episodes of trigeminal neuralgia. Opioids are usually not needed for the management of pain, but in extreme cases may become necessary. If these modalities do not relieve your pain, your pain is probably due to trigeminal nerve compression, most often by one of your arteries. Your surgeon may refer you to a neurosurgeon for surgical treatment.

Other Affected Areas

Pain in your mouth and face can come from your teeth, jaws, your temporal mandibular joints, your muscles involved in chewing, and from your salivary glands. Your nose and sinuses can also be a source of pain. Another source of pain is trigeminal neuralgia, which is a pathological state involving your trigeminal nerve. A diagnosis of pain coming from your teeth or jaws can be diagnosed accurately. If you have had recent dental work, hypersensitive teeth from an abscessed nerve root or from a cracked tooth may be localized. This type of pain is aggravated by warm coffee, cold tea, or candy. If your tooth is only cracked, it can cause pain when you bite into something, especially a piece of hard candy. (J.D. Loeser. *Bonica's Management of Pain*. n.p.: Lippincott Williams and Wilkins, 2001) If you have tooth decay that involves the pulp, it can aggravate your pain, but cold can relieve your pain. When the pulp tissue dies, your pain will subside. When you have these symptoms, seek attention from your dentist.

If you develop an abscess and if your abscess becomes severe, you may need surgical drainage of this abscess and antibiotic therapy. An infection from your tooth could spread to other tissues in your mouth and to your neck. If the situation causes you to have significant swelling around the throat, especially your airway, you may have trouble breathing. Your airway can be compromised so severely that you could die.

You are probably aware of a term called a "dry socket." This happens usually after a tooth extraction. It is not uncommon following extraction of one of your wisdom teeth. This dry socket is actually a localized inflammation of the bone where your tooth was removed. This pain can start two or three days after your tooth was removed and can last approximately two weeks.

You can also develop pain that comes from your salivary glands. Your parotid gland as well as other salivary glands can be a site of infection. Furthermore, a small stone can block your parotid duct. Your gland toward the bottom of your face and upper neck can swell. Your pain will increase at the sight or smell of food. Sometimes your swelling and pain can decrease after you eat but can recur following another meal. If your stone remains in the duct, it may have to be removed surgically.

You can experience pain that is called atypical facial and oral pain. This type of pain may be related to psychiatric problems. An example of atypical facial pain is phantom tooth pain in which a tooth has been pulled but the individual still reports complaints of pain in the area of the extracted tooth. If you have phantom tooth pain, your dentist may provide you with fillings or different treatments, none of which will provide you with significant relief in most instances. Your dentist may even extract neighboring teeth. If you have diabetes or have some vitamin deficiencies, you can develop a syndrome that causes you to have a burning mouth as well as a burning tongue. (J.D. Loeser. *Bonica's Management of Pain*. n.p.: Lippincott Williams and Wilkins, 2001) Sometimes psychogenic factors can give you a pain syndrome of this type. Your doctor and dentist will do a thorough physical examination, including x-rays. In many instances, a psychiatric consultation is indicated. Usually the tricylic antidepressants such as Elavil will decrease your pain if you have these symptoms.

If you worry a lot, anxiety can cause chronic facial pain. This type of pain can also be associated with a major life change. If you or someone in your family has become ill or if there has been a death in the family or acute stress, you may develop facial pain. You may also have an increased heart rate as well as headaches and breathing difficulties. With an anxiety reaction, you may notice excessive perspiration. Relaxation techniques can help you manage this type of pain. Relaxation techniques such as meditation, yoga, and biofeedback can help you relieve your pain. Some tranquilizers can also help you with this problem as well. If you have more severe psychiatric conditions, you may also have pain.

Schizophrenia and hypochondriasis or other emotional problems can also cause you to suffer facial pain. As with many of the other pain syndromes in this book, there is no one definable treatment for facial pain, especially atypical facial pain. Your health-care provider will obtain a complete history and do a thorough physical examination with the possibility of other tests before initiating definitive treatment. With this information in mind, you can be an extreme help to your health-care provider by keeping an accurate diary of your pain symptoms.

A stroke can also cause you to have pain in your facial area. Be aware that coronary artery disease can also cause you to have facial pain. If you suffer from this type of pain, nitroglycerin can sometimes relieve it. Remember that the pain from a heart attack can go into your jaw. If you have jaw pain without chest pain or pain in your shoulder or arm, your doctor might fail to consider a heart attack as the cause. If you have had a whiplash injury, one of the nerves off of your cervical spine can send nerve branches to the skin over the angle of your lower jawbone. This type of pain can cause you to have significant sharp pain. On occasional local anesthetics and steroids can be used to decrease this pain. You can have facial pain that has been called atypical facial pain or facial pain of a psychological origin. This type of pain is usually associated with psychiatric symptoms. It can be seen in malingers as well as drug abusers.

Diagnosing a Facial Pain

Diagnosis of oral pain can be difficult. (J.D. Loeser. *Bonica's Management of Pain*. n.p.: Lippincott Williams and Wilkins, 2001) Pain in your mouth and face is common. It is fortunate that in most cases the cause of your pain can be easily determined. However, the anatomy of the area around your face and throat is complex. This is the reason why a diagnosis can be difficult for your doctor. When you have pain in your mouth as well as in your face, the pain comes from nerves that branch off of your brain. These nerves are called cranial nerves. One common cranial nerve frequently involved as a cause of your facial nerve is a major nerve called the trigeminal nerve, which has three branches: ophthalmic, maxillary, and mandibular. Other nerves can also cause you to experience facial pain. Your facial nerves, glossopharyngeal nerve, your vagus nerve, and some cervical nerves go to various parts of your mouth areas and facial areas and can cause you to experience pain.

Your mouth and face receive a lot of pain fibers. As with other pain syndromes, your doctor will obtain a thorough history from you before examining you. This information is extremely helpful in making a diagnosis of your pain. If your pain is coming from a nerve, usually your pain is sharp and stabbing. On the other hand, if your pain is coming from your muscles, it is usually continuous and dull. Pain from your blood vessels is usually of a throbbing nature.

You must explain to your doctor the effect of your pain on your ability to work and perform social activities. If you are suffering from sleep deprivation, tell your doctor. You should try to remember what happened when you developed the pain. Keep a diary of the duration of your pain, how frequently it occurs, and what causes your pain to subside. Also note whether emotional stress worsens your pain. Tell your doctor what treatments in the past have helped your pain if you have had a previous history of this pain. Tell your doctor if you have nasal congestion or if you are producing excessive tears from your eyes. Your doctor will do a complete examination and may obtain blood and urine samples from you. X-rays will be done when indicated. On occasion you may need an MRI to attempt to diagnose the cause of your symptoms.

Treatment for Facial Pain

As you can see TMJ and other facial pains can be relatively mild or they can be totally disabling. In the majority of instances, facial pain can be adequately controlled.

Sometimes an injection of a numbing medicine with steroid into this painful area can decrease the pain. If you have had a previous traumatic event or have had some tissue removed surgically, pathological changes may occur in the area of your trigeminal nerve. Sometimes your trigeminal nerve can compress blood vessels in your face. This can be the cause of a sensation of throbbing pain. If you are younger than 40 years of age, you may develop trigeminal neuralgia, which may be related to an underlying disease such as multiple sclerosis (MS) or a tumor. Another type of pain is glossopharyngeal neuralgia. This type of pain has trigger areas around your tonsils or the back of your throat or even at the base of your tongue. The injection of local anesthetics and steroids will not usually provide you with long-term pain relief. These types of neuralgias usually require the use of anticonvulsant medications.

Carbamazepine has been used for years for the treatment of trigeminal neuralgia, but now a new anticonvulsant medication, gabapentin (Neurontin) can be helpful in alleviating your pain.

Sometimes a radiofrequency heat lesion can be used to destroy the area where your nerves come from your brain to your face. Your neurosurgeon can do surgery within your brain to get your blood vessels away from parts of your trigeminal nerve. In these previous pain conditions, there were no abnormal central nervous system signs. However, you can have facial pain associated with abnormal central nervous system signs. This can be as a result of trauma, infection of bone in your face, or tumors.

For Men

- Steroid injections can help reduce inflammation in your facial joints and muscles.
- Your doctor can inject numbing medications in your painful areas to reduce your pain.
- Anticonvulsant medications prescribed by your doctor such as Carbamazepine and Neurontin can help alleviate your facial pain.
- In extreme cases, your doctor can perform radiofrequency heat lesion to destroy the area where your nerves come from your brain to your face in order to relieve your pain.
- Tricyclic antidepressant medications prescribed by your doctor can help relieve your symptoms of pain, as well as serve as an antidepressant. Different doses will be given depending on which it is being used for.

For Women

- Steroid injections can help reduce inflammation in your facial joints and muscles.
- Your doctor can inject numbing medications in your painful areas to reduce your pain.
- Anticonvulsant medications prescribed by your doctor such as Carbamazepine and Neurontin can help alleviate your facial pain.
- In extreme cases, your doctor can perform radiofrequency heat lesion to destroy the area where your nerves come from your brain to your face in order to relieve your pain.
- Tricyclic antidepressant medications prescribed by your doctor can help relieve your symptoms of pain, as well as serve as an antidepressant. Different doses will be given depending on which it is being used for.
- Aromatherapy may help release chemicals in your body that reduce the amount of pain impulses that reach your brain.
- Because of sex differences with respect to the effect of estrogen as well as progesterone on the absorption, metabolism and elimination of medications, drug dosing may fluctuate in the female patient depending on whether or not the female is pre- or post-menopausal. The physiological changes that occur during the menstrual cycle can affect the responses of a drug in the female body. You must discuss the effects of your drug with your doctor because the effect of your drug may decrease during menses.

Chapter 23
Understanding Angina

Chest pain in both men and women can be serious. Even though minor medical conditions can cause you to have chest pain, if you are having a heart attack, it can be potentially fatal. (L.M. Tierney, et al. *Current Medical Diagnosis and Treatment*. New York: McGraw Hill, 2001) (T.E. Andreolli, et al. *Cecil Essentials of Medicine*. n.p.: W.B. Saunders, 1997) For this reason, do not take any chest pain lightly. To be safe, seek medical attention whenever you experience significant chest pain.

In this chapter, you will learn about the heart condition angina, as well as its association with heart attacks and coronary artery disease. Also, angina and another chest pain syndrome, cardiac syndrome x, are compared. You will learn how hormones play a role in the symptoms of angina between men and women, as well as how it is diagnosed and treated.

Not Just Chest Pain

If your heart muscles do not obtain enough oxygen, some of your heart muscle can become injured and even some of the muscle can die. This can lead to some dysfunction in the remainder of the muscle that is trying to pump blood out of your heart to the rest of your body. The injured muscle can't pump blood efficiently if at all. You can develop *angina* or a *myocardial infarction*. Angina is pain in the center of your chest and is usually relieved by rest. Anginal chest pain in men may spread to the jaws and arms. Numbness and pain radiating from the chest into the left arm is especially characteristic of anginal pain in men. In women with a decrease in oxygen to the heart muscle for some reason, symptoms of angina pain include pressure in the center of the chest accompanied by pain in the neck or arms. (L.M. Tierney, et al. *Current Medical Diagnosis and Treatment*. New York: McGraw Hill, 2001) (T.E. Andreolli, et al. *Cecil Essentials of*

Medicine. n.p.: W.B. Saunders, 1997) Angina or heart pain occurs when the demand for blood by the heart exceeds the supply of the arteries.

A myocardial infarction (heart attack) or death of a segment of your heart muscle occurs following interruption of the blood supply to the heart muscle. A heart attack can cause sudden severe chest pain. There is a danger that your heart could go into an irregular heartbeat called an arrhythmia. (L.M. Tierney, et al. *Current Medical Diagnosis and Treatment*. New York: McGraw Hill, 2001) (T.E. Andreolli, et al. *Cecil Essentials of Medicine*. n.p.: W.B. Saunders, 1997) If you have a severe arrhythmia, your heart can stop, which is referred to as a cardiac arrest. If you have interruption of the blood flow going to your heart, you can have irreversible injury to your heart muscle. This injury usually begins within 20 minutes from the time of the loss of blood flow to your heart muscle. Therefore, if you think that you are having a heart attack, contact your local emergency room or your doctor. If your pain is severe, go directly to your emergency room by ambulance.

The extent of your heart muscle injury is related to the amount of obstruction that you have in your heart vessels. It is also related to the length of time that your heart muscle is without blood flow. You will probably have other vessels in your heart that supply your heart muscle. This is called collateral circulation. (L.M. Tierney, et al. *Current Medical Diagnosis and Treatment*. New York: McGraw Hill, 2001) (T.E. Andreolli, et al. *Cecil Essentials of Medicine*. n.p.: W.B. Saunders, 1997) This collateral circulation can get some blood flow to your muscle that is without blood flow. When your heart muscle is without oxygen and when your heart muscle dies, the electrical conduction of impulses through the muscle is decreased or stopped. This is the mechanism by which your heart develops abnormal heart beats.

It is a diagnostic problem for your doctor to determine whether you are suffering from chest pain from your heart or from another structure. You need to be aware that not all chest pain is heart related pain. Pain in your chest can also come from pneumonia, cancer, or pleurisy (an inflammation of the lining of the lung). Diseases of the esophagus can also cause you to have chest pain, as can shingles.

You have probably heard of or read about angina pectoris. Angina pectoris is chest pain that results from decreased oxygen from your heart muscle. Angina pectoris is usually pain under your breastbone.

You may perceive discomfort instead of pain or pressure. The pain, if it is present, or the pressure can radiate to your neck or arm which is usually the left arm. Shortness of breath may also be reported. Angina pectoris is usually elicited by physical exertion. Occasionally psychological stress can cause you to have angina pectoris. The stress can cause your heart rate to increase, which increases your oxygen demand. If you are worried about an impending speech that you have to give, this could cause you to have anxiety with an increase in your heart with the possibility of developing angina. Climbing stairs can also cause you to have angina pectoris if you have some obstruction of your arteries that supply blood to your heart muscle. You may develop angina when you awake in the morning. Exposure to cold air can also cause angina. You could even develop angina after meals. Angina comes on quickly and can last for up to 15 minutes. It usually resolves with rest or with nitroglycerin.

The figure that follows shows a heart with the aorta, pulmonary artery, vena cava, and coronary blood vessel labeled. These areas are involved in the heart conditions such as angina, heart attacks, and coronary artery disease that are discussed in this chapter.

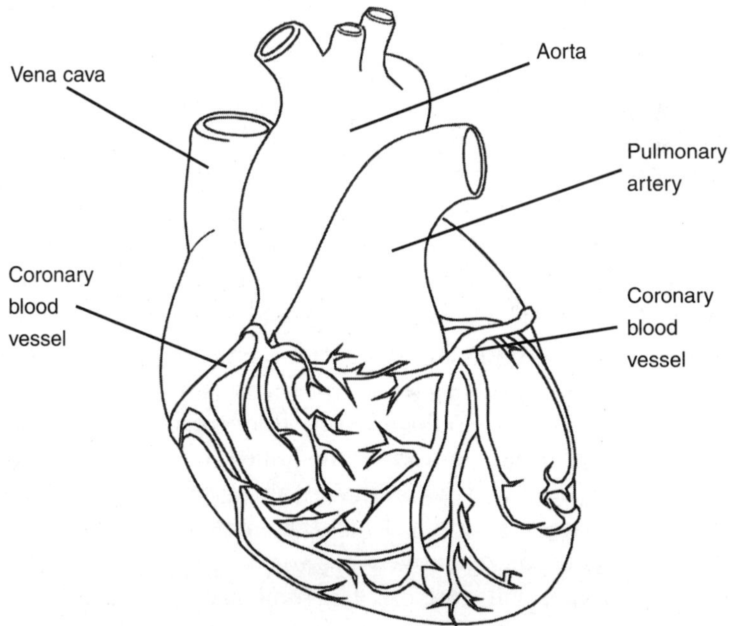

Areas of the heart involved in heart conditions.

Understanding Angina Chest Pain

To understand the mechanics of chest pain associated with angina attacks, you need some basic knowledge of coronary heart disease. Coronary heart disease is the major cause of death in not only the United States but also in most industrialized countries. Coronary artery disease can cause you or one of your family members to have a sudden stoppage of his or her heart. Coronary artery disease can be a cause of angina. Over time coronary artery disease can also cause you to have a heart attack (myocardial infarction). There has been a decrease in the number of deaths from coronary artery disease over the past three decades. This is probably related to the treatment of high blood pressure with medication as well as surgical treatments. Lifestyle changes such as diet, exercise, and stopping smoking tobacco can decrease the incidence of coronary artery disease. (L.M. Tierney, et al. *Current Medical Diagnosis and Treatment*. New York: McGraw Hill, 2001) (T.E. Andreolli, et al. *Cecil Essentials of Medicine*. n.p.: W.B. Saunders, 1997)

Coronary heart disease is usually related to atherosclerosis, which can occur in your heart arteries as well as other arteries throughout your body. Atherosclerosis is a buildup of fat and other materials in the walls of arteries that causes them to become narrowed. This entity is caused by many factors. If you are over 60, a man, and have a family history of coronary artery disease, you are prone to develop this disease. If you are hypertensive and have an elevated cholesterol and smoke, you are at a higher risk for developing atherosclerosis. If you are obese and have a sedentary lifestyle, your risk for atherosclerosis is increased. (L.M. Tierney, et al. *Current Medical Diagnosis and Treatment*. New York: McGraw Hill, 2001) (T.E. Andreolli, et al. *Cecil Essentials of Medicine*. n.p.: W.B. Saunders, 1997)

At first, you will develop a buildup of a type of "bad" cholesterol called low-density lipoproteins (LDL) in the walls of your blood vessels around your heart. These low-density lipoproteins eventually can calcify. This calcification will narrow the lumen, or diameter of your blood vessels, causing a decrease in the amount of blood that can pass through them. This is similar to calcium building up in your plumbing in your residence. If you repetitively deposit calcium in your pipes, eventually your pipes will close off. The same analogy is true for the blood vessels in your heart. When you have a deposit of calcium in your blood vessels, your heart will still pump blood through these vessels. It takes a decrease in the diameter of your blood vessels by approximately 70 percent to decrease your blood flow.

Many diverse factors lead to the progression of atherosclerosis. Increasing age and a family history of coronary artery disease may predispose you to develop this entity. The male sex is an important risk factor for developing coronary artery disease and for having a heart attack, but coronary heart disease is also the leading cause of death in women over 50 years of age. Women will generally have their symptoms approximately 10 years later than men. The risk of coronary artery disease increases with the use of birth control pills and with the onset of menopause. However, the risk of coronary artery disease could be increased with hormone therapy following the onset of menopause.

If you have an elevated blood pressure, you are also at risk for developing coronary artery disease. In fact, hypertension is a major risk factor for developing this disease. If you have a family history of hypertension or if you are beginning to increase your blood pressure, you may need to change your lifestyle. You will need to stop smoking. If you are obese, you will need to decrease your weight. Sodium restriction is important for the control of your hypertension, which can ultimately decrease coronary artery disease. Aerobic exercise is also necessary to decrease your risk for developing coronary heart disease. Exercise is extremely important if you have risk factors for developing coronary artery disease. Smoking is another factor that can cause you to be at a high risk for developing coronary artery disease.

You are probably aware that your cholesterol level must not be allowed to become elevated because it can increase your risk of developing coronary artery disease. If you have high levels of low-density lipoprotein cholesterol, you have an elevated chance of developing coronary heart disease. If your cholesterol is elevated, your doctor will help you reduce your cholesterol with both diet and with pharmacologic management. You must monitor your diet for fat intake. You must significantly decrease your intake of saturated fats. If you eat out a lot at fast-food restaurants, calculate the amount of fat present in the foods that you are consuming. The total fat grams will be listed on the package of the food that you are consuming. Fast-food restaurants also list the fat content of their food in the restaurant and on their websites. Strive to decrease your fat intake. Your doctor can tailor a proper diet for you. However, you must follow this diet. You are probably beginning to realize that you can do things to decrease your chance of developing angina and decrease your chance of having a heart attack.

Plaques (deposits of fat and calcium in your blood vessels) are usually the most common causes of obstruction to blood flow in your arteries around your heart, but other factors can also cause obstruction of blood flow in your heart. Vegetations, small growths that can develop on the valves in your heart from infections, can extend up to your coronary arteries and cause them to become blocked. Diseases such as rheumatoid arthritis can affect the caliber of your coronary arteries.

You must be aware that if you have had or need radiation therapy for cancer treatment, that radiation therapy can cause you to have coronary artery disease. Cocaine use has become more and more prevalent in the United States. However, cocaine use can make the arteries in your heart to go into spasm. Cocaine can accelerate the deposition of fat and calcium in your blood vessels, which can cause you to have angina as well as a heart attack.

Sometimes a decrease in the blood flow in your arteries around your heart can lead to decreased blood flow to the heart muscle tissue, and a decrease in oxygen to your heart will cause a possible injury to your heart muscle. Your heart muscle is dependent upon a balance of oxygen supply as well as demand. At rest, your heart should receive adequate oxygen or you may complain of chest pain. However, if you run a mile or run up steps, the oxygen demand to your heart muscle is increased. The blood vessels that deliver the blood carrying oxygen to your heart must provide your heart muscle with an adequate blood flow. If your blood vessels are narrowed, your heart cannot get enough blood carrying oxygen to your heart muscle. As a result, some of your heart muscle could become injured and die. This is what happens to your heart muscle when you suffer a heart attack (or myocardial infarction, MI). If you are doing any exercise or aerobic activity and if you develop chest pain, stop the activity that you are doing *immediately*.

You will usually develop chest pain when your heart oxygen demand exceeds the supply of oxygen that your blood vessels are supplying to your heart. Usually if your heart begins beating faster, the increase in oxygen demand is met by an increased blood flow in your arteries around your heart. The small arteries around your heart muscle will increase their diameter to provide your heart with more oxygenated blood. If your vessels cannot dilate, your heart will not receive enough oxygen and you will experience pain in your chest. (L.M. Tierney, et al. *Current Medical Diagnosis and Treatment*. New York: McGraw Hill, 2001) (T.E. Andreolli, et al. *Cecil Essentials of Medicine*. n.p.: W.B. Saunders, 1997) Fat and calcium within your heart vessels will restrict the amount of blood that goes to your heart.

Diagnosis Differences in Men and Women

Men may have chest pain with radiation of pain to their left arm. A recent study of women finds that fatigue and sleeplessness are accurate predictors of an impending heart attack. Exhaustion, sleep deprivation, and nausea were frequently seen in women who were having impending heart attacks. Fatigue and sleeplessness are warning signs for heart attacks in women. It is thought that this research will alter the way doctors diagnose and treat women who are likely to suffer heart attacks. The appearance of fatigue and sleeplessness with nausea and vomiting in addition to women's heart attack risk factors should alert the doctor that a woman needs to be thoroughly examined for the possibility of a heart attack. Furthermore, women should not ignore these warnings. (R.B. Fillingham. *Sex, Gender, and Pain*. n.p.: IASP Press, 2000)

It is not uncommon for women workaholics to have heart attacks. If you are a woman under a lot of stress and you have severe exhaustion but can't sleep and develop nausea as well as sweating, you should go to a hospital emergency room. You must note that in this study that was recently released, 43 percent of the women who had heart attacks and were surveyed did not have any chest pain during their heart attacks. (Arkansas Democrat Gazette, 2004) However, more than 70 percent of the women who had heart attacks reported feeling unusual fatigue. These new findings differ from the previous findings that chest pain was the most important symptom for identifying heart attacks in both men and women. Other, previously discounted symptoms such as fatigue, sleeplessness, nausea, anxiety, and shortness of breath are important signs of heart disease as well.

In this study, 48 percent of women reported sleeplessness, whereas 42 percent reported shortness of breath. Thirty-five percent of women in the study complained of anxiety. These symptoms interfered with the daily activities of the women in the study. The study was sponsored by the National Institute of Nursing Research. It involved 515 women. The women in the study were mostly Caucasian. These women had been diagnosed with a heart attack within the previous six months prior to entering the study. The results of this study indicate that women should be thoroughly checked for coronary artery disease.

Women, however, should look beyond the results of this study and look at other risk factors such as whether they smoke, are overweight, or have high cholesterol levels. Furthermore, diabetes and a family history of heart disease can make them prone to heart attacks as well. The results of this study are important because numerous studies have shown that men on the other hand experience chest pains before a heart attack. There are physiologic differences between men and women that may account for these differences in symptoms associated with a heart attack.

Hormones are different for men and women, and women have smaller arteries that supply their heart muscles. These physiologic differences may account for the differences in heart attack symptoms. You need to realize that heart disease is the number one killer of women as well as men in the United States. When woman have a heart attack, they are more likely to die than men. They are also more likely to have a repeat heart attack within a year as opposed to men.

According to the American Heart Association, approximately 6.3 million men and 6.6 million women have histories of heart attacks. (L.M. Tierney, et al. *Current Medical Diagnosis and Treatment*. New York: McGraw Hill, 2001) (T.E. Andreolli, et al. *Cecil Essentials of Medicine*. n.p.: W.B. Saunders, 1997) In the year 2000, more than 500,000 people died from heart disease.

The results of this study that we described are important because usually we think of angina as chest pain. Different types of angina have been described that can occur in both men and women. Stable angina is angina that is chronic and is usually caused by physical activity or emotional stress. Stable angina is usually heart-related pain relieved by rest or nitroglycerin. Unstable angina, on the other hand, can increase with rest. Other types of unstable angina can occur at low activity levels. Unstable angina may not be responsive to nitroglycerin. Sometimes you can develop spasms of your arteries that supply your heart muscle. This type of spasm is called Pinzmetal's angina and can be relieved frequently with nitroglycerin. Stable angina is a term used to describe pain that is predictably caused by narrowing of coronary arteries and a given stress to your heart. For example, walking two flights of stairs or chasing a bus for half a block. The pain is predictable in terms of its severity, how long it lasts, and what brings about relief (such as a single tablet of nitroglycerin placed under the tongue). On the other hand, unstable angina describes a new pattern of pain not previously experienced, for example, pain previously felt after a flight of stairs is now suddenly experienced at rest. Unstable angina is a medical emergency that should be immediately evaluated by a doctor.

As you can see, an adequate and accurate history of your pain is extremely important for your doctor. If you are suffering from angina or suffering a myocardial infarction, an adequate history can help your doctor make an accurate diagnosis so that you can receive the appropriate treatment. I recommend that you write down all of your symptoms. Write down what you were doing when your pain occurred. If you are having only anxiety and fatigue, write down what you were doing before the onset of your symptoms. Remember that other symptoms of other medical problems can be confused with angina pectoris. Pain that remains in one area, is not referred to other areas, and is stabbing and fleeting is usually not angina pectoris, but it is very important to remember that all chest pain can be a sign of a heart attack or angina and should be urgently evaluated by a doctor, especially that which has never before been experienced or is associated with nausea and vomiting, sweating, fatigue, or shortness of breath. Your doctor will do a physical examination on you. Your heart rate and blood pressure can be normal, although heart pain will often cause an increase in heart rate and blood pressure. You can have an irregular heartbeat. Sometimes your doctor will hear a new heart murmur that was not present before your angina attack. In many instances during an angina attack your EKG, a tracing of the electrical activity of your heart, will show signs of cardiac injury. However, it is also possible that your EKG can be completely normal, and this finding does not rule out heart attack or angina.

If you are having chest pain and your EKG appears normal, your doctor may do an echocardiogram or administer radioactive dye and do a heart perfusion study. Your doctor may take a sample of your blood to have it analyzed for any elevations of your heart enzymes. If you have heart muscle damage, the injured tissue will release chemicals. If these so-called heart iso-enzymes are increased, this may be a sign that you are having a heart attack. If you have a history of risk factors for coronary artery disease and if your symptoms are stable, your doctor may do a pharmacologic stress test. A dobutamine echocardiogram study may also be done. You will be given a drug that will increase your heart rate. You will be monitored with a continuous EKG to see if there are any changes on your EKG that suggest decreased perfusion to your heart muscles. Occasionally your cardiologist may want to do a coronary angiogram, which is a test that uses a dye to assess the extent of your coronary artery disease.

Cardiac Syndrome X vs. Angina

A chest pain syndrome that may be more prevalent in women is an entity called syndrome X. (R. Melzack and P. Wall, *Handbook of Pain Management a Clinical Companion of Textbook of Pain*, New York: Churchill Livingstone, 2003) If you have this syndrome, you may have an exaggerated response of the small arteries that go to your heart muscles. This exaggerated response is constriction of the diameter of your arteries. When this happens, you have decreased blood flow going to your heart. Usually women that suffer from this illness have a generalized increase in their body pain overall. This disease is undergoing further research at the present time.

As mentioned previously, women can have myocardial infarctions without having any chest pain. This can also be true in men. (L.M. Tierney, et al. *Current Medical Diagnosis and Treatment*. New York: McGraw Hill, 2001) (T.E. Andreolli, et al. *Cecil Essentials of Medicine*. n.p.: W.B. Saunders, 1997) In other words, painless myocardial infarctions can occur in both sexes. These painless myocardial infarctions are usually discovered on routine EKGs. As stated, women need to be educated as to the symptoms based on evidence obtained from studies including men and women. You must know that women have significantly greater back and jaw pain when it does occur as well as nausea and vomiting than men when they present with symptoms of acute coronary syndromes. If you have these symptoms, you may be having a heart attack and you must seek medical attention immediately. Men have more chest pain as well as sweating when they are having a heart attack. Essentially men and women can experience the same symptoms, but the proportions of the symptoms are more prevalent in women than men.

The prevalence of the cardiac syndrome X is higher in women when compared to men. Estrogen deficiency has been shown to play a major role in the origin of cardiac syndrome X. Estrogen has properties on blood vessels that can increase the diameter of the blood vessels. (L.M. Tierney, et al. *Current Medical Diagnosis and Treatment*. New York: McGraw Hill, 2001) (T.E. Andreolli, et al. *Cecil Essentials of Medicine*. n.p.: W.B. Saunders, 1997) The results of this study demonstrate that the blood vessels in your heart can be modified by sex hormones. A further study reveals that an estrogen deficiency contributes to the development of angina and that in women this angina can be treated with estrogen supplements.

Current Research Findings

Men are more likely to be hospitalized for unstable angina than women. In the year 2000, one study by cardiologists in one area reported there were approximately 30,000 hospitalizations for men and approximately 16,000 hospitalizations for women of a similar age. The reason for this data is being examined.

Research has demonstrated a smaller proportion of women who suffer from angina have coronary artery disease than men who have angina. At one time it was thought that these findings contributed to the perception that chest pain was less serious in women. However, we now know that chest pain is serious in both men and women.

Research continues to demonstrate that heart disease, which has not always been considered a serious problem for women, is now a serious problem for women. With more women smoking today, the incidence of heart disease has risen. Approximately 240,000 women in the United States die from heart disease each year. Heart disease is the second-leading killer of women under age 55. (L.M. Tierney, et al. *Current Medical Diagnosis and Treatment*. New York: McGraw Hill, 2001) (T.E. Andreolli, et al. *Cecil Essentials of Medicine*. n.p.: W.B. Saunders, 1997) Cancer is the primary reason why women die. However, by age 55 heart disease causes more deaths in women than cancer. Did you know that one out of two American women will die of heart disease or stroke? Just like men, women should not smoke. Men and women should be aware of their blood pressures, cholesterol levels, and their blood sugar levels.

Studies have shown that if women control their weight and work with their doctor to control their blood pressure and modify their lifestyle, they can minimize the risk of heart disease and minimize the risk of having a heart attack. Be aware that if you are overweight, you run the risk of having an elevated blood pressure. The elevated blood pressure can cause you to have a heart attack. The problem in this country is that obesity is increasing and is near epidemic. Almost 50 percent of adults in the United States are overweight. Furthermore, about 30 percent of the youth in the United States are overweight. These findings suggest that more individuals will develop high blood pressure and eventually more individuals will develop coronary artery disease and one can expect that there will be more deaths related to myocardial infarction.

Women have not been included in research studies done on the heart until recently. The reason for this was that most premature heart attacks occurred in men before age 55. Women who develop heart disease at older ages were not included in the studies. Furthermore, researchers eliminated women in their earlier studies because it was thought that women's hormones could alter the results of the studies on the incidence of heart attacks and deaths. The good news is that there have been inclusions of women in studies of coronary artery disease following the institution of the Women's Health Initiative about 10 years ago.

Studies are being done to evaluate hormone-replacement therapy for the prevention of heart disease. It is known that estrogen does affect the caliber of the arteries that go to your heart and also affects the muscles in the walls of your arteries. Estrogen may also have an effect on your blood's ability to clot. If your blood clots too readily, you can have stoppage of the blood flow in your coronary arteries. The estrogen hormone may have an affect on your body's ability to form clots. Estrogen therapy can be associated with a stroke and the risks of this therapy must be discussed with your physician.

Aspirin can affect your body's ability to clot and, if you are having angina or if you suspect that you are having a heart attack, aspirin can be lifesaving. Current studies are being done examining the effects of nutrients for the prevention of heart disease.

A new and important study has been recently released. In this study a synthetic compound that consists of "good cholesterol" given through the veins reduced coronary artery disease in one to two months. Cleveland Clinic cardiologists describe this as a liquid Drano for coronary arteries. This drug is still investigational but does give promise if you are suffering from coronary artery disease. This drug administered through your veins can remove substances that have built-up in your arteries. It can also remove fatty buildups from your bloodstream. The study demonstrates that high-density lipoproteins can improve your body's ability to eliminate deposits from your coronary arteries. Research is continuing with this new drug.

Treatment for Angina

Remember that angina (heart pain) is not a heart attack. Angina is your body's warning to you that something is wrong and only means that some of your heart muscle is not getting enough blood temporarily. Angina does not mean that your heart muscle is suffering permanent damage. A heart attack, on the other hand, occurs when the blood flow to your heart muscle is suddenly and permanently cut off. This will cause damage that is usually permanent to your heart muscle. If you have angina, it means that you have an underlying coronary heart disease. When you have an angina attack, you are at an increased risk of having a heart attack.

Your angina is treated by controlling your risk factors. (L.M. Tierney, et al. *Current Medical Diagnosis and Treatment*. New York: McGraw Hill, 2001) (T.E. Andreolli, et al. *Cecil Essentials of Medicine*. n.p.: W.B. Saunders, 1997) This includes decreasing your blood pressure if you are hypertensive. It also means that you should stop smoking cigarettes. If your cholesterol is elevated, you must follow your doctor's instructions to reduce the cholesterol and take any cholesterol-lowering drugs that your doctor may prescribe. If you are overweight, strive to exercise and reduce the fat in your diet. If you take these steps, you will reduce the possibility that you will have a heart attack. Do not overdo physical activity. Use alcohol only in moderation, if at all. If angina occurs after eating a large meal, avoid large meals and avoid foods that leave you feeling stuffed. Angina can be controlled by medications.

Even though physical activity is helpful to you in most instances, in people with pre-existing heart disease physical exercise can precipitate a heart attack and should only be conducted under the direction of your doctor.

Remember if you have unstable angina or chest pain at rest, you will probably need hospitalization for intensive medical therapy. Aspirin and heparin can be given to decrease the clotting factors of your bloodstream. If you have angina, these drugs can decrease the progression of angina to a heart attack. If you suspect that you are having a heart attack, seek immediate medical attention. Most deaths associated with an acute heart attack occur during the first hours following the onset of the heart attack.

Call your emergency medical service if you suspect that you are having a heart attack. Most emergency medical technicians can recognize the symptoms of a heart attack. You will require oxygen.

Nitroglycerine and morphine will be administered to you. If your heart rate is abnormal, these professionals can treat your abnormal heart rate as well. Your EKG can be sent by telemetry by your emergency medical technician to a local emergency room so that the emergency room doctor can make a diagnosis of your heart rhythm and recommend any treatments that may be immediately necessary. It is important that blood is restored to your heart muscle. Sometimes your blood flow to your heart muscles can be increased by administering therapy to you that will break up blood clots in your heart blood vessels. Streptokinase is one drug that can be used in this situation. You will be confined to bed for 24 to 36 hours. You will be placed in a cardiac care unit. Your activities will be gradually increased. There are enzymes that are released into your bloodstream when you have heart muscle damage. These enzymes will be monitored by your treating doctor.

Nitroglycerin is a commonly prescribed drug for the treatment of angina. Nitroglycerin will relieve your angina pain by making your blood vessels going to your heart wider. The increased blood flow will permit more oxygen to go to your heart. This increased oxygen will keep up with the demand of your heart. You should take nitroglycerin when you have the onset of discomfort.

Other medicines such as beta blockers can be used to slow your heart rate and decrease the contraction of your heart muscle. This will conserve oxygen. Propanolol (Inderal) is an example of a beta blocker. Calium channel blockers (Verapimil) affect the calcium in your muscle cells. Calcium channel blockers such as Verapamil can decrease the incidence of you having angina as well as a heart attack.

If medication fails to control your angina, coronary artery bypass surgery is sometimes necessary. A blood vessel is grafted onto your blocked artery. This allows your blood flow to bypass the blockage so that blood can go to your heart muscle to provide your heart muscle with needed oxygen. Your surgeon can use an artery inside your chest or take a vein from your leg.

Another treatment that can be used to increase your artery size is called balloon angioplasty. This involves insertion of a catheter that has a tiny, tiny balloon on the end of it into an artery either in your arm or your leg. The balloon is inflated briefly to widen your vessel in places where your arteries are narrow.

Work with your doctor to develop an exercise plan. A physical therapist can work with you and observe you while you are doing some exercise. You may start with a 5-minute walk and increase your exercise 5 minutes per week until you reach a 30-minute walk.

The diagnosis and treatment of angina is extremely important because there are more than 500,000 deaths in the United States related to coronary artery disease every year. Over 1 million new and repeat cases of heart attack occur each year. (L.M. Tierney, et al. *Current Medical Diagnosis and Treatment*. New York: McGraw Hill, 2001) (T.E. Andreolli, et al. *Cecil Essentials of Medicine*. n.p.: W.B. Saunders, 1997) Approximately 44 percent of these patients die. Almost 13 million individuals who have angina or a heart attack are still living. The number of men and women living are almost equal. Since 1990, the death rate from coronary artery disease has actually decreased. More than 6 million people in the United States suffer from angina. Another study was done that revealed that 400,000 new cases of stable angina occur each year. The incidence of angina is greater in women than men. Furthermore, the incidence of angina in women over age 20 was highest in African American women followed by Mexican American followed by Caucasian women. The same is true for racial differences in men.

If you have persistent angina that is refractory to treatments, your pain-medicine doctor could place a catheter in your epidural space. This device is called a dorsal column stimulator. It provides electrical current to the back of your spinal cord. This current could decrease your chest pain. It is used frequently in Europe for angina that is refractory to other treatments.

Another type of procedure that can increase your blood flow is called a stent. A stent is a surgical procedure, but it is a minor procedure compared to open heart surgery. Stents are implanted through your veins with a catheter. The stent expands when it is placed. The stent will provide better blood flow at the location of your artery where the blood flow is decreased. Your chest wall is not opened to have this procedure done. Stents that are being used currently are coated with heparin to prevent clotting within the stent. The purpose of the stent is to permanently hold your blood vessel open. This procedure like placement of the balloon into your coronary arteries is a relatively safe procedure and can be extremely effective.

For Men

- *Stop* Smoking! Smoking increases your risk of coronary artery disease.

- If you are obese, you should make dietary changes to decrease your cholesterol and weight.
- Nitroglycerin and other vasodialator medications will make the blood vessels going to your heart larger, therefore increasing the amount of oxygen that your heart receives.
- If your heart rate is too fast, your doctor may prescribe beta blockers, such as Propanolol, to slow your heart rate and decrease the contraction of your heart muscle to help conserve oxygen.
- Your doctor may prescribe you a calcium channel blocker, such as Verapamil, to decrease your incidence of having angina or heart attack.
- Exercise regimens prescribed by your doctor may be necessary to strengthen your heart muscles.
- Surgical interventions such as coronary artery bypass surgery, balloon angioplasty and stent placement may be needed to improve blood flow to your heart if medications are not successfully treating your condition.

For Women

- *Stop* Smoking! Smoking increases your risk of coronary artery disease.
- If you are obese, you should make dietary changes to decrease your cholesterol and weight.
- Nitroglycerin and other vasodialator medications will make the blood vessels going to your heart larger, therefore increasing the amount of oxygen that your heart receives.
- If your heart rate is too fast, your doctor may prescribe beta blockers, such as Propanolol, to slow your heart rate and decrease the contraction of your heart muscle to help conserve oxygen.
- Your doctor may prescribe you a calcium channel blocker, such as Verapamil, to decrease your incidence of having angina or heart attack.
- Exercise regimens prescribed by your doctor may be necessary to strengthen your heart muscles.
- Surgical interventions such as coronary artery bypass surgery, balloon angioplasty and stent placement may be needed to improve blood flow to your heart if medications.

Chapter 24
Understanding Complex Regional Pain Syndrome

Reflex sympathetic dystrophy (RSD) can be a devastating entity for you, especially if it is not diagnosed and treated within a timely fashion. Reflex sympathetic dystrophy usually affects one of your extremities (arms or legs) but can also affect your face. Reflex sympathetic dystrophy is now called *complex regional pain syndrome.*

In this chapter, you will learn about your sympathetic nervous system and how it relates to complex regional pain syndromes. You will learn the differences between RSD and causalgia, another complex regional pain syndrome, but the pain conditions associated RSD will be discussed more in-depth. The three phases of RSD and its diagnosis will be discussed. You will also learn about your treatment options and current research findings.

Pain and Reflex Sympathetic Dystrophy

Reflex sympathetic dystrophy is serious, painful, and potentially disabling. Pain associated with this entity is throbbing, burning, or aching. (R. Harden, et al. *Complex Regional Pain Syndrome.* n.p.: IASP Press, 2001) You can have pain just to the touch. You can have swelling of your extremity as well as either warmth or coldness depending on the phase of your RSD and sweating. Your hair may grow faster on the extremity with RSD at first, only to slow down as the disease progresses. Your extremity will sweat and can turn color. The nails in your affected limb can grow faster on the extremity that suffers from reflex sympathetic dystrophy.

Reflex sympathetic dystrophy usually occurs following an injury. However, a heart attack or stroke can cause you to have reflex sympathetic dystrophy. It can be seen in the knee as well as in the shoulder. (R. Harden, et al. *Complex Regional Pain Syndrome.* n.p.: IASP

Press, 2001) In a study of reflex sympathetic dystrophy, 40 percent of the cases followed an injury to a muscle or a nerve. Simple bruises or sprains can trigger reflex sympathetic dystrophy. Fractures accounted for 25 percent of reflex sympathetic dystrophy cases. Twenty percent of the RSD patients were postoperative on an arm or leg, whereas 12 percent occurred after a heart attack. Three percent occurred after a stroke. Approximately 37 percent of patients in the study had emotional disturbances at the time of the onset of the reflex sympathetic dystrophy.

It was once thought that reflex sympathetic dystrophy was an emotional problem. However, studies have shown that many people do not suffer from emotional problems at the time of onset of reflex sympathetic dystrophy. (R. Harden, et al. *Complex Regional Pain Syndrome*. n.p.: IASP Press, 2001) Would you become anxious or depressed if you had constant severe pain that decreased your daily activity and disrupted your sleep? To prevent you from having permanent disability, treatment needs to be started immediately. Treatment usually consists of oral medications as well as injection therapy by an anesthesiologist using local anesthetics. Steroids may also be used effectively to treat RSD. If your symptoms persist, sometimes you will need surgery to remove the offending nerves causing your pain.

As you can see, reflex sympathetic dystrophy can be potentially disabling. If you have any of the signs or symptoms of complex regional pain syndrome mentioned in this chapter, you should notify your doctor. Remember that early diagnosis and treatment can significantly improve your outcome. Further research in the exact cause of this disease and the appropriate treatment continues.

Your Sympathetic Nervous System

If you have had reflex sympathetic dystrophy, it may have been called another condition. Only recently have scientists throughout the world come together at an International Association for the Study of Pain meeting. These scientists devised a term to describe reflex sympathetic dystrophy that is now called complex regional pain syndrome. At one time it was called post-traumatic sympathetic dystrophy, algodystrophy, Sudeck's atrophy, transient osteoporosis, and post-traumatic vasomotor syndrome. The shoulder/hand syndrome was also used to describe reflex sympathetic dystrophy following a heart attack or a stroke. If you sustained actual nerve damage, your reflex sympathetic dystrophy is called causalgia.

A previous definition of causalgia was referred to the syndrome associated with known nerve injury, whereas reflex sympathetic dystrophy included those patients whose pain and associated symptoms were followed by a variety of causes. (R. Harden, et al. *Complex Regional Pain Syndrome*. n.p.: IASP Press, 2001) Injury associated with causalgia was more severe, whereas that associated with RSD was relatively minor. Now reflex sympathetic dystrophy is referred to as complex regional pain syndrome I, whereas causalgia is referred as complex regional pain syndrome II. Causes of both of these syndromes include fractures as well as dislocations.

Reflex sympathetic dystrophy and causalgia were originally described by Dr. Mitchell, a neurologist during the Civil War. He noted that some soldiers who had injuries to their hands or feet developed a syndrome that consisted of burning pain, pain to the touch over the skin of the in-jured extremity, shiny skin, and skin that had different colors consisting of either redness or a blue cyanotic color. Blue or cyanotic discoloration usually occurs when skin or other tissues do not get enough blood and oxygen. Mitchell also noted that the pain in the extremity was out of proportion to the injury. For example, if you sustained a sprain to your ankle, you would expect to have some pain. However, if you develop reflex sympathetic dystrophy, the pain is excruciating and unbearable. Mitchell noted the onset of reflex sympathetic dystrophy following gunshot wounds. (R. Harden, et al. *Complex Regional Pain Syndrome*. n.p.: IASP Press, 2001) The exact cause of reflex sympathetic dystrophy remains under investigation.

It was originally hypothesized that if your sympathetic nervous system became hyperactive, this hyperactivity was at least one of the causes of reflex sympathetic dystrophy. Your sympathetic nervous system is one component of your autonomic nervous system. The other component of your autonomic nervous system is called the parasympathetic nervous system. Your autonomic nervous system regulates your circulation and your breathing as well as your stomach and bladder functions. You have no control over your autonomic nervous system. This distinguishes it from your peripheral nervous system which is usually under your control.

Because it is thought by some medical clinicians that your sympathetic nervous system can have some role in the onset of reflex sympathetic dystrophy, you must have a basic understanding of this system in order to understand reflex sympathetic dystrophy. Your sympathetic nervous system fibers emerge from your mid-back part of your spinal cord. On the other hand, your parasympathetic fibers come from your brain stem as well as your lower sacral areas. Your sympathetic nervous system sends sympathetic nerve fibers to the blood vessels in your head and neck as well as to your skin and muscles in your arms and legs. These fibers also go to your heart, your lungs, and your esophagus.

Furthermore, fibers can go to your stomach, pancreas, liver, gallbladder, and your intestines. Your kidneys, ureter, uterus, bladder, and prostate can all be affected. (R. Harden, et al. *Complex Regional Pain Syndrome*. n.p.: IASP Press, 2001) In your extremities, sympathetic fibers go to your blood vessels as well as your sweat glands and hair follicles. Remember that we said that your hands and feet can sweat profusely if you have reflex sympathetic dystrophy and the hair on your arms and legs can grow faster or fall out. Your sympathetic nerve fibers can restrict circulation in certain areas of your body.

Your sympathetic nervous system can also change the chemical environment of your muscle tissue as well as your other nervous system tissue and will make the small pain fibers in these different tissues sensitive. You must also realize that your sympathetic nervous system is linked to emotional states. Therefore, your sympathetic nervous system plays an important role in the psychological aspects of pain. Sometimes if your doctor blocks your sympathetic nerve pathways, you can have some relief of your reflex sympathetic dystrophy. (R. Harden, et al. *Complex Regional Pain Syndrome*. n.p.: IASP Press, 2001) When you have an injury to your extremity, for example, you will have pain im-pulses that go to your spinal cord as well as your brain. The impulses that are going to your spinal cord and brain are initiated by pain fibers in your tissue. These pain fibers are both enhanced and inhibited at all levels of your brain and spinal cord. Your tissues produce pain-producing as well as pain-enhancing chemicals. This causes your nerves to transmit pain impulses onto your spinal cord and ultimately to your brain. However, in your spinal cord you have chemicals that can stop or attenuate the pain impulses.

You also have what are called descending pathways, which are essentially nerves with chemicals that decrease the transmission of pain signals before they reach your brain. To modulate your pain, there must be checks and balances within your nervous system. Remember that pain is a warning to your brain that something is wrong at a particular place in your body. However, your body has normal mechanisms to lessen your pain. When you suffer from reflex sympathetic dystrophy, your pain-producing chemicals and nerves are much stronger than the aspects of your nervous system that are able to decrease the pain. Over time the part of your nervous system that decreases your pain becomes unable to function properly. At this time, your pain becomes overwhelming and disabling.

Chemical substances in your tissues activate your pain fibers. These chemicals cause your blood vessels to increase their diameter. When this happens, you will have warmth in your painful area as well as redness and increased temperature. As your blood vessels enlarge, you may also have swelling in your tissue. Chemicals such as acetychloline, potassium, and serotonin can stimulate pain in your tissues. However, when these chemicals are in your brain or spinal cord they do not cause pain. Histamine in your tissues can also be a chemical that can cause you to have pain. However, histamine is being used in creams to decrease your pain in your skin and muscles. Further studies have shown that the release of histamine into your spinal cord can decrease your pain as well. The mechanisms by which histamine either cause pain or help relieve pain remain to be studied and elucidated.

Prostaglandins are also released if you have injury to your tissue. As mentioned previously, prostaglandins themselves do not produce pain; when they are around pain nerves, however, they sensitize these nerves to pain. Prostaglandins can intensify any inflammation that you may have and increase the action of bradykinin on your nerve endings. *Substance P* in your tissues can be a cause of significant pain. It is important for you to realize that there are many pain producing chemicals especially in reflex sympathetic dystrophy. You will note later in this chapter that different drugs are administered for the treatment of reflex sympathetic dystrophy. The reason for this polypharmacy is that many chemicals combine to cause you pain associated with your reflex sympathetic dystrophy. If you have increased sweating associated with reflex sympathetic dystrophy, this implies that your sympathetic nervous system has become overactive. (R. Harden, et al. *Complex Regional Pain Syndrome*. n.p.: IASP Press, 2001) However, if your reflex sympathetic dystrophy persists over time, you will notice that your sweating in your hands or feet can significantly decrease. It is believed that with chronic reflex sympathetic dystrophy that the sympathetic reflexes do not remain active.

RSD—Prolonged Pain After Injury

In 1916 a surgeon described that reflex sympathetic dystrophy pain could be relieved by surgically removing some of the sympathetic fibers that innervate the affected extremity. This surgeon also noted that patients who had his procedure had some pain relief and had decreased sweating and improvement in their skin color. This surgeon then thought that the sympathetic nervous system was involved in the etiology of reflex sympathetic dystrophy. In 1995, another doctor described another method using a scope for the removal of sympathetic nerve fibers that innervate your limb that has RSD, and this has became a standard treatment for reflex sympathetic dystrophy.

Over time the treatment of reflex sympathetic dystrophy included repetitive sympathetic blocks or removal of the sympathetic nerves, either surgically or by chemicals such as phenol. Sympathetic blocks involve placing a local anesthetic around the bundles of nerves which exist outside of your central nervous system. These nerve bundles which are called ganglia are in your neck as well as your lower back. The ganglion in your neck influences your arm pain while your ganglia in your lower back influences RSD pain in your leg.

These procedures for many years have been the standard treatment for reflex sympathetic dystrophy. Finally, doctors who regularly treat reflex sympathetic dystrophy critically evaluated the effectiveness of these procedures. It is now known that temporary relief can occur with these procedures, but long-term results are poor. It is possible that these procedures have only survived time as a standard treatment for RSD because of the lack of more effective therapy. Furthermore, for years research on reflex sympathetic dystrophy was lacking because it was thought that this entity was mainly of a psychological origin.

Early description of reflex sympathetic dystrophy included injuries without obvious nerve damage. Causalgia, on the other hand, was the description given to symptoms of reflex sympathetic dystrophy where a nerve had been actually injured, such as in a gunshot wound that was described by Dr. Mitchell during the Civil War.

Sprains and strains can also be a cause of these syndromes as well as bursitis and tendonitis. Arthritis can also cause either reflex sympathetic dystrophy or causalgia. If you are a female and have had a mastectomy, you may develop reflex sympathetic dystrophy. If one of the veins in your legs has been occluded, you may also develop reflex sympathetic dystrophy. After placement of a cast on your arms and legs, you may develop reflex sympathetic dystrophy and/or causalgia. Some individual have developed these syndromes following the onset of shingles. Head injuries and strokes can also cause you to have reflex sympathetic dystrophy or causalgia.

A rare but devastating form of reflex sympathetic dystrophy can occur after a tooth extraction. Heart attacks can be associated with reflex sympathetic dystrophy of your upper arms. Painful reflex sympathetic dystrophy–like symptoms can occur around your perineum (the area between the anus and urinary outlet) following surgery around this area. Remember that sympathetic nerve fibers go to all parts of your body and, therefore, all parts of your body can be affected. The problem with reflex sympathetic dystrophy is that in many instances it is either overdiagnosed or underdiagnosed. A consensus conference, therefore, was held by doctors and scientists from all over the world during proceedings of the International Association for the Study of Pain. These individuals have compiled the diagnostic criteria for complex regional pain syndrome. The results of their meeting stated that complex regional pain syndrome describes a variety of painful conditions. The painful conditions must exceed the duration of the expected clinical course of the inciting event. For example, if you sustain an ankle sprain, your pain should be gone in several weeks. If your pain becomes severe and remains for several months, this suggests that you may have a complex regional pain syndrome. The problem with the two types of complex regional pain syndrome is that they can progress over time.

For you to be diagnosed with RSD, you should have the following happen:

- An initiating traumatic event to your tissue.
- The onset of spontaneous pain with excruciating pain to the touch as well as pain to a noxious stimulus that lasts longer than expected. Your pain must be global. For example, if you have injured your hand, you may have an injury to one of the nerves in your hand. For example, your ulnar nerve will give you pain or numbness in your last two fingers of your hand. This is the definition of a *neuritis,* which means inflammation of a nerve. This is not RSD. RSD means that the whole hand (global) is painful and not just in the distribution of one nerve.

- Evidence of swelling of your extremity, either an increase or a decrease in your skin blood flow as well as alterations in the color of your skin and sweating. (R. Harden, et al. *Complex Regional Pain Syndrome*. n.p.: IASP Press, 2001)
- The diagnosis of RSD must be excluded by the existence of other conditions that could account for the degree of your pain and dysfunction. For example, arthritis and inflammation can give you pain that is similar to that of reflex sympathetic dystrophy.

For you to be diagnosed with causalgia, also known as complex regional pain syndrome II, you will have the above mentioned symptoms but you should also have a documented nerve injury. Furthermore, for the diagnosis of both of these entities, you should have documented temperature changes noted on the skin over the area of your reflex sympathetic dystrophy. Remember that the diagnosis of CRPS cannot be made if you do not have pain. This is because CRPS is a pain syndrome by definition. Most of the time your pain will be of a burning nature. Your pain will develop after a traumatic event or after immobilization such as casting. Your pain will be on one side. Only rarely can reflex sympathetic dystrophy spread to another extremity. The onset of your symptoms usually occurs within a month from your surgery or trauma. You do not have reflex sympathetic dystrophy if you have anatomical, physiological, or psychological conditions that would cause your pain and dysfunction in your affected extremity. Remember that infection or arthritis are diseases that can mimic the symptoms of RSD. These entities can cause you to have significant pain. If you have behavioral problems, your behavioral problems can be a cause of pain.

If you become extremely anxious, you can have sweating associated that one normally sees in reflex sympathetic dystrophy. If you have complex regional pain syndrome, light touch or deep pressure should cause you pain. Cold applications to your skin can worsen your pain. Movement of your joints can also cause pain. You skin should be shiny. Your nails should grow faster on the side of the reflex sympathetic dystrophy. At first your hair will grow faster on the side of your reflex sympathetic dystrophy but eventually your hair pattern will decrease and you may even lose hair in this area. Tremors or spasms should be noted on the side of your reflex sympathetic dystrophy. If you have complex regional pain syndrome, you should also have complaints of stiffness at the joints where your fingers meet your hand or where your toes meet your foot. Remember that the complex regional pain syndrome is usually overdiagnosed. Unfortunately, some doctors will call shoddy surgery RSD. This condition is rare. However, when it does occur, it must be treated immediately. If you have any of these symptoms mentioned in this chapter, notify your doctor.

Following surgery, reflex sympathetic dystrophy is a difficult entity to diagnose and treat. Studies on reflex sympathetic dystrophy, for example, following hand surgery can vary from less than 1 percent to 15 percent of all patients. As previously stated, reflex sympathetic dystrophy is often accompanied by dysfunction of your sympathetic nervous system, which results in changes in the blood flow to your skin of your affected limb. It was noted in 1946 that reflex sympathetic dystrophy needs to be diagnosed early because the treatment is more effective if you have an early diagnosis. In other words, early treatment positively affects your outcome. Blockade of your sympathetic nervous system is most effective for the treatment of your complex regional pain syndrome if it is performed within the first four to six weeks from the onset of your symptoms. These blocks become less effective the longer you wait to treat your complex regional pain syndrome.

After surgery, the clinical diagnosis of RSD is often delayed because RSD can resemble normal postoperative states. If you have had hand surgery, for example, you can expect to have pain, swelling, and loss of function as well as the other symptoms associated with reflex sympathetic dystrophy. However, these symptoms should be gone by six weeks. At one time, it was thought that a three-phase bone scan was useful for the diagnosis of complex regional pain syndrome. Studies were done as early as 1981. Individuals also used the three-phase bone scan for monitoring the progress of RSD. This imagery is related to the distribution of a radioactive isotope throughout the body, and a nuclear medicine doctor will note the distribution of this radioactive isotope in the affected extremity. The distribution of the radioactive isotope is dependent upon blood flow as well as the activity of the bone. The problem with this test is that it has not been shown to be as good as previously assumed. Furthermore, if your three-phase bone scan is negative, this does not mean that you do not have reflex sympathetic dystrophy. A study in 2001 found that the three-phase bone scan was positive in only 53 percent of the individuals studied. Furthermore, it was published in 1999 that the three-phase bone scan is of little value in monitoring the course of the treatment of your complex regional pain syndrome. (P.P. Raj. *Practical Management of Pain*. St. Louis: Mosby Yearbook, 1992) A three-phase bone scan may be effective for staging the early or late forms of RSD. Magnetic resonance imaging (MRI) can aid in the diagnosis of RSD by identifying swelling in the center of your bone. This bone marrow edema is characteristic of complex regional pain syndrome. This study is more reliable than a three-phase bone scanning or plain x-ray exams.

In 2002, it was reported in a medical journal that skin temperature differences in the arms and legs are extremely useful for the diagnosis of complex regional pain syndrome. (R. Harden, et al. *Complex Regional Pain Syndrome*. n.p.: IASP Press, 2001) Contact and infrared thermography have both been recommended for the diagnosis of reflex sympathetic dystrophy, but the problem with thermography is that it can be influenced not only by skin blood flow but also by the temperature of the room environment as well as by your muscle and your deep tissue metabolism. A new method called laser Doppler imaging has been shown to be effective for the diagnosis of complex regional pain syndrome. This is a new entity and is not readily available in most medical centers or doctors' offices. It is a noninvasive procedure that takes no more than 10 minutes for your evaluation. It measures your skin blood flow. This laser doppler is important because the results of this study is influenced by your superficial blood flow. Your superficial blood flow is under the control of your autonomic nervous system. Other studies are being developed, which include plethsmography and capillaroscopy. Another device to evaluate reflex sympathetic dystrophy is called the quantitative pseudomotor axon test. This test is time-consuming and is currently available only in several academic centers. However, the results of this test are accurate.

Three Phases of RSD

There are different phases of reflex sympathetic dystrophy. (P.P. Raj. *Practical Management of Pain*. St. Louis: Mosby Yearbook, 1992) A test that measures all three of these phases is necessary. The only one to date that will detect all three phases is the laser Doppler device. After you have sustained an injury to your extremity, the blood vessels to your extremity become bigger. This allows more blood flow to go to your extremity. Your hand or foot will, therefore, feel warm and may appear to be red. This phase usually occurs within the first month of your injury. A three-phase bone scan at this time will demonstrate increased isotope activity in your extremity, which indicates phase I reflex sympathetic dystrophy.

As your RSD progresses, the blood vessels to your extremity will decrease in size. (P.P. Raj. *Practical Management of Pain*. St. Louis: Mosby Yearbook, 1992) They go from the enlarged diameter to a normal appearing diameter. This is phase II. A three-phase bone scan will, therefore, appear normal at this time. A laser Doppler study, on the other hand, will reveal an abnormality of your sympathetic nervous system. You will have some swelling at this time as well as global pain around and sweating of your extremity as your sympathetic nervous system becomes overactive. This phase can progress on to phase III. During this phase, your blood vessels become extremely small and you have decreased blood flow to your hand, foot, or your affected extremity. This will cause your skin to become cold. By this time, you will notice that your skin has become shiny and that the sweating in your hand or foot may have increased. A three-phase bone scan at this time can detect a significant decrease in your blood flow to your extremity. Your treating doctor should try and prevent you from progressing through these phases.

As stated previously, an early diagnosis and treatment will prevent this progression to the worst phase. (P.P. Raj. *Practical Management of Pain*. St. Louis: Mosby Yearbook, 1992) After you have reached phase three of reflex sympathetic dystrophy, the disease is irreversible. The success rate for phase I is extremely high, which does decrease as you progress to phase II. This is the reason why you should keep an accurate and thorough pain diary. Your symptoms of your pain will provide some suggestion to your doctor as to what phase of reflex sympathetic dystrophy you are in. In all the phases, you will need an occupational therapy evaluation to attempt to desensitize the pain in your skin and to preserve normal range of motion in your hand, foot, arm, leg, and so on.

Current Research Findings

A recent study from the Netherlands published in 1993 noted symptoms and signs of complex regional pain syndrome. Pain was noted in 84 percent of individuals longer than 12 months. Ninety-one percent had temperature differences in their extremities after 12 months. Recurrence with exercise was noted in 97 percent of patients. Fifty-five percent continued to have swelling after 12 months. Muscle spasms were noted in 42 percent of individuals. Sweating was noted in 40 percent of patients. Nail growth continued in 52 percent of individuals, whereas hair patterns were present in only 35 percent of patients. Be aware that on rare occasions RSD can spread into more than one extremity. This observation suggests that an individual may have a predisposition to develop RSD. If you have chronic RSD, you can have skin infections associated with persistent swelling of your skin as well as blood vessels that can spontaneously rupture. You may have a change in skin pigmentation and your fingernails or toenails on the affected extremity can become clubbed. The frequency of reflex sympathetic dystrophy shows a peak of the incidence of this entity around 50 years of age. However, you must be aware that both children and elderly individuals can develop RSD. (P.P. Raj. *Practical Management of Pain*. St. Louis: Mosby Yearbook, 1992)

The distribution of RSD between men and women is almost equal for individuals younger than 50 years of age. However, for those over 50 years of age there is a predominance of reflex sympathetic dystrophy noted in women. Even though some investigators have questioned the existence of the sympathetic nervous system's influence on the pain associated with reflex sympathetic dystrophy, there is clinical evidence that this influence does actually exist. This led investigators to describe two types of pain. One is sympathetically maintained pain which is pain associated with chemicals released by the sympathetic nervous system. The other type of pain is sympathetically independent pain, which is not associated with the chemicals liberated by the sympathetic nervous system into the bloodstream. Other types of pains can be responsive to sympathetic blockade. This type of blockade with a local anesthetic can even decrease pain associated with peripheral nerves. Sympathet-ically maintained pain usually has a decrease in your pain component following a sympathetic block. Sympathetically maintained pain can be seen in other entities besides reflex sympathetic dystrophy. It may be seen in neuropathies, phantom limb pain, and shingles as well as neuralgias.

The onset of reflex sympathetic dystrophy can occur at any time following a traumatic event. (P.P. Raj. *Practical Management of Pain*. St. Louis: Mosby Yearbook, 1992) It was thought at one time that RSD could occur without any trauma. This is no longer thought to be true. There is a case report of reflex sympathetic dystrophy beginning one year after a fracture occurred.

Exact causes of reflex sympathetic dystrophy continue to be studied. As stated previously, it is thought that there is a sympathetic nervous system component that causes you to have pain when you develop reflex sympathetic dystrophy. Your nerve ending develop an abnormal sensitivity to the chemicals that are liberated by your sympathetic nerve fibers. If you have had a nerve injury, your nerve will attempt to regrow and will sprout small sensory pain fibers. Sometimes as your nerves attempt to grow together, the area where they come together can be extremely painful. This can cause an extremely painful area called a *neuroma*. This neuroma is sensitive to the chemicals released by your sympathetic nervous system.

Most medical investigators report that over time the sympathetic nervous system becomes less involved in the maintenance of reflex sympathetic dystrophy syndrome. As mentioned earlier in this chapter, you can have reflex sympathetic dystrophy that does not involve a nerve injury. In 1996, it was reported that the peripheral nervous system as well as the central nervous system is involved in the progression of RSD. With this type of pain, your pain receptors may be stimulated by both sympathetic nervous system biochemicals such as norepinephrine or through the release of prostaglandins. Prostaglandins will sensitize your nerve endings to other substances that are in your tissues. The prevalent theory is that pain associated with reflex sympathetic dystrophy is mediated by prostaglandins.

Because many individuals have no decrease in their pain when they have sympathetic blocks in both reflex sympathetic dystrophy and causalgia, many investigators question the existence of any sympathetic involvement in these pain syndromes. In 1995, it was proposed that inflammation with the release of prostaglandins function was the cause of pain in both RSD and causalgia. Furthermore, evidence indicates an inflammatory basis for the loss of bone mass that occurs in reflex sympathetic dystrophy.

More recent studies have determined that the COX-2 enzyme may be responsible for the pain associated with reflex sympathetic dystrophy. This is the reason why many doctors today treat reflex sympathetic dystrophy with the new COX-2-inhibiting drugs such as Vioxx or Celebrex. Furthermore, there may be an interaction between COX-2 enzyme and stimulation of the sympathetic nervous system. Even though your injury usually occurs in your arms or legs, there can be distorted information processing within your spinal cord. In other words, changes in your spinal cord can occur secondary to your nerve injury in your arms or legs. Small inhibitory nerves in your spinal cord, called internuncial neurons, may be ineffective if you develop reflex sympathetic dystrophy.

In addition to your central nervous system (composed of your brain and spinal cord) as well as your peripheral nervous system, which is composed of nerves outside of your brain and spinal cord, you also have a sympathetic nervous system. Studies have shown that females are more vulnerable to sympathetically mediated pain than males. The chemicals that are involved which cause you to have reflex sympathetic dystrophy are potentially affected by your sex hormones. It is believed that your hormone status at the time of your trauma is important for the development of the pain associated with reflex sympathetic dystrophy.

Treatment for Complex Regional Pain Syndrome

The effects of reflex sympathetic dystrophy on the central processing in your central nervous system may be the basis for the spread of reflex sympathetic dystrophy to your other extremities. Many recommendations for the treatment of reflex sympathetic dystrophy and causalgia exist. Because there are so many different treatments proposed, you should be aware that no single treatment is superior to the others. Remember that no treatment for complex regional pain syndrome is consistently successful. It is known that early recognition and active treatment of the complex regional pain syndrome improves your outcome. For example, injections of local anesthetics around your sympathetic nervous system can alleviate your symptoms of reflex sympathetic dystrophy long term. (P.P. Raj. *Practical Management of Pain*. St. Louis: Mosby Yearbook, 1992) These types of injections must be done early in the onset of your symptoms of reflex sympathetic dystrophy. The injections can be done in your stellate ganglion, which provides sympathetic fibers to your arms, or the injections can be done in the lumbar sympathetic ganglion, which supplies sympathetic fibers to your legs.

Because disuse of your extremities can contribute to the onset of reflex sympathetic dystrophy, your doctor will institute occupational therapy for you. This type of therapy emphasizes range of motion. As stated previously, the new COX-2-inhibiting drugs can be helpful in decreasing your pain associated with complex regional pain syndrome.

A Clonidine patch can be used to decrease your pain. This patch is usually used to treat high blood pressure. However, the patch does decrease the sympathetic nervous system chemicals that can be released if you have reflex sympathetic dystrophy. The patch is usually worn for one week before it is changed.

Steroids administered by mouth have been shown to be effective for the treatment of reflex sympathetic dystrophy. Steroids will decrease inflammation caused by prostaglandins. If your pain is severe, your doctor will probably prescribe a narcotic drug for you. Depending on the severity of your pain, your doctor will prescribe a mild narcotic such as Darvocet or a stronger narcotic such as Methadone. Anticonvulsive medications can be helpful in decreasing your pain. Gabapentin (Neurontin) is frequently used now for the treatment of pain associated with your complex regional pain syndrome.

Narcotic medications administered into your spinal fluid can help decrease your pain. Sometimes a morphine pump, which sends a narcotic into your spinal fluid, needs to be implanted to control your RSD pain. Clonidine, which is frequently administered by a patch over your skin, can also be administered into your epidural space for the control of your pain.

Antidepressant medication such as amitriptyline has also been shown to be effective in the management of pain associated with reflex sympathetic dystrophy and causalgia. Amitriptyline increases certain chemicals in your central nervous system that are helpful in decreasing the amount of pain that reaches your brain.

Implantation of a wire attached to a battery into your epidural space can also provide you with significant pain relief. This apparatus is called a dorsal column stimulator.

Psychological intervention is also helpful; because of the severity of the pain associated with reflex sympathetic dystrophy, you can develop fear, anxiety, and depression. Psychological intervention including the use of biofeedback and sometimes hypnosis can successfully be used to treat your pain.

For Men

- Early in your symptoms of RSD, your doctor can inject local anesthetic near your ganglion to relieve pain in your sympathetic nervous system.

- Local long-acting anesthetic injections may be needed in your areas of discomfort to help relieve your pain.
- Steroids can help reduce inflammation caused by prostaglandins.
- Your doctor may prescribe narcotic medications such as morphine and Clonidine to help control your pain.
- Antidepressant medications prescribed by your doctor can increase certain chemicals in your central nervous system that are helpful in reducing the amount of pain impulses that reach your brain.
- Some RSD patients may require psychological therapy, such as biofeedback, to help treat the fear, anxiety, and depression they may feel because of their pain condition.

For Women

- Early in your symptoms of RSD, your doctor can inject local anesthetic near your ganglion to relieve pain in your sympathetic nervous system.
- Local long-acting anesthetic injections may be needed in your areas of discomfort to help relieve your pain.
- Steroids can help reduce inflammation caused by prostaglandins.
- Your doctor may prescribe narcotic medications such as morphine and Clonidine to help control your pain.
- Antidepressant medications prescribed by your doctor can increase certain chemicals in your central nervous system that are helpful in reducing the amount of pain impulses that reach your brain.
- Because of sex differences with respect to the effect of estrogen as well as progesterone on the absorption, metabolism and elimination of medications, drug dosing may fluctuate in the female patient depending on whether or not the female is pre- or post-menopausal. They physiological changes that occur during the menstrual cycle can affect the responses of a drug in the female body. You must discuss the effects of your drug with your doctor because the effect of your drug may decrease during menses.
- Aromatherapy may help release chemicals in your body that reduce the amount of pain impulses that reach your brain.
- Some RSD patients may require psychological therapy, such as biofeedback, to help treat the fear, anxiety, and depression they may feel because of their pain condition.

Chapter 25

Understanding HIV Infections and Pain

Do you know anyone who has or had AIDS? This disease can be very painful. The acquired immune deficiency syndrome (AIDS) is known to be caused by the human immunodeficiency virus (HIV). Pain from other diseases and infections can be worsened by the HIV virus and AIDS. It is important for you to understand how AIDS is developed and what complications can come about in someone with this devastating and debilitating syndrome. (C.J. Carpenter, et al. "Antiretroviral Therapy in Adults," *JAMA* 283 [2000]: 381-389) (JAMA Patient Page. "Drug Treatment Options for HIV," *JAMA* 280 [1998]: 106-113) (R.W. Simms, et al. "Fibromyalgia Syndrome in Patients with Human Immunodeficiency Virus," *American Journal of Medicine* 92 [1992]: 368-374) (L.M. Tierney, et al. *Current Medical Diagnosis and Treatment*. New York: McGraw Hill, 2001) (T.E. Andreolli, et al. *Cecil Essentials of Medicine*. n.p.: W.B. Saunders, 1997) Although it has many facets, pain resulting from AIDS and HIV can be controlled.

What Is a Virus?

To understand AIDS, you should know what a virus is and how a virus is replicated. A virus is a biological particle that is composed of a genetic material called DNA or RNA and a protein. A virus is not considered to be a living organism. Viruses are organisms that are essentially between living and nonliving things. Viruses can take over the genetic machinery of a cell or cells that they infect. By taking over the whole cell that they infect, they ultimately control the genetic machinery of the cell. The genetic machinery directs the cell's fate.

A virus can replicate itself within a host cell or do nothing once it infects the host cell. When a virus replicates itself in a host cell, thousands or even millions of copies of itself can be released from the cell and then go on to infect other cells. HIV, for example, can enter your body from unsafe sex practices or contaminated blood, enter your cells, and make millions, billions, and even trillions of copies of itself that go on to infect other cells in your body. A virus, therefore, is a highly effective means of causing you to develop and have an infection. A virus will consist of either RNA or DNA that is encased in a protein outer coat, which is called a capsid. If the virus gets into your body, it can cause a disease unless it is attacked by your antibodies. A virus that causes a disease is called virulent. If the virus gains entrance into your body but does not cause a disease, it is called a temperate virus. It is not clearly understood why a virus will be temperate or virulent.

Viruses are not considered living organisms, as previously stated. The cells in your body reproduce naturally. A virus, on the other hand, can reproduce only by invading one of your cells. The virus then uses your chemicals and other structures within your cell, referred to as genetic material, to make more viruses. A virus cannot reproduce unless the virus is able to invade one of your cells. The virus in your cells acts essentially like a parasite. If the virus is outside of your cell, it is the lifeless particle that has no control of its movement. It is spread randomly through the wind, in water, food, by blood, or by body secretions.

With respect to HIV, blood and body secretions are important mechanisms by which this virus spreads from one person's body into someone else's body. (C.J. Carpenter, et al. "Antiretroviral Therapy in Adults," *JAMA* 283 [2000]: 381-389) (JAMA Patient Page. "Drug Treatment Options for HIV," *JAMA* 280 [1998]:106-113) (L.M. Tierney, et al. *Current Medical Diagnosis and Treatment*. New York: McGraw Hill, 2001) (T.E. Andreolli, et al. *Cecil Essentials of Medicine*. n.p.: W.B. Saunders, 1997)

The science of virology is relatively new. A virus was first isolated in 1935. Electrophoresis is now used to examine different properties of a virus. Electrophoresis is a process that separates molecules based on their electrical charges. Different types of viruses exist depending upon the genetic material that it contains.

HIV, which is the causative virus of AIDS, is very complex. HIV has two strands of RNA inside of it. These two RNA strands are surrounded by two layers of a protein. A layer of fatty substances surround the inner proteins. Proteins with sugar chains attached to them are located within the fatty layer. The protein sugar complex on the fatty layer forms the outer coat of the virus.

Viruses in general are classified as DNA viruses or RNA viruses, depending on whether RNA or DNA is within the viral structure. In other words, a virus contains either RNA or DNA, but never both. The difference between an RNA virus and a DNA virus is the fashion in which they change the genetic machinery of the cell that they infect. When the virus is inside of your cell, a DNA virus usually produces new RNA, which in turn makes more viral proteins. On the other hand, the DNA from the virus that has infected your cell may join the DNA of your cell and then direct the synthesis (creation) of more new viruses. An RNA virus works in a different fashion. An RNA virus can enter your cell and make new proteins directly. The polio virus is an RNA virus.

You need to know that in a normal, nonviral cell such as a cell in your skin or muscle, DNA is needed to make RNA. The HIV virus is a different type of virus, called a retrovirus. In a retrovirus, RNA makes DNA with the help of an enzyme. This new DNA then makes new RNA. The RNA then makes the proteins that become part of new viruses. Now that you understand what a virus is, you need to understand what a vaccine is. Vaccines can be important for the treatment of HIV and AIDS.

What Is a Vaccine?

In 1881, Louis Pasteur grew a weakened form of the rabies virus. He knew that if he could inject a weakened form of the virus he could help the body to use its mechanisms to fight the rabies virus and prevent it from replicating. If you are given a weak form of a virus, you will not have the symptoms normally associated with a virus such as fever and chills. Louis Pasteur showed that a single injection of a weak virus could provide you with future immunity from a normal infectious virus. Following injection of a weak form of a virus into your body, your body will construct antibodies to destroy not only the weakened virus (vaccine) but also the strong infectious form (virulent form) of the virus.

Louis Pasteur's original experiment is the basis of the development of vaccines to combat viral infections. When a virus, such as HIV or any other virulent virus attacks one of your cells, first the virus attaches to your cell. The virus will attach itself to the outer membrane of your cell at an area called a receptor site. When the virus attaches to your receptor site, the virus will release an enzyme that weakens a spot on the wall of your cell membrane. After the virus has weakened the outer wall of your cell, it will then inject the RNA from itself into your cell through the hole in your cell wall. Sometimes the whole virus can go right through the hole in your cell wall without just injecting its RNA. When the virus is inside of your cell, the HIV complex can make RNA, which in turns makes DNA. The DNA can then take complete control of your cell. The DNA can tell your cell to make new DNA, which is an RNA that is needed to make new viruses.

When the new viruses are made, an enzyme is released that destroys the outer wall of your call. When this wall is destroyed, the new viruses that have been made within your cell are now released into your body. These viruses will go to infect different cells of different tissues within your body at this time. As this process progresses, you can see how you can develop a viral infection. You develop fever, chills, joint pain, muscle pain, and so forth.

The HIV Virus

Be aware that when the new virus is made from the original virus, your cell that was infected by the virus will then be destroyed. You need to also know that when a new virus infects your cell, it does not cause immediate cellular destruction. Remember that a temperate virus does not cause a disease immediately. Therefore, even though a virus is within your cell or cells, it may take time for it to do any damage to your cell.

This example is the reason why HIV can be present in the body for some time before causing symptoms. HIV is classified as a retrovirus, as stated previously. The majority of the other viruses that commonly cause people to become sick are either DNA or RNA viruses. A retrovirus more commonly infects animals.

Most viral infections are contracted from particles in the air or from touching infected individuals. The retrovirus that can cause AIDS can be transmitted by one of three means:

- Exposure to infected blood products
- Sexual contact with infected people
- An infection from a mother to her baby

The infection with this virus appears within two to six weeks following infection. Early symptoms of infection with HIV are much like flu symptoms and include muscle pain, joint pain, headaches, as well as a sore throat and fever. (L.M. Tierney, et al. *Current Medical*

Diagnosis and Treatment. New York: McGraw Hill, 2001) (T.E. Andreolli, et al. *Cecil Essentials of Medicine*. n.p.: W.B. Saunders, 1997)

Antibodies to the HIV virus develop in your body within three to six months of your infection. Later symptoms, which take up to 10 years to develop, as those of AIDS, result from the destructive effects of HIV on your immune system and are characterized by unusual types of pneumonia, cancer, central nervous system infections, and other problems.

Changes in your immune system will eventually occur after you have been infected with the HIV virus. After the HIV virus enters your cell, the virus can set up a chronic infection in which new virus particles are constantly produced. You may develop some antibodies to the virus. When the level of your body's antibodies decreases, you can develop AIDS. Progression to AIDS, which is a syndrome following infection with the virus, can begin with a low red blood cell count. Other factors can be necessary for you to contract the HIV infection and for the development of progression to AIDS.

Other Factors Associated with HIV

There are four high-risk groups for developing AIDS, as follows:

- Homosexual and bisexual men
- Hemophiliacs and transfusion recipients
- Intravenous drug abusers
- Children born to infected mothers

Homosexual and bisexual men account for approximately 37-40 percent of the reported cases of AIDS in the United States. (L.M. Tierney, et al. *Current Medical Diagnosis and Treatment*. New York: McGraw Hill, 2001) However, this number is increasing. The majority of women with AIDS in the United States are in childbearing years. The number of individuals with AIDS does not take into account the high number of HIV-infected asymptomatic women. Remember that an HIV infection takes time to develop AIDS. The risks for a woman to expose herself to the HIV virus are through unsafe sex practices, intravenous drug use, and transfusions. A significant number of HIV-infected women have given birth to HIV-infected babies.

There is speculation that pregnancy can accelerate the disease progression of HIV. If you are pregnant and have HIV, you may develop symptoms two to three years after the delivery of your baby. This rate of AIDS development is faster than for homosexual men or intravenous drug users; approximately 40 percent of asymptomatic carriers of the virus in these categories will develop AIDS. The AIDS virus will decrease your lymphocytes, which are cells that normally exist in your bloodstream. Lymphocytes are important mediators of your immune system. These cells help fight the development of various diseases. The average time of onset of your viral infection to development of AIDS varies months to years with a mean time of approximately 10 years.

Health-care providers can not test an individual for HIV without permission. To check you for an HIV infection, your doctor must obtain an informed consent from you. Informed consent is a legal requirement and means that your doctor must inform you that you will be tested for HIV. You must sign an agreement that gives your doctor the right to do this test. Without your informed consent, your doctor is violating your patient rights. Informed consent is required in most states before you can be tested for HIV.

If you received blood products between 1987 and 1995, you are at an increased risk of developing AIDS. If you have active tuberculosis, you run a higher risk of contracting the HIV virus. If you are a health-care worker who performs invasive procedures such as starting intravenous catheters, surgery, and so on, you are at a risk of being exposed to the virus as well. It is not the invasive procedure itself that poses the risk for HIV, but the risk of a dangerous blood exposure while performing such a procedure. Furthermore, if you are a health-care provider and have had a needle stick, you again run the risk of exposure to the virus. If the needle puncture produces minimal blood exposure, the chance of you becoming infected is rare. If you are in any of these higher-risk categories, you should have your blood tested for the virus.

The name for the initial viral test performed is ELISA (enzyme-linked immunoabsorbent assay). If you have a positive screening test using ELISA, the infection with the HIV complex is confirmed with a repeat ELISA test as well as another test called a Western blot test. A doctor will usually not report a positive ELISA test to you until your Western blot test has been confirmed to be positive.

If you are pregnant and have been infected with the HIV virus, the incidence of a premature birth is increased as well as mental retardation of your baby. You also run the risk of having a low-birth-weight baby. Otherwise, there is no evidence that the HIV virus affects the outcome of your pregnancy if you have no symptoms. Remember that if you have been infected by the HIV virus and do give birth, your baby has a chance of developing AIDS.

Because HIV can be transmitted sexually, if you are positive for the virus you should be screened for other sexually transmitted diseases such as gonorrhea and syphilis. You may need to be tested for the hepatitis virus as well as Chlamydia infection. If you have the HIV virus, you should be immunized with some vaccines for other diseases.

You can develop a pneumococcal infection, which can cause pneumonia. It is recommended that you receive a pneumococcal vaccine. (L.M. Tierney, et al. *Current Medical Diagnosis and Treatment*. New York: McGraw Hill, 2001) (T.E. Andreolli, et al. *Cecil Essentials of Medicine*. n.p.: W.B. Saunders, 1997) Revaccination after five years should be considered. You should also have the hepatitis B virus vaccine. HIV-infected individuals are at a higher risk of becoming carriers of the hepatitis B virus after having an acute hepatitis B virus infection. You may also need to be tested for the hepatitis C virus.

Causes of Pain Associated with AIDS

You should realize now that HIV is a serious infection. When AIDS becomes prevalent, you can develop significant pain with multiple causes.

HIV virus infection is characterized by a deterioration of your body's immune system. This deterioration in your immune system will cause you to develop AIDS. Cells in your immune system are disabled and are killed during the infection. You have important immune cells in your body called CD4+T. During the HIV infection, the number of these cells progressively declines. When these cells fall to a critical level, you are vulnerable to infections as well as cancers.

The HIV virus induces AIDS by causing the death of the CD4+T cells in your body. (T.E. Andreolli, et al. *Cecil Essentials of Medicine*. n.p.: W.B. Saunders, 1997) These cells are important for the normal function of your immune system. The AIDS virus also interferes with their normal function. When this happens, your ability to fight other infections is diminished. HIV virus is called a slow virus. This means that the course of infection with the HIV virus has a long interval between the initial infection and the onset of the AIDS symptoms.

Here are some of the conditions that HIV/AIDS can cause:

- Fever and night sweats
- Loss of appetite
- Nausea and vomiting
- Chest pain related to pneumonia
- Chronic sinus infection with headache
- Tumor on your spinal cord
- Meningitis with neck pain and headaches
- Painful lesions in your mouth
- Hepatitis with abdominal pain
- Burning or piercing pain in your arms or legs

(C.J. Carpenter, et al. "Antiretroviral Therapy in Adults," *JAMA* 283 [2000]: 381-389) (JAMA Patient Page. "Drug Treatment Options for HIV," *JAMA* 280 [1998]: 106-113) (R.W. Simms, et al. "Fibromyalgia Syndrome in Patients with Human Immunodeficiency Virus," *American Journal of Medicine* 92 [1992]: 368-374) (L.M. Tierney, et al. *Current Medical Diagnosis and Treatment*. New York: McGraw Hill, 2001) (T.E. Andreolli, et al. *Cecil Essentials of Medicine*. n.p.: W.B. Saunders, 1997)

After you are infected by the HIV virus, in two to four weeks you will have flulike symptoms. The HIV virus is unique in that it escapes your body's immune responses. Once infected, you can progress to AIDS in an average of 10 years. Combinations of three or more anti-HIV drugs called highly active antiretroviral therapy can delay the progression of the HIV disease for prolonged periods. As your body's immune system is overwhelmed, increased quantities of the virus enter your bloodstream from your cells that were infected. With the increased use of agents for erectile dysfunction, there have been increases in sexual activity among older adults. With this increase in sexual activity, the number of HIV and AIDS cases has increased drastically.

This virus can cause you to have a *neuropathy*. A neuropathy is a lesion in your nerves in your body that are outside of your spinal cord and brain. AIDS can cause you to have a painful neuropathy. Neuropathy associated with AIDS can be intermittent or constant. The pain can vary in severity from mild to severe. The pain can be burning, shooting, aching, or stabbing. It is believed that the HIV virus can cause nerve damage, which is the cause of your neuropathy. You can develop headaches from an HIV virus meningitis. Also you can have abdominal pain related to gastrointestinal disease and chest pain related to pneumonia.

The Risk of Other Infections

The use of receiving an influenza vaccine is if you have AIDS is controversial. There is a chance that this vaccine could promote HIV replication for up to three months following your vaccination. You should also be considered for a vaccination against the Haemophilus influenza pneumonia. If you have the HIV virus, you run the risk of being infected with the varicella zoster virus. If you are exposed to chicken pox or shingles, you may need an antiviral medication. You should have a tuberculosis test in addition to the other recommended tests. This test is called a PPD test, which is a protein extract from cultures tuberculin bacteria. This test will tell if you have been in contact with tuberculosis. It takes 48 to 72 hours for this test to become positive. If you have a positive test, you should receive tuberculosis treatment, which consists of treatment with an antituberculin drug or drugs. (C.J. Carpenter, et al. "Antiretroviral Therapy in Adults," *JAMA* 283 [2000]: 381-389) (JAMA Patient Page. "Drug Treatment Options for HIV," *JAMA* 280 [1998]: 106-113)

If you have been infected with the HIV virus, you run the risk of other bacterial infections. You can develop a bacterial infection causing purple colored lesions around your skin. You can also develop gastrointestinal infections as well as pulmonary infections. You can develop a salmonella infection as well as bacterial pneumonia. Bacterial pneumonias occurs frequently in HIV-infected patients. These bacterial pneumonias can be a result of a streptococcus pneumonia or an H. influenzae pneumonia. Some of these infections can be resistant to antibiotics. If you have syphilis and are HIV infected, treatment failures are common. You need to know that syphilis can affect your central nervous system. When this happens, your doctor will do a spinal tap to diagnose whether you are developing neurosyphilis. You are at a risk of developing not only tuberculosis but you are also at risk for developing a fungal infection in addition to all of the other diseases described.

A common fungal infection is candidiasis. This fungus can affect your mouth, esophagus, and your vagina (if you are a woman and have HIV). These fungal infections are common in HIV-infected individuals. The severity of a fungal infection as well as the other diseases mentioned depends on your degree of suppression of your immune system. Oral and vaginal fungal infections usually respond to topical therapies. You can also develop a fungal infection of your central nervous system. The cryptococcus neoformans fungal infection is the most common cause of central nervous system fungal infections in patients who have developed AIDS.

You can develop headaches as well as fever and have significant changes in your mental status. To make this diagnosis, your doctor will do a spinal tap on you. Your doctor will measure your spinal fluid pressure by placing a needle into your spinal fluid to see whether you are having excessive pressure on your brain. You may need repeated spinal fluid taps followed by removal of some of your spinal fluid to decrease any pressure that could be affecting your brain.

Some fungal infections are more prevalent in certain areas of the United States. You can also develop a histoplasmosis fungal infection if you live around the Ohio Valley, although this type of infection is not limited to this area. You can develop a fever, weight loss, and an enlargement of your liver and possibly your spleen. This fungus can affect your bone marrow and decrease some of your blood cells.

Another fungal infection that is prevalent in the southwestern United States that can cause you problems is the coccidioides immitis. This fungal frequently affects the lungs. Aspergillosis is another fungus that can infect you. When these different organisms affect your body, you can have generalized pain, including muscle pain, joint pain, and headaches. If you have increased pressure in your spinal fluid that is compressing your brain, you can have severe headaches. Of course, with pneumonia, you will expect to have chest pain associated with a bacterial or fungal infection.

One of the leading causes of death in individuals with AIDS is the pneumocysdis carinii pneumonia. This is the most common infection in AIDS patients and is the leading cause of death in this patient population. Not only does this disease affect your lungs, it can affect other parts of your body as well.

If you have AIDS, you can also develop tumors associated with AIDS. These tumors include Kaposi's sarcoma as well as Hodgkins and non-Hodgkins lymphoma. Another type of infection that you can develop is a protozoan infection. Protozoa is an infectious agent. You can develop a parasite infection caused by a protozoa. Protozoa will get into your cells. When inside your cells, protozoa will use what it needs from your cell so that the protozoa can survive. Protozoa is composed of one cell. They are microscopic in size but are larger than a virus. The protozoa can multiply within your body.

A protozoa infection example is toxoplasma gondii, which can cause a serious infection of your central nervous system. You can present to your health-care provider with a severe headache as well as other abnormalities of your nervous system. Cryptosporidium is an infection that can give you chronic diarrhea. Usually this parasite can be observed in your stool. Other protozoeal infections can cause you to have chronic diarrhea as well. Another protozoa that can cause generalized infections in your body is the strongyloides protozoa.

Differences in Men and Women

Gender differences between men and women are noted. With respect to AIDS, women's bodies differ from men's bodies. Drug companies are doing studies to see whether there is any evidence that women respond differently to the AIDS drugs. A study at Johns Hopkins revealed that women were progressing to AIDS at the same rate as men but it only took half the viral infection that it took to infect men.

It is now known that there are gender differences in HIV. (L.M. Tierney, et al. *Current Medical Diagnosis and Treatment*. New York: McGraw Hill, 2001) (T.E. Andreolli, et al. *Cecil Essentials of Medicine*. n.p.: W.B. Saunders, 1997) A study in Kenya revealed that women were often infected by multiple virus variants as opposed to men. In other words, the HIV infecting the men appeared to be of one type of HIV virus, whereas women have several different variants of the virus. It was speculated that the virus was mutating faster in women than in men. Women naturally have more cells in their bodies that recognize and attack the HIV virus. It is thought that women's stronger immune response than men to the virus could force the virus to mutate or it is possible that women have a greater infection of the virus than men. In other words, women probably get a larger dose of the virus when they are infected than men. If women are infected with more versions of the HIV virus, this could mean that they would react differently to different drugs or to different vaccines. Women who are infected with the smaller number of the HIV virus became sick at the same rate as did men.

Current Research Findings

It has been reported recently by the American Civil Liberties Union that there are civil rights violations against individuals who have HIV and AIDS. (*Arkansas Democrat Gazette,* 2003) The ACLU related that individuals are being fired, rental agreements are destroyed, and they receive inadequate care when they relate that they have HIV or AIDS. It is estimated that 900,000 people in the United States have AIDS or HIV. They are denied medical treatment and are discriminated against in their workplace. They have difficulty getting into nursing homes as well.

In New York, an AIDS mortality rate per 10,000 persons age 15 to 64 was studied. AIDS was among the five leading causes of death for men age 25 to 54 and the leading cause of death for men age 30 to 39. For women AIDS was the fourth leading cause of death for women age 25 to 29 and the second leading cause of death for women age 30 to 34. Premature mortality was noted to be 10 percent in men age 15 to 64 and 3.6 percent for women. (*The New York Times,* 2003)

Condom use has been recommended as a method to prevent HIV transmission. According to the Ovid Medline website (a subscription-based service), a study published in 1989 revealed that 62 percent of men used condoms to prevent HIV virus transmission, whereas only 17 percent of women purchased or used condoms to prevent AIDS transmission. Public health professionals have been concerned about the devastation caused by HIV and AIDS in the developing world. It is estimated that 10 percent of people in South Africa are infected with HIV. These rates are higher in other African countries. In Africa, for some reason, the HIV virus passes from women to men at a higher rate of efficiency than is observed in the West. In the year 2000, then President Clinton declared the world AIDS epidemic a threat to U.S. national security.

It is estimated that if 1 million people in the United States now have HIV or AIDS, approximately 500,000 of them are either untreated or undiagnosed. Drugs for the treatment of AIDS are constantly being developed. (T.E. Andreolli, et al. *Cecil Essentials of Medicine*. n.p.: W.B. Saunders, 1997) Essentially, AIDS has gone from being an immediate sentence of death to a chronic manageable disease. Currently Russia has the fastest growing epidemic of AIDS, thought to be because of intravenous drug use. Epidemics are now beginning in China. The rate of AIDS cases and deaths did slow down, which was attributed to successful antiretroviral therapy. The problem with some of the drug therapy is that some individuals either develop a resistance to the drugs or they experience side effects from the drugs and stop taking them.

With the increased use of agents for erectile dysfunction, there have been increases in sexual activity among older adults. With this increase in sexual activity, the number of HIV and AIDS cases has increased drastically. The problem that has arisen in the United States is that many adults over age 50 are not protecting themselves against AIDS. Some of these individuals do not think that they are at risk for HIV infection. The incidence of AIDS in individuals over 50 continues to increase in the United States. In women over 50, the number of new AIDS cases more than doubled between 1991 and 1996. In older men, the increase was similar.

An effective vaccine against HIV infection continues to be researched. (C.J. Carpenter, et al. "Antiretroviral Therapy in Adults," *JAMA* 283 [2000]: 381-389) (JAMA Patient Page. "Drug Treatment Options for HIV," *JAMA* 280 [1998]: 106-113) That one "magic bullet" remains to be developed. Some of the vaccines currently being studied provide protection for some individuals but not all. Two anti-HIV drugs have been shown to cause death in some pregnant women. These drugs are stavudine and didanosine. Between 1991 and 1995, there was a 63 percent increase in women diagnosed with AIDS.

The increase in HIV infection in men was noted in younger women who date older men. It has been shown that young women are less likely to insist that older men wear condoms during sexual intercourse. When HIV and AIDS was first made known in the 1980s, it was a disease of gay men as well as a disease of people who had received blood transfusions or individuals who shared needles for injecting drugs. An increasing number of women with AIDS has been reported, and the exposure to the HIV virus was through heterosexual sex.

A current public health movement in the United States now exists with an intention of reducing a woman's risk of HIV infection. Prevention of HIV in women is being emphasized. As you can see from this chapter, the HIV infection with a progression to AIDS is a devastating disease. However, as new treatments are being discovered, if you have the HIV infection, your quality of life will be greatly improved. You must, however, remember that the drugs to treat AIDS are extremely powerful drugs but they do not render a cure for the HIV infection.

We all need to comprehend the worldwide AIDS epidemic. We need to do whatever we can to address this epidemic and attempt to make a difference where we can.

Treatment for HIV and AIDS

Your pain can be treated with *narcotic* drugs as well as *antidepressants* and *anticonvulsant* medications such as Neurontin. Mexilitine, an anticonvulsant medication, may also help to control your pain. Exercise therapy is sometimes beneficial for the management of your pain. It is believed that exercise can increase your body's endorphins, which in turns helps to manage your pain. HIV-related pain becomes increasingly severe as the disease progresses. Drugs used to treat the HIV infection can cause neuropathic pain. It is estimated that 30 percent of the neuropathic pain syndromes suffered by individuals who have the HIV disease are caused by drugs to attack the HIV virus. Neuropathic pain in the HIV-infected patient in most instances can be adequately controlled.

In treating AIDS-related pain, your doctor should direct attention to your emotional distress, your depression, and anxiety, which can also be seen if you suffer from AIDS.

New therapies and increased knowledge in the causes of pain associated with the HIV virus has given HIV-infected individuals an increased quality and duration of life that several years ago would have been totally unimaginable. Overall the AIDS incidence and mortality have continued to decline, probably because of new therapies, especially antiviral therapies. However, for women the benefits have been shown to be less than for men. It has been reported that there is gender-based discrimination in the treatment of women with HIV infections. It is also reported that there is insufficient attention to the medical community's response to women's HIV risks.

For Men

- Exercise therapy will help release endorphins that can help inhibit your pain.
- Prescriptions such as anticonvulsants, antidepressants, and narcotics should be taken to relieve your symptoms of pain.
- Be aware that new therapies are constantly evolving for HIV and the treatment of its pain. Keep educating yourself on these new discoveries and talk with your doctor about them to see if they will be beneficial in helping relieve your pain.

For Women

- Exercise therapy will help release endorphins that can help inhibit your pain.
- Prescriptions such as anticonvulsants, antidepressants, and narcotics should be taken to relieve your symptoms of pain.
- Be aware that new therapies are constantly evolving for HIV and the treatment of its pain. Keep educating yourself on these new discoveries and talk with your doctor about them to see if they will be beneficial in helping relieve your pain.

Chapter 26

Understanding Raynaud's Disease and Phenomena

Maurice Raynaud was a French doctor who died in 1881. He described a syndrome wherein the skin of the fingers or toes of some of his patients became white in color or blue in color, and these patients complained of moderate to severe pain after exposure to cold temperatures or as a result of emotional stress. Raynaud described his patients as complaining of burning pain, numbness, swelling in their extremities, as well as excessive sweating. This condition is now called Raynaud's disease. (J.A. Spittell. "Diagnosis and Management of Occlusive Peripheral Arterial Disease," Curr Probl Cardiol 15 [1990]: 1-35) (D.S. Sumner. *Hemodynamics for Surgeons*. n.p.: Grune & Stratton, 1975)

Diseases that contribute to Raynaud's disease or phenomena include obstructive arterial disorders, vascular disorders, and scleroderma. Drug intoxications as well as some cancers and neurological entities can cause Raynaud's disease. Furthermore, thermal or occupational trauma, especially vibration trauma, can also cause Raynaud's disease. Raynaud's disease is a vascular pain. It is also a complex form of pain. Raynaud's disease can last a few minutes to hours. The average length of attack is 5 minutes to 60 minutes.

This chapter will teach you about vascular diseases, their many causes, risk factors, and current treatment methods. You will learn about Raynaud's disease and other diseases related to it, as well as what the diagnosing criteria are. Current research findings and treatment options are also discussed.

What Are Vasospastic Diseases?

Vascular pain in general can be divided into three categories:

- Arterial pain
- Pain due to dysfunction of the capillaries in your tissue
- Pain related to pathology of your veins

Arterial pain, which originates in your heart vessels, is discussed in Chapter 22. Pain coming from your arteries can be a result of different diseases such as atherosclerosis, which is a buildup of fat and calcium within the inside of your arteries. You may have a thrombosis, which is a stoppage of blood in your small arteries. You can also have inflammation of your arteries. If you have a decreased blood flow going to your heart muscles, you will have heart pain called angina pectoris. This is the result of decreased oxygen to your tissue, which is called ischemia.

If you have no blood flow at all to your heart muscle and if your heart muscle dies, you will suffer a heart attack or a myocardial infarction. You have blood flow that normally goes to your legs. If your arteries are occluded, you will not have adequate blood flow going to your legs. This will cause you to have pain in your lower extremities, especially in your calves (for example, when you walk). If you have decreased blood flow going to your legs, you will have pain, aches, cramps, and occasionally some numbness in your leg muscles. These symptoms are noted mostly during exercise such as walking. Furthermore, these symptoms are usually relieved by rest. The severity of pain following exercise such as walking can help your doctor determine the severity of this syndrome. The more clogged up your arteries are, the more pain you will experience with minimal exercise. For example, if you are able to walk 100 yards without pain, this demonstrates much less severity than if you can only walk 15 yards before you develop pain in one or both legs.

If your major arteries in your abdomen are occluded with plaque, you may develop pain in your abdomen. You should remember that the tissues in your legs need oxygen. When you exercise, your leg muscles have a higher oxygen demand than when you are at rest. If your blood flow to your muscles and nerves in your legs is decreased, your tissues do not receive adequate oxygen. The supply of oxygen to your tissues is low while your body's demand for oxygen is high. This imbalance in your tissue oxygen will cause you to have leg pain.

You can have obstruction of both your arteries and veins of your limbs. When this happens you have what is called Burger's disease. This disease is caused by swelling of the small arteries and veins in your extremities. (J.A. Spittell. "Diagnosis and Management of Occlusive Peripheral Arterial Disease," Curr Probl Cardiol 15 [1990]: 1-35) (D.S. Sumner. *Hemodynamics for Surgeons*. n.p.: Grune & Stratton,

1975) The painful symptoms that you note are a result again of decreased oxygen flow to your tissues. When your blood supply is decreased, which happens in Burger's disease, your oxygen to your tissue is significantly decreased. You will develop pain in the calves of your legs. If the oxygen deficit is extremely low, your nerves to your legs will suffer injury. This nerve injury will cause you pain as well as lack of oxygen to your extremity muscles. If your pain is severe, you may not experience relief with rest. If your tissues are deprived of oxygen for a long time, you can develop ulcerations in your skin and also develop gangrene.

Another problem with your blood vessels that can cause you to have pain is Takayasu's syndrome. This syndrome is due to inflammation or swelling of your small arteries of the upper part of your body, including your eyes. It occurs more in young girls as well as young women. More than 60 percent of individuals complain of weakness and fever as well as joint pain and pain in the upper extremities. (J.A. Spittell. "Diagnosis and Management of Occlusive Peripheral Arterial Disease," Curr Probl Cardiol 15 [1990]: 1-35)

When this pain occurs, you will soon develop the pain around the arteries that are inflamed. This disease can progress to even cause you to have angina pectoris. If this angina pectoris progresses, you may have a heart attack as well.

Temporal arteritis is another inflammation of the large arteries, especially around your temples. Inflammation of one or both of these arteries can cause you to have a significant headache. It can also involve other branches of your carotid artery. Temporal arteritis occurs usually if you are over 55 years of age.

Temporal arteritis is more common in women than in men. Occasionally if you have temporal arteritis you will have headaches that are occasionally unbearable. Your headache will begin over your involved arteries. As stated, the pain mostly begins about your temples. However, this disease can also affect your occipital arteries. These are the arteries that are toward the back of your head and approximate an area where the back of your skull meets your neck. You may have tenderness to touch over the swollen and inflamed arteries. The areas around your inflamed arteries are extremely sensitive to firm touch. You may even have decreased blood flow to your jaw muscles. Therefore, when you chew you may have significant pain in your jaw muscles. Temporal arteritis can affect arteries in multiple locations throughout your body. You may develop a flulike syndrome with generalized muscle pain as well as fever and weakness. The muscle pain can progress and involve your neck, shoulders, and pelvis as well as your legs. The arteries are usually affected on both sides of your body. This will cause a decrease of blood flow to your organs, resulting in significant pain. Your small arteries throughout your body are called arterioles.

Sometimes the diameter of your arterioles can significantly decrease. This change in your vessel diameter is called vessel constriction. Your fingers and toes may change color. With a decrease of oxygen to your tissues, you will experience a burning pain. With a prolonged decrease in blood flow to your tissues, you may develop abnormal shocking sensations in your extremities including your fingers and toes.

Erythemalgia is a syndrome that can affect both your arms and your legs. (J.A. Spittell. "Diagnosis and Management of Occlusive Peripheral Arterial Disease," Curr Probl Cardiol 15 [1990]: 1-35) (D.S. Sumner. *Hemodynamics for Surgeons*. n.p.: Grune & Stratton, 1975) The temperature in your extremities will be elevated and you will have redness in either your arms or legs. Along with the change in color, you will have burning pain as well as tingling in your extremities. Sometimes you will experience swelling in your hands and feet. Usually this disease affects your legs. However, it can also affect your arms. This entity is usually seen if you are exposed to an increased temperature. When you experience the pain, it can last for a few minutes up to hours. This type of pain in this syndrome can be associated with diabetes. Sometimes sympathetic blocks such as described in Chapter 17 can help decrease the pain associated with your erythemalgia. Patients have reported complete relief of their pain following sympathetic blocks. This observation led scientists to question whether this disease is related to reflex sympathetic dystrophy.

Types of Raynaud's Disease

You have seen different diseases that decrease blood flow to tissues and cause pain. Raynaud's disease is a disorder of your fingers, toes, nose, ears, and sometimes your tongue. When you have symptoms, you will suddenly experience a decrease in your blood flow to these areas. You will have color changes of your skin, especially on your fingers and toes, with exposure to cold or emotional stress. As stated previously, cold on your face can also cause changes in your fingers and toes. Many people use the term Raynaud's disease to include Raynaud's phenomena. This disease is classified as one of two types: primary and secondary. Secondary Raynaud's disease is also called Raynaud's phenomena.

Primary Raynaud's disease has no underlying medical problem and is mild and causes fewer complications than secondary Raynaud's disease. Approximately 50 percent of people diagnosed with Raynaud's disease are primary Raynaud's disease and 50 percent are Raynaud's phenomena. Women are five times more likely than men to develop primary Raynaud's disease. Most patients develop Raynaud's disease before age 40. Be aware that 30 percent of individuals with primary Raynaud's disease progress to secondary Raynaud's disease. Approximately 15 percent of individuals with primary Raynaud's disease do improve. The secondary Raynaud's disease or Raynaud's phenomena is essentially the same as primary Raynaud's disease but secondary Raynaud's disease occurs in individuals who have predisposing factors.

We have mentioned the associated diseases that you can have if you have secondary Raynaud's disease. Primary Raynaud's disease can be later classified as a secondary Raynaud's disease after a predisposing underlying disease has been diagnosed. This observation is seen in 30 percent of patients. A secondary type of Raynaud's disease is more complicated and severe. This type of Raynaud's disease is more likely to worsen. We have mentioned diseases that can predispose you to secondary Raynaud's disease, including scleroderma, SLE, rheumatoid arthritis, and polio. For some reason, herniated discs and spinal cord tumors as well as cerebrovascular accidents and polio can progress to Raynaud's disease.

Causes of Vasospastic Diseases

The syndromes that we have mentioned are related to lack of oxygen to tissue. If you have decreased oxygen to your tissue, you will develop pain. The pain may be intermittent or it can be constant. Your pain will be constant if the oxygen flow to your muscles and nerves in your extremities is severely compromised. If you have decreased blood flow to your muscles, you will have areas in your muscles that are painful. These painful areas will mimic myofascial trigger points. If you have decreased blood flow to your tissues as well as inflammation and release of *prostaglandins*, your pain can become severe.

Cold Temperatures

In the 1800's Raynaud described a condition in which fingers and toes became cold and painful following exposure to cold temperatures or as a result of emotional stress. Consequently, Raynaud's phenomena refers to symptoms of decreased blood flow in the fingers and toes. Eighty percent of individuals who have Raynaud's disease are female. Usually Raynaud's disease occurs before age 35. The prevalence in the general population in the United States approaches 5 percent for this disease. If you have Raynaud's disease, usually you have normal arteries. The painful symptoms that you experience with this disease are again related to a decrease in oxygen to your tissues. Usually these symptoms are reversible. Sometimes if you have underlying systemic diseases, you can develop Raynaud's disease.

In your fingers, toes, nose, and ears, you have small blood vessels or arteries that transmit blood and oxygen to your tissues. If you have Raynaud's disease, these vessels become extremely small. This is called *vasoconstriction.* When your Raynaud's disease crisis is over, your blood vessels will appear normal.

If your hands become cold, you may develop Raynaud's disease. If you live in a cold environment and have to shovel snow off of your walkway, your hands will become cold. If your hands or your feet become cold, this will cause the internal diameter of your blood vessels to decrease. When this happens, your blood vessels can vaso constrict, causing you to have significant pain. As your extremities become colder, the blood flow to your fingers, toes, ears, and nose can completely stop. As your toes and fingers become warm again, your blood vessels reopen. It is recommended that you dress warmly to avoid extreme cold exposure.

Cold on your face can also trigger Raynaud's phenomena in your hands. This observation suggests that there is an abnormality in your area of your brain that controls temperature regulation. (J.A. Spittell. "Diagnosis and Management of Occlusive Peripheral Arterial Disease," Curr Probl Cardiol 15 [1990]: 1-35) (D.S. Sumner. *Hemodynamics for Surgeons*. n.p.: Grune & Stratton, 1975) This will develop pain in your veins. You can have inflammation in one of your veins. Sometimes this inflammation can decrease the blood flow in your vein. Your vein can be red and tender as well as firm to touch. You may develop pain at rest. If you have a stoppage of blood in your veins, it can form a clot. You may develop pain in your calf muscle noted when you bend your foot up toward the ceiling. You may develop pain in your muscles and tendons in the leg that has the occlusion of blood flow in the vein. If the blood flow in your vein has returned, you can still have pain that remains in your legs. You can also develop pain in your muscles that mimics myofascial trigger points.

Any time that you have an effect on the blood flow to any of your tissues caused by the syndromes that was mentioned, you can develop reflex sympathetic dystrophy. The reason for this development of this potentially disabling disease is unknown. If reflex sympathetic dystrophy occurs, your skin will become shiny and you will develop sweating in your hands or on the soles of your feet. Your bone density will decrease. This is due to the lack of blood flow to your bones. When your bone blood flow decreases, minerals and calcium do not reach the bone. Your bone will become weak as a result. This can make you prone to fractures of your bone. Your muscles may shrink in size and you may even develop tremors. Sometimes sympathetic blocks with local anesthetics performed by your anesthesiologist can relieve these painful symptoms.

Sickle Cell Disease

Sometimes abnormalities in blood cells can include an onset of pathology in your arteries and veins and cause you to have pain. Sickle cell disease can cause you to have pain all over your body. This pain can be severe. The sickling cells can stop blood flow to your blood vessels. As a result, you have generalized lack of oxygen to all of your tissues and this can cause severe pain. Sickle cell disease is inherited. Sickle cell disease is more prevalent in African Americans. In Africa, the sickle cell gene gave advantage to individuals because it would resist infection caused by malaria. This is the reason why the disease is prevalent in populations of African descent. The deposition of sickle cells, as previously mentioned, decreases blood flow to your tissues. This causes a painful crisis to the majority of your organs.

If you have sickle cell disease and if you have a painful crisis, you will note the development of severe pain. The frequency of the pain occurs most in the third and fourth decades. Cold and infection can induce you to have a sickle cell crisis. Furthermore, dehydration and alcohol consumption can cause you to have a crisis as well as exposure to low-oxygen tension. You can have pain in different parts of your body. Chest pain can occur. This is usually accompanied by a fever. You back, legs, and stomach may also develop significant pain.

If you have pain in your abdomen, this pain can mimic appendicitis. The sickle cell–related pain can last from hours to even weeks. You can have a gradual or sudden onset of pain. You can have decreased blood flow to your bone. This will cause some tissue death in your bone. You can have pain in your joints as well as swelling. This pain is severe enough to cause you to experience depression.

Treatment of this disease is usually the administration of either steroids or nonsteroidal anti-inflammatory drugs. If your pain is severe, your doctor may prescribe narcotic medications until your crisis subsides. If you have infection as a cause of your sickle cell crisis, you may require antibiotics. Because of the depression associated with this entity, you may need to have a psychological evaluation as well as the administration of antidepressant drugs.

Bleeding in Your Joints and Muscles

Hemophilia is a disorder of your blood's ability to form a clot. You can have spontaneous bleeding into your joints. Not only can you have bleeding into your joints, you will also have swelling of your joints including your knees, ankles, elbows, and shoulders. The bleeding into your joints will cause your joints to swell. If you have persistent bleeding into your joints, you will eventually have decreased range of motion of your joints. This restriction will make it difficult for you to move about.

Be aware that you can also have bleeding into your muscles. This bleeding will cause you to have the immediate onset of pain. It becomes worse as you try to move the muscle that has suffered the bleed. Your forearm muscles are frequently involved from a hemophiliac-related bleed. You can injure the nerves that go to your hand. The bleeding will enter your forearm and compress the nerves that go to your hand. You should not be given aspirin or any nonsteroidal anti-inflammatory drugs other than possibly the COX-2 inhibitors, because nonsteroidal anti-inflammatory drugs can make your bleeding worse.

Multiple Myeloma Cancer

Vascular-related pain can also be associated with multiple *myeloma.* If you have myeloma, you will have a malignant formation of your plasma cells. Plasma cells are antibody producing cells found in bone forming tissue as well as in your lungs and your abdomen. This increase in your plasma cells can affect your organs and cause you to have painful symptoms. Usually bone pain is the most common pain noted involving multiple myeloma.

The bone pain associated with this entity involves primarily the back. If you have multiple myeloma, your pain is usually worse at night and is made worse by movement. This disease can destroy your bone. With significant destruction of your bone, your bone can collapse. If the bones in your spine collapse, the collapsed bone can injure your spinal cord. With injury to your spinal cord, you can lose control of your bowel and your bladder and even become paralyzed.

Multiple myeloma can be an extremely painful entity and is usually treated by a medical specialist who deals with cancer called an oncologist. While oncologists know how to treat cancer, they may not know how to adequately treat your cancer pain. Oncologists sometimes request the help of a pain medicine specialist to help manage their patient's cancer pain. You should now be aware that any type of pathology that will decrease the blood flow to your tissue can cause you to have significant pain.

Connective Tissue Disorders

Raynaud's disease can also be associated with connective tissue disease. This disease can be related to connective tissue diseases such as scleroderma, systemic lupus erythematosus, rheumatoid arthritis, dermatomyositis, and polyarteritis. These are all connective tissue disorders. Connective tissue is the supporting tissue or framework of your body. It is formed of different substances that contain different kinds of cells.

Vibration Trauma and Repetitive Motion Movements

Vibration trauma associated with chainsaws and jackhammers can predispose you to developing Raynaud's disease. (P.M. King. *Sourcebook of Occupational Rehabilitation.* New York: Plenum Press, 1998) Repetitive motion movements that can cause carpal tunnel syndrome can also predispose you to develop Raynaud's disease. Electrical shocks and persistent exposure to extreme cold can also lead to the development of Raynaud's disease. The prevalence of Raynaud's phenomena in the general population can be up to 15 percent of the population.

If you work with vibratory tools such as jackhammers, you are prone to Raynaud's disease. (P.M. King. *Sourcebook of Occupational Rehabilitation.* New York: Plenum Press, 1998) The problem is that this aspect of Raynaud's disease will be permanent even if you stop working with a vibratory tool. This is an industrial disease and is eligible for workmen's compensation benefits in most states. In some instances, Raynaud's disease is so mild that it is no more than a nuisance, whereas sometimes you can have severe enough pain to require you to take narcotic medications.

Risk Factors

The exact cause of Raynaud's disease remains speculative. It can be caused by hyperactivity of your sympathetic nervous system. Furthermore, it could be caused by your body's increased sensitivity to chemicals that are circulating in your bloodstream. There are receptors on your blood vessel walls. Some of these receptors are called alpha receptors. With the stimulation of these receptors, the internal caliber of your blood vessels can significantly close. If you have an increased number of these receptors on your blood vessels, you could develop Raynaud's disease.

You need to be aware that there are three phases of Raynaud's disease. When you are first exposed to cold, your small arteries contract and your fingers, toes, ears, or the tip of your nose and tongue become pale and white. This observation occurs because you are deprived of blood. Remember if you have an increased blood flow to your tissues, the tissue will appear red. After your oxygen is deprived, your blood vessels will expand. It is the veins that expand most. The veins carry blood that has minimal or no oxygen. This will give your blood a bluish tint. The area of the low-oxygen-carrying blood will appear blue. The area also feels cold to touch. When your arteries begin to dilate, the blood flow is increased. Oxygen is increased and your tissue color will appear normal. Putting your extremities in a warm environment will cause your blood vessels to expand. As the blood vessels expand, you may experience a throbbing pain.

As previously stated, females are more likely to develop Raynaud's disease than males. (R. Melzack and P. Wall, *Handbook of Pain Management a Clinical Companion of Textbook of Pain*, New York: Churchill Livingstone, 2003) Studies are now being done attempting to correlate Raynaud's disease with caffeine consumption as well as some dietary habits. The predisposition to develop Raynaud's disease may be genetic. Risk factors for developing Raynaud's disease do differ between males and females. Smoking is associated with Raynaud's disease only in males. Alcohol abuse can be associated with Raynaud's disease only in women. These observations tell you that there must be different mechanisms that influence the onset of Raynaud's disease.

Menopause and changes in your sex hormones can alter your blood flow to minimal levels in your digits as well as your ears and nose. If you have adult onset diabetes mellitus, your blood vessels may not dilate normally. Some individuals with diabetes are, therefore, prone to develop Raynaud's disease. Be aware that extreme cold will cause the muscles in the walls of your small arteries to contract. If you have a decrease in blood flow to your tissues, you have decreased oxygen as we have reiterated which will cause you pain. However, if you do suffer from Raynaud's disease, the amount of constriction of your arteries is extreme as compared to others who do not have Raynaud's disease. If you have Raynaud's disease, you will have a more severe constriction of your blood flow. Remember that anxiety and emotional distress can increase the activity of your sympathetic nervous system, which causes your blood vessels to constrict as well.

If you live in a cold area, wear a hat that covers your ears or wear earmuffs. If you are sensitive to cold, use drinking glasses that are insulated. You must also wear gloves before putting your hands into a freezer. The thermal regulatory control of your skin blood flow is vital to the maintenance of your normal body temperature. The sympathetic nervous system controls your skin blood flow. If you are exposed to cold, your sympathetic nervous system will cause your vessels to constrict.

You can have other predisposing factors to cause you to have Raynaud's disease. Living in a cool, damp climate can predispose you to Raynaud's disease. Hypertension can also have an effect as well as excessive sweating.

If you have a history of migraine headaches, you have an increased incidence of developing Raynaud's disease. Operating any machinery that vibrates can make you subject to Raynaud's disease; and if your fingers are subject to continuous physical stress such as typing or if you are a professional pianist, you can develop Raynaud's disease as well.

Rare symptoms of Raynaud's disease can occur as well. (J.A. Spittell. "Diagnosis and Management of Occlusive Peripheral Arterial Disease," Curr Probl Cardiol 15 [1990]: 1-35) (D.S. Sumner. *Hemodynamics for Surgeons*. n.p.: Grune & Stratton, 1975) There has been a case reported of a 38 year old female who had Raynaud's disease in her right upper extremity but also developed Raynaud's disease in her right nipple. She would develop pallor around the nipple and her pain on occasion would become unbearable.

If your Raynaud's disease is severe and chronic, you will develop deep ulcers in your skin. If your Raynaud's disease persists, you may develop gangrene, which can cause you to have an amputation of your affected digits. If you sustain a cut to your hands or your feet, notify your doctor if the cuts do not heal in a reasonable time. The treatment for Raynaud's disease can include calcium channel blockers, drugs that increase the caliber of your blood vessels. Your doctor will decide what treatment will best suit you. You should take vitamin C as well as E. Garlic has been shown in some noncontrolled studies to be effective.

Other Diseases Associated with Raynaud's

Your connective tissue can be classified as dense or loose. Adipose tissue is an example of lose connective tissue. Connective tissue can be elastic. Cartilage and bone are connective tissues. Your blood can be regarded as a connective tissue. For some reason that is not totally known, connective tissue diseases can be associated with Raynaud's disease. For example, Raynaud's phenomena is seen in 90 percent of patients with scleroderma, 30 percent of patients with rheumatoid arthritis, and 30 percent of patients with Sjogren's syndrome. (J.A. Spittell. "Diagnosis and Management of Occlusive Peripheral Arterial Disease," Curr Probl Cardiol 15 [1990]: 1-35) (D.S. Sumner. *Hemodynamics for Surgeons*. n.p.: Grune & Stratton, 1975) Scleroderma is essentially a disorder of a smooth muscle. This is a connective tissue disease that can be associated with esophageal reflux because of the effect of smooth muscle in your esophagus.

Scleroderma also affects your skin. By definition, it is called "hard skin." It is uncommon. Scleroderma is classified according to the degree of your skin thickening. Scleroderma is most common in adults. However, it can be seen in children. The hallmarks of scleroderma are light skin and Raynaud's phenomena.

Scleroderma is a generalized disorder of the small arteries as well as the connective tissue. Not only can your gastrointestinal tract be affected but also your lungs, your heart, and your kidneys. Most all patients who have scleroderma have Raynaud's disease. Patients with scleroderma can have pallor of the digits following cold exposure or emotional stress. Your fingers and toes can turn blue followed by redness in addition to burning pain and tingling. Raynaud's phenomena associated with scleroderma can affect your toes, fingers, ears, nose, and even your tongue. You can get gangrene in your fingers and toes and end up with an amputation. Swelling can be seen over your hands and feet. Over time, thinning of your skin can occur. The thinning of your skin is easily noted over joints. Usually scleroderma begins before age 40 and is more common in females. Approximately 80 percent of scleroderma patients are females.

Scleroderma can affect the kidneys and cause you to have kidney failure. Scleroderma can also affect your heart and cause some arrhythmias around your heart. You may need an echocardiograph if you have chest pain. This test can reveal some thickening around the outer wall of your heart. You will have muscle pain as well as joint pain if you have scleroderma. You will have stiffness in the morning. Systemic lupus erythematosus is a disease of unknown cause. It can also be associated with Raynaud's disease. Systemic lupus erythematosus (SLE) is caused by your body's production of antibodies that injure the tissues of some of your organs in your body. The symptoms can come and go. You may have a rash develop on your face. However, SLE can be life threatening if it involves your internal organs. SLE can cause you to have failure of your kidneys or hemorrhage as well as a pulmonary disease.

If you suffer from *vasculitis* (inflammation of your blood vessels) you can develop Raynaud's symptoms. Usually SLE occurs between ages 16 and 55. SLE occurs more frequently in women. (J.A. Spittell. "Diagnosis and Management of Occlusive Peripheral Arterial Disease," Curr Probl Cardiol 15 [1990]: 1-35) (D.S. Sumner. *Hemodynamics for Surgeons*. n.p.: Grune & Stratton, 1975) It is more prevalent in African American as well as Asian women. The triggering of your antibodies to attack your tissue is unknown. In some individuals, ultraviolet light can trigger the disease. This disease is usually inherited. This disease is caused by your antibodies. If your antibodies are deposited in your kidneys, you can have irreversible kidney damage. Antibodies can attack your red blood cells as well as your platelets. If your platelets become low, you can develop bleeding problems. If you have SLE, you will develop fatigue as well as muscle pain and arthritis. These symptoms can disappear only to come back at a later time. The rash that you develop over your face looks like a butterfly shape. Individuals with SLE are prone to develop Raynaud's disease. There is no known cure for SLE. Your generalized pain in your joints will be treated with analgesics. Approximately 30 percent of individuals with SLE will develop Raynaud's disease associated with SLE.

Arthritis is another disease that associated with Raynaud's disease. Rheumatoid arthritis is a chronic inflammatory disease that affects various organs. However, rheumatoid arthritis mostly affects the joints between your bones. You will notice changes in your hands, feet, elbows, neck, and so on. No one knows why rheumatoid arthritis occurs. It can be due to a accumulation of some of your white cells caused by a substance in your bloodstream. Rheumatoid arthritis will cause invasion of your cartilage, and your cartilage will be degraded and also your bone will be affected by rheumatoid arthritis. Rheumatoid arthritis is destructive. Inflammation and pain can occur around your tendons as well. Rheumatoid arthritis affects 5 percent of Native Americans. Otherwise, the rheumatoid arthritis affects between 1 to 2 percent of the population. Because Raynaud's disease is associated with rheumatoid arthritis, occasionally you may need sympathetic blocks with local anesthetic. Rheumatoid arthritis can affect your skin, eyes, lungs, and heart as well as your nervous system. Rheumatoid arthritis can also affect the arteries that supply blood to your heart muscle.

Dermatomyositis is an inflammatory disease that can affect your muscle. You will have muscle pain and tenderness. This disease is accompanied by a rash. The rash occurs on your upper eyelids. You may have some swelling around your eyes as well. You can have redness about the knuckles of your fingers. This disease can affect almost any organ system in your body. You can have involvement of the muscles of your fingers and toes. The muscles in your legs can become weak. This disease, like SLE, can be caused by an abnormality in your immune system. Raynaud's phenomena can become prominent if you have dermatomyositis. Your muscles will become weak. The diagnosis of this disease can be done by taking samples of your muscle.

Polyarteritis nodosa can also be associated with Raynaud's disease. This disease is caused by inflammation or swelling of the walls of your blood vessel. This disease can affect blood vessels of any size as well as in any location. It usually occurs between ages 40 and 50. Men are affected more than women. Your kidneys can be affected. If the disease progresses, you can develop kidney failure. This disease can affect your arteries going to your heart and can cause you to have a heart attack. It may cause abdominal pain and bleeding. This disease can affect your nervous system as well. It can cause you to have weakness as well as loss of sensation. As stated previously, it can be associated with rheumatoid arthritis.

Raynaud's disease can also be associated with *carpal tunnel syndrome*. The carpal tunnel syndrome causes one of the nerves at your wrist (median nerve) to be trapped and compressed. You can develop burning pain and tingling in your hand. Usually this affects the first three fingers of your hand. The symptoms usually occur at night. Sometimes if you shake your hand, the pain will go away. Not only can Raynaud's phenomena be associated with carpal tunnel syndrome, but other disorders can be associated with the carpal tunnel syndrome as well, including rheumatoid arthritis, gouty arthritis, and trauma.

If you have a *thoracic outlet syndrome*, you may develop Raynaud's disease as well. Like carpal tunnel syndrome, the thoracic outlet syndrome compresses nerves. The nerves from your spinal cord that go to your arms must pass through an outlet between your neck and shoulders. This outlet can be compressed by one of your ribs or by bone, muscles, or other tissues. You can have abnormal sensations in your fingers called parathesias. You may develop weakness of your hand muscles. Sometimes surgery can help this syndrome. If you have this syndrome, you may also be prone for Raynaud's phenomena as well. Be aware that pressure caused by crutches can compress nerves and vessels that go throughout your arms to your hands and fingers. Chronic use of crutches can contribute to the onset of Raynaud's phenomena.

In spite of all these diseases associated with Raynaud's disease, there is no reliable method of provoking Raynaud's phenomena. In other words, there may be some time during a day, month, or year that you develop the symptoms associated with Raynaud's phenomena.

Diagnosing Raynaud's Disease

The diagnosis of Raynaud's disease involves several components. The first component is that color changes must occur during the attacks provoked by cold or emotional stress. Another criteria is that these episodes must occur for at least two years. If you have no disease that decreases your blood flow to your tissues, the third criteria is that the attacks must occur in both the hands and the feet. Another criteria is that there should be no other cause for these episodes.

A diagnosis of Raynaud's disease can be confirmed by a cold stimulation test. The temperature of your fingers and toes is taken. Your hand and/or your foot is then placed in a container of ice water for 20 seconds. After your extremity is removed from the water, your temperature is immediately recorded. Your temperature is taken every five minutes until it returns to a normal baseline level. Normal individuals recover their temperature within 15 minutes. If you have Raynaud's disease, it will take you longer than 20 minutes to reach your baseline temperature.

We mentioned laser Doppler scanning, which is used to determine skin blood flow in Chapter 17. The laser Doppler scanning is now helpful for the diagnosis of Raynaud's disease. Blood flow can be measured around your fingers and toes. Laser Doppler scanning is usually correlated with your finger blood pressure. Skin blood pressure results can determine diagnosis of Raynaud's disease more accurately than the laser Doppler study. The laser Doppler study can be useful as well.

There are no good laboratory tests that will give you a diagnosis of Raynaud's disease. Currently there is no known way to prevent the development of Raynaud's disease. As a result, there is no known cure for this disease.

Current Research Findings

According to the National Library of Medicine website, www.NLM.gov, a study published in 2003 from England reported that gingko biloba extract can be useful in decreasing the symptoms associated with Raynaud's disease. The number of attacks per week was decreased with this remedy.

A newer drug is being studied for the treatment of Raynaud's syndrome. This drug is isosorbide mononitrate. A drug has been studied using laser Doppler flometry. The isosorbide mononitrate was shown to be effective in the treatment of the symptoms associated with Raynaud's disease in 19 women. This is a small study.

Further research needs to be carried out to evaluate the effects of this drug compared to a placebo control. As you now see, Raynaud's disease can fluctuate from being a mild nuisance to a severe disabling disease that can result in loss of fingers or toes. Research continues in diagnosis and treatment of this disease. If you suspect that you are developing Raynaud's disease, seek medical attention from a doctor knowledgeable in the diagnosis and treatment of this disease.

Treatment for Raynaud's Disease and Phenomena

Since ancient times, Chinese medical texts have described problems of hands and feet as a result of severe cold. Chinese doctors have prescribed herbal remedies. Sometimes bitter orange and honey-baked licorice can be of benefit according a traditional Chinese medicine specialist. If you want to utilize Chinese herbal medicine for the treatment of your Raynaud's disease, consult a specialist in this field. Fish oil supplements may possibly decrease some of the symptoms associated with mild Raynaud's disease. It is believed that this effect is due to the anti-inflammatory property of the fish oils.

Avoid triggers that cause you to develop Raynaud's disease. Keep your extremities warm. Use layered clothing. Use rubber gloves or mittens under your regular gloves. Regular gloves allow heat to escape in extremely cold weather. If you are inside, wear socks as well as comfortable shoes. You should not smoke or use any tobacco products. Also avoid the use of any vibrating tools. You must learn to manage your stress. Regular exercise can increase blood flow to your tissues and reduce stress. Relaxation techniques and biofeedback may be of extreme benefit to you if you suffer from Raynaud's disease.

Vitamin E, magnesium, and fish oils can be of some benefit. Herbal medicines are currently being studied to determine their effects on the treatment of Raynaud's disease. Cayenne pepper and ginger may possibly enhance circulation to your painful areas. Again, further research is indicated for the effective herbal medicines on the prevention of Raynaud's disease.

If you have primary Raynaud's disease, your prognosis is much better than if you have secondary Raynaud's disease. If you have secondary Raynaud's disease, your prognosis depends on the severity of the other conditions that were mentioned such as scleroderma and so on.

Pain can be associated with Raynaud's phenomena. Nicotine can decrease the internal diameter of the vessels in your body. A class of drugs used to treat hypertension called beta blockers can also be associated with Raynaud's phenomena. The exact reason for this observation remains unclear at present. Beta blockers can decrease your heart rate as well as your strength of contraction of your heart muscles. Side effects of beta blockers can result in cold extremities. This may be the reason that you can develop Raynaud's phenomena.

A class of drugs called ergots is used for the treatment of migraine headaches. This class of drugs can also be used for vascular headaches as well as cluster headaches. An example of this drug is Wigraine. This drug can cause constriction of your blood vessels. A decrease in the blood flow and oxygen to your tissues can precipitate Raynaud's phenomena. Any drug that stimulates the sympathetic nervous system, such as dopamine, can cause your blood vessels in your body to constrict. An example of a sympathetic stimulating drug is dopamine.

Dopamine can be used to increase the strength of your heartbeat if you have had heart failure. However, drugs that stimulate your sympathetic nervous system also constrict your blood vessels. Raynaud's phenomena have been associated with use of drugs that stimulate your sympathetic nervous system.

When you have a sympathetic injection with a local anesthetic in your sympathetic nerves, the blockade of your sympathetic fibers to your arteries will cause your arteries to become bigger in diameter. This will increase the blood flow to your painful tissues, which in turn increases the oxygen to your nerves and muscles as well. This is the mechanism why sympathetic blocks can decrease your pain. If you have a decrease in blood flow to the tissues we have described, chemicals in your body that cause pain are released. *Histamine, kinins,* 5-Hydroxytriptamine, and *substance P* are released. Substances will transmit pain to your spinal cord, which will eventually reach the pain-processing center in your brain.

For Men

- Stop smoking! Smoking is associated with Raynaud's disease in men. Smoking also constricts your blood vessels, depriving you of oxygen and causing pain.
- Avoid vibrating tools such as jackhammers and jigsaws. Repetitive motion movements can predispose you to carpal tunnel syndrome and Raynaud's disease.
- Avoid any triggers that cause your pain, such as extreme cold.
- Stay warm by dressing in layers. Be sure to wear gloves if you are outside. It is important to keep your skin temperature warm and regulated. If your skin becomes cold, your sympathetic nervous system will cause your blood vessels to constrict which can cause you pain.
- Perform relaxation and biofeedback techniques to reduce your stress level.
- Regular exercise can increase blood flow to your tissues and reduce stress.
- NSAIDs such as ibuprofen may reduce any swelling and pain that you have.

- Take any medications as prescribed by your doctor.
- Injections of local anesthetic into your sympathetic nerves may relieve some of your pain.

For Women

- Stop drinking alcohol! Alcohol use is associated with Raynaud's in women.
- Stop smoking! Smoking constricts your blood vessels, depriving you of oxygen and causing pain.
- Avoid vibrating tools such as jackhammers and jigsaws. Repetitive motion movements can predispose you to carpal tunnel syndrome and Raynaud's disease.
- Avoid any triggers that cause your pain, such as extreme cold.
- Stay warm by dressing in layers. Be sure to wear gloves if you are outside. It is important to keep your skin temperature warm and regulated. If your skin becomes cold, your sympathetic nervous system will cause your blood vessels to constrict which can cause you pain.
- Perform relaxation and biofeedback techniques to reduce your stress level.
- Regular exercise can increase blood flow to your tissues and reduce stress.
- NSAIDs such as ibuprofen may reduce any swelling and pain that you have.
- Take any medications as prescribed by your doctor.
- Injections of local anesthetic into your sympathetic nerves may relieve some of your pain.

Chapter 27
Understanding Shingles

Have you ever been to a nursing home and noticed a patient fidgeting and walking around a room or an individual shrieking trying to escape his or her pain? If you have experienced this scenario, you are probably aware of a painful entity that is called shingles. This infectious disease is caused by a virus that causes herpes zoster and affects some of the nerves that go into the spinal cord.

One or more nerves can be affected. Usually the shingles pain stays on one side of your body. Sometimes shingles will affect your lower extremities. The virus is called *varicella zoster.* Chicken pox is caused by the same virus that will cause you to have shingles. (R.B. Smith, et al. *Anesthesia and Pain Control in the Geriatric Patient.* New York: McGraw Hill, 1995) (J.F. Loeser. "Herpes Zoster and Postherpetic Neuralgia," *The Journal of Pain* 25 [1986]: 149-152)

In this chapter, you will learn about the virus that causes shingles and its associated pain. Several options for controlling your shingles pain will be covered, including alternative therapies, topical analgesics, oral medications, physical therapy, anesthetic injections, nerve blocks, electrical stimulation, neurolitic blocks, and a narcotic pump. Since shingles more commonly occurs in geriatric patients, it is important to recognize the effects that some medications and methods of treatment may have on older individuals.

The Varicella Zoster Virus

This virus will remain in the area that connects your spinal nerve and your spinal cord. This area is called your dorsal root ganglia. This virus typically reactivates when people are older than 50. This reactivation usually occurs after your immune system has been weakened, usually by another viral infection such as the flu or common cold. If you have cancer, you may be prone to develop shingles as well.

Sometimes there is no known reason why you develop shingles. If you have had contact with an individual who has had chicken pox, there is a chance that you could develop shingles. However, this scenario is rare. You need to be aware that shingles does not increase during seasonal chicken pox outbreaks. When the virus is reactivated in your dorsal root ganglia, it goes along your nerves to your nerve endings. The virus at this time will cause your skin to develop lesions. You need to be aware that any part of your *central nervous system* can be affected by this virus. In rare cases, this virus can even affect your brain; this is called an encephalitis. The virus has been reported in some cases to affect the sympathetic ganglia as well, which can cause severe burning pain. This will cause you to have symptoms that mimic reflex sympathetic dystrophy.

If you have Hodgkin's disease, you risk developing shingles. If you have a history of cancer of your breasts, lungs, or gastrointestinal tract, you run an increased risk of developing shingles. Early reports indicated that men and women were affected at the same rate. However, more recent studies have reported that men are affected more frequently than women. (R.B. Smith, et al. *Anesthesia and Pain Control in the Geriatric Patient.* New York: McGraw Hill, 1995) (J.F. Loeser. "Herpes Zoster and Postherpetic Neuralgia," *The Journal of Pain* 25 [1986]: 149-152)

Following chicken pox, antibodies are made in your body to fight the chicken pox virus. This is the reason why you usually do not get chicken pox again. If your immune system is compromised for any reason, however, your body's ability to combat the virus is greatly reduced. This is the reason why you may develop shingles. If your immune system appears to be attacked, your body will immediately fight the shingles virus.

After you have had the onset of shingles, you may develop *postherpetic neuralgia.* This is a chronic pain syndrome that occurs following the onset of shingles. When you have the onset of shingles, you will have blisters as well as burning sensations in your skin where the infected nerves run. When you develop postherpetic neuralgia, which can persist for years, however, your skin lesions usually heal. If you are between the ages of 40 and 60, the chances of you developing postherpetic neuralgia are 20 percent. If you are over 60 years of age, your chance of developing postherpetic neuralgia will increase to 50 percent. Postherpetic neuralgia is a difficult entity to treat.

Postherpetic neuralgia can cause you to have agonizing pain as well as suffering. Some individuals have even committed suicide to escape this terrible pain. Sometimes you can develop burning pain associated with the herpes zoster virus. However, it may be some time before your skin lesions appear.

Before you develop a skin rash, the diagnosis of herpes zoster is difficult to make. After your skin lesions erupt, the diagnosis is easier to make. If you have pain in your mid-back, you may be incorrectly diagnosed with a coronary artery disease or pneumonia. If your doctor wants to confirm your diagnosis, the virus should be isolated from your pustules no later than seven days after they erupted. (R.B. Smith, et al. *Anesthesia and Pain Control in the Geriatric Patient.* New York: McGraw Hill, 1995) (J.F. Loeser. "Herpes Zoster and Postherpetic Neuralgia," *The Journal of Pain* 25 [1986]: 149-152)

If you are suffering from postherpetic neuralgia, you may have difficulty with sleep because of your torturous pain. Your activities will be decreased. As a result of continuous pain, loss of sleep, and the inability to socialize, you may easily become depressed. Your postherpetic neuralgia may be confused with other medical diseases. However, you must keep a documented history of your shingles onset. You must tell your doctor if you have had lesions on your skin. By the time you see your doctor, you may still have the skin lesions or you may have scarring of your skin. The problem with the postherpetic neuralgia is that it can affect your central nervous system, which includes your spinal cord and brain.

Be aware that if you have severe burning pain that develops on one side of your body, you may or may not have a skin eruption but you can have shingles. Sometimes the lack of a skin eruption confuses doctors as to whether you actually have the onset of shingles, because skin lesions are so common. If you do develop skin eruptions, the lesion will begin as redness. The redness over your skin will turn to blisters. The blisters can form pus. Eventually these lesions on your skin break down. A crust then forms. If your skin, in addition to your nerves, is affected by the virus, you may develop scars as well as loss of skin pigment about the infected site. (R.B. Smith, et al. *Anesthesia and Pain Control in the Geriatric Patient.* New York: McGraw Hill, 1995) (J.F. Loeser. "Herpes Zoster and Postherpetic Neuralgia," *The Journal of Pain* 25 [1986]: 149-152)

Be aware that the virus can travel to your eyes. If you or anyone in your family has developed shingles and begins to complain of eye pain, this is a medical emergency. You must contact an ophthalmologist immediately. If left untreated, you may be blinded by the virus. The incidence of shingles is approximately 4 to 5 cases per 1,000 people. The chance of you developing shingles increases with your age. Usually when you have a viral infection, you will build up antibodies in your body that will help to fight the virus. The problem with shingles is that you do not appear to have developed antibodies to this virus that caused the initial episode of shingles. In other words, you run the risk of developing shingles after your initial case of shingles has resolved.

As mentioned previously, shingles may be preceded by other events. Be aware that psychological stress can also trigger the onset of shingles. If you have a history of a prolonged use of steroids, you may also be prone to develop shingles. For reasons yet unknown, the Caucasian race appears to have a higher incidence of shingles than other races.

Your chest will be most affected by shingles. Nerves that come off of your spine at your mid-back are called *thoracic nerves*. These thoracic nerves may be affected by the virus, causing an outbreak of shingles in your chest. Your chest is most commonly affected (50 percent of individuals who develop shingles experience chest effects). A nerve coming off of your brain that distributes branches to your face called the trigeminal nerve is the next most common nerve affected. Next the nerves off of your neck (called the *cranial nerves*) are affected, followed by the nerves coming off of your spinal cord that go to your legs (called the *lumbar nerves*). As you can see, shingles can affect nerves all over your body.

Different types of laboratory tests are available to diagnose acute herpes zoster. As noted previously, virus recovery from your tissue and blood can provide a rapid diagnostic tool for early diagnosis. Occasionally, the virus can be recovered from the back of your throat. Different types of diagnostic tests that use various stains are available. After these scrapings are stained, they may show diagnostic material in your cells. Many doctors advocate taking a small amount of your tissue (called a punch biopsy) so that they can do an examination under a specialized, high-powered microscope called an electron microscope. This is an extremely reliable test and it can provide a diagnosis of whether you have the herpes zoster virus before you develop blisters on your skin.

Shingles Pain

Be aware that not every patient who develops shingles has severe, incapacitating pain. You may only complain of itching. On the other hand, you may complain of the most horrible pain that you could ever imagine. Your pain can be either constant or it can be intermittent. It is the constant, severe, horrible pain that predisposes individuals to suicide to escape this torment. The problem with this disease is that you could have excruciating pain to the touch. This poses a problem if you are trying to sleep. You would have difficulty lying on a mattress without having severe pain. It is interesting to note if those younger than 50 years of age rarely develop prolonged pain after the acute onset of shingles. You also need to know that if you are over 50 years of age and develop shingles that your pain is usually worse (and that your postherpetic neuralgia pain is also worse than for individuals who are younger than 50 years of age). (R.B. Smith, et al. *Anesthesia and Pain Control in the Geriatric Patient.* New York: McGraw Hill, 1995) (J.F. Loeser. "Herpes Zoster and Postherpetic Neuralgia," *The Journal of Pain* 25 [1986]: 149-152)

After you have been diagnosed with shingles, your doctor will probably treat you with antiviral agents. Acyclovir, famciclovir, and valacyclovir can be used for the treatment of your viral infection. Antiviral medications are used to decrease the intensity and duration of your shingles and are used to prevent the chronic pain associated with postherpetic neuralgia. Be aware that you can still have the onset of postherpetic neuralgia even after treatment with these antiviral agents. Pain associated with postherpetic neuralgia can be described as aching, burning, or stabbing. (R.B. Smith, et al. *Anesthesia and Pain Control in the Geriatric Patient.* New York: McGraw Hill, 1995) (J.F. Loeser. "Herpes Zoster and Postherpetic Neuralgia," *The Journal of Pain* 25 [1986]: 149-152) The worst pain is pain that is triggered by light touch such as clothing, bathing, or lying on a mattress. Sometimes cold weather or cold water can worsen your pain. Postherpetic neuralgia is a dreaded complication of shingles.

If you develop shingles and if your pain lasts longer than six weeks after your skin lesions have disappeared, you have developed postherpetic neuralgia. Be aware that a certain proportion of individuals who develop postherpetic neuralgia will improve over time with no treatment. If you have postherpetic neuralgia, the chances are that you will have improved by 12 months. Approximately 30 percent of individuals who develop postherpetic neuralgia still complain of pain after one year. Two percent of individuals who suffer from postherpetic neuralgia will have pain longer than five years.

Anxiety and depression are psychological factors that can affect your shingles as well as your postherpetic neuralgia. As mentioned previously, stress can play an important role in the development of both shingles and postherpetic neuralgia. Psychological stress in some instances can decrease your immune system, making you prone to develop shingles. Many individuals who have abnormal behavioral patterns will become preoccupied with their pain. Usually these individuals are critical of health-care providers who have tried to help them relieve their pain. These individuals may also have narcotic tolerance.

Another problem associated with shingles and postherpetic neuralgia is *myofascial pain.* When you are in severe pain, many times you will guard your body to keep it from changing any position that could worsen your pain. With any alteration in your body posture, you may compress muscle tissue, which in turn can lead to a myofascial pain syndrome. Usually the virus affects the nerves that transmit pain as well as other sensations. However, be aware that this virus can also go to the nerves that go to your muscles. Post-mortem examinations have been done on individuals who died from postherpetic neuralgia. Pathologic lesions were found in the nerves as well as the nerve's entry into the spinal cord. Two types of nerves conduct pain. One nerve is a larger nerve that conducts sharp, stabbing pain, whereas the other nerve is a small nerve that conducts burning pain.

It appears that postherpetic neuralgia affects the smaller nerves that cause you to have severe, burning pain. For some reason, on occasion your sympathetic nervous system can become overactive. (R.B. Smith, et al. *Anesthesia and Pain Control in the Geriatric Patient.* New York: McGraw Hill, 1995) (J.F. Loeser. "Herpes Zoster and Postherpetic Neuralgia," *The Journal of Pain* 25 [1986]: 149-152) This over activity of your sympathetic nervous system can cause blood vessels that are going to your tissue to decrease their diameter (constrict). This will cause your tissue to have a decrease in its blood flow. The decrease in blood flow decreases oxygen as well as nutrients to your tissue. This lack of tissue oxygen can cause you to have pain. The decreased oxygen can cause release of pain-producing chemicals at the nerve endings in your tissues. The lack of oxygen to your nerves can affect the larger nerves that transmit the stabbing pain. It appears that your smaller nerves that cause burning pain are resistant to a decrease of oxygen in their tissue. Some larger nerve fibers in your body transmit touch. Stimulation of these fibers can decrease the amount of pain impulses from pain fibers that reach your brain. Only so many impulses can be processed by your spinal cord. By stimulating your larger nerves by touch, theoretically you can decrease the number of pain impulses that reach your brain.

A significant problem associated with postherpetic neuralgia is that these large nerves can be damaged and actually disappear. When these nerves are gone, there are no impulses to fight the burning impulses transmitted by the small nerves called *C fibers*. Sometimes as your nerves are being damaged by the virus that causes postherpetic neuralgia, these nerves can become hyperirritable, causing you to suffer significant pain. You must understand that this virus can injure and destroy the nerves that it affects. When your nerves become injured, they can develop areas of sensitivity at the site of nerve destruction. These sites can become hyperirritable and as a result can cause you to have significant, horrible pain. These injured nerves, as they attempt to heal, can develop sprouts. It is these sprouts that can become extremely sensitive. These sprouts of hypersensitivity can occur at any location on your nerve. Studies have shown that these nerves can conduct spontaneous pain impulses. (R.B. Smith, et al. *Anesthesia and Pain Control in the Geriatric Patient.* New York: McGraw Hill, 1995) (J.F. Loeser. "Herpes Zoster and Postherpetic Neuralgia," *The Journal of Pain* 25 [1986]: 149-152) This increase in nerve electrical activity can recruit other pain transmitting nerves around your lesion. In other words, there can be a magnification of the amount of pain (because the pain is combined) that you will suffer.

A potential problem exists for you in that some family members or even some doctors do not believe that you are suffering severely. Doctors who do not frequently treat postherpetic neuralgia can be reluctant to give strong analgesic medications. These doctors think that over time you may become addicted to narcotic medications. As stated previously in this book, if you are suffering from severe, significant pain, you have only a minimal chance of becoming addicted to a narcotic. Be aware that severe pain can have significant adverse effects on your body. It can increase your blood pressure, your pulse, and even decrease your immune system. Your blood vessels can decrease in their caliber. All of these changes can ultimately affect your heart as well as your kidneys and your psychological make-up. Therefore, you and your doctor must decide whether you are to be prescribed a narcotic pain medication.

Remember that both pain medication and chronic suffering can have adverse effects on your body. Most pain-medicine doctors believe that your pain should be managed appropriately. If you follow your pain-medicine doctor's instructions, your chances of becoming addicted are extremely small.

When you have the acute herpes zoster attack, your pain is usually localized to the affected nerves. You may have a fever as well as weakness and fatigue. At this time, your pain could be shooting, dull, or even burning. Your skin eruptions usually occur approximately four days later. As stated previously, the herpes zoster virus can go not only to your sensory nerves but also to the nerves that go to your muscles. As a result, the muscles that are in your chest can be paralyzed. Also muscles in your arms or legs can be paralyzed if the virus is in these nerves. You may not have paralysis, but you will experience weakness. Usually your weak muscle symptoms are reversible. If you have the initial stage of the viral infection, you are suffering viral replication. This means that the virus in your system is replicating rapidly. Your immune system is usually depressed. As the disease progresses, your immune system should be able to fight the virus. As you go into a third phase, your body will continue to fight the virus with your antibodies. However, it is at this time that you could have permanent nerve changes.

Shingles recurs in 8 percent of individuals. Usually the shingles will occur at the same site affected previously. After you have developed crusts, these lesions will fall off in five to six weeks. After they have fallen off, they will leave an irregular scar. You may not have any feeling around the scar. If you have suffered from postherpetic neuralgia for six months, the chance of a complete cure is remote. As discussed previously, you can have pain associated with postherpetic neuralgia, but you can also have dysesthesias. These are uncomfortable, unpleasant sensations but are not true sensations. (R.B. Smith, et al. *Anesthesia and Pain Control in the Geriatric Patient.* New York: McGraw Hill, 1995) (J.F. Loeser. "Herpes Zoster and Postherpetic Neuralgia," *The Journal of Pain* 25 [1986]: 149-152)

Many patients describe them as "yucky." However, these funny and unpleasant sensations can progress to painful sensations with a stimulus such as a cold breeze. You need to realize that the virus associated with herpes zoster can be extremely destructive. It can cause nerve as well as tissue damage and bleeding into your tissues. Your nerves where they join the spinal cord can become extremely swollen, and bleeding can occur within the nerves. Significant nerve damage can occur within two weeks. After you have sustained nerve damage, your nerve tissue may be replaced by a scar.

As noted earlier in this chapter, herpes zoster can be associated with a loss of your larger fibers that conduct sensation. Older patients in general have a loss of these larger fibers. Therefore, when they develop postherpetic neuralgia their pain can be more severe than a younger individual who has a greater number of these large pain fibers. Remember, the initial stage of the infection is a viral replication. The virus duplicates itself rapidly. This is the reason why an antiviral medication must be administered as early as possible after the diagnosis has been made to decrease the rate of this replication. Not only is the virus recovered from blisters, it can also be recovered from the bloodstream. Occasionally, the virus can get into the fluid that surrounds your spinal cord and ultimately cause you to have meningitis.

Treatment for Shingles

As you can see from reading this chapter, the management of acute herpes zoster as well as postherpetic neuralgia presents a challenge for both you and your doctor.

Doctors of different specialties treat shingles. You may be treated by your primary-care doctor or a dermatologist. You may have to go to an emergency room because of severe pain and be treated by that doctor. You may also be referred to a pain-medicine specialist. Psychologists are also valuable in the management of your pain. All of these health-care providers can significantly help you manage your pain. You may find that each of these providers uses a different modality for the treatment of your pain. This is not to say that any one of these treatments is entirely wrong nor does it mean that any of these methods provided by different health-care providers are entirely correct.

Assessing Your Shingles Pain

Herpes zoster is a potentially complex, painful condition and usually requires a team health-care approach with you as a team member for the management of your pain. Most doctors agree that the antiviral medications need to be started soon after the diagnosis of shingles has been made. Most health-care providers agree that you need analgesics. The type of analgesic will depend on the severity of your pain. For example, if your pain is mild, you may need only a nonsteroidal anti-inflammatory drug for the management of your pain. If your pain is moderate, a mild analgesic such as Ultracet or a mild narcotic such as Darvocet or Tylenol with codeine may suffice for the management of your pain. If your pain becomes excruciating, these medications will not provide you with any significant pain relief. At this time, you may require more potent opioid medication such as Percocet or Vicodin. If these stronger narcotic drugs do not provide you with relief, you may require the administration of a strong opioid medication such as morphine.

Before providing you with any of these medications, your doctor will take a history from you and examine you. This is why it is important for you to keep an accurate history of your pain progression or regression. It would not be advantageous for you if your pain was only mild and your doctor prescribed you a strong narcotic medication such as morphine. On the other hand, if your pain is severe and excruciating, you will not receive much relief from an aspirin. Your doctor may refer you to a psychologist for biofeedback treatment or hypnosis. These modalities give you some control over your pain and eliminate the need for narcotic analgesics. If you have developed postherpetic neuralgia, avoid stressful situations that may worsen your pain. Avoid situations that cause you significant anxiety and/or depression. If you live in a cold environment, dress warmly.

Using Alternative Therapy to Relieve Shingles Pain

Some alternative therapy such as aroma therapy can deviate your attention temporarily away from your pain. (B. Goldberg. *Alternative Medicine, The Definitive Guide*. Berkeley: Celestial Arts, 2001) Because your body can cause you to guard against further pain, you may develop muscle cramps. Aroma therapy or deep breathing exercises with concentration on relaxing may relax your tight muscles. These modalities will not rid you of your pain but can decrease your pain so that you will not be dependent upon oral medications such as strong narcotic medications to control your chronic pain. If your pain is only mild, try to avoid narcotic medications altogether.

Treating Shingles in Geriatric Patients

If you are elderly, you also have a predisposition to depression. Pain management in elderly individuals is unique because you may present with multiple underlying medical problems in addition to your pain problem. This makes the management of your postherpetic neuralgia challenging. The correct diagnosis must be made before any treatment is initiated. If you are taking multiple drugs, remember that drugs can interact. Therefore, an accurate diagnosis must be made prior to initiating pain management.

As you age, your body will respond differently to different drugs. (R.B. Smith, et al. *Anesthesia and Pain Control in the Geriatric Patient.* New York: McGraw Hill, 1995) Furthermore, the distribution of the drugs in your body will change. Elderly individuals in nursing homes may have difficulty communicating their pain. This lack of communication can make it extremely difficult for a pain-management doctor or a primary-care doctor to manage a painful postherpetic neuralgia syndrome. If you are a family member of an elderly individual, help your relative's doctor by providing that doctor with a detailed history of the onset, duration, and severity of the postherpetic neuralgia.

If you are elderly, you may have a disruption in your normal activities of daily living. If you have severe postherpetic neuralgia on top of this decreased activity, you may be totally devastated. If you are elderly, it is important for you to have range of motion around your joints. If you have severe pain, however, it is difficult for you to do range of motion. This will cause your joints to become stiff. If you can't sleep, you will become fatigued. You may become irritable, which may strain family as well as spousal relationships.

Shingles and postherpetic neuralgia are common in elderly individuals. If you are elderly, you may have a decrease in your body's antibody levels. If you are elderly and because you can have more pain associated with postherpetic neuralgia than younger individuals, your doctor will treat you aggressively. In addition to antiviral agents, your doctor may prescribe steroids. Lotions, different types of patches, nonsteroidal anti-inflammatory drugs, antidepressants, and muscle relaxants may all be needed to control your pain. You may even need injections of numbing medicines into your nerves. Placement of local anesthetics around your sympathetic nerves may be of benefit in reducing your pain, especially if the injection is done soon after the onset of your pain.

Topical Analgesics

Topical agents are frequently used to treat shingles pain. These agents accelerate the healing of your skin and can decrease the pain associated with the shingles virus. However, topical anesthetics administered at the time that you develop shingles will not affect the development of postherpetic neuralgia. Compresses or Burrow's solution or calamine lotion placed directly over your painful site can decrease the pain associated with acute herpes zoster.

A relatively new patch has been developed for the treatment of shingles. This patch has proven to be extremely useful in the management of shingles and postherpetic neuralgia pain. A local anesthetic called lidocaine is placed within a patch system. The lidocaine is placed within an adhesive. The adhesive binds to your skin. The lidocaine that is in this patch is dispersed through your skin and travels to your painful, hyperirritable nerve endings. When this drug reaches your nerve endings, it calms your painful nerves. Note that this patch will not cause you to have numbness throughout your skin. If you are numb, you could injure the tissue. You may lie on the tissue not knowing that you are injuring your tissue. This is the reason why you do not want to be numb for any length of time throughout your skin.

You should only wear the lidocaine (Lidoderm) for 12 hours. Take the patch off after 12 hours and reapply it again in 12 hours. The medicine in the patch, lidocaine, is also a heart medication. If you have too much of the drug, it could slow or stop your heart. There is no danger of this happening when you wear the patch properly. You should not wear more than three of these patches at any one time. If you are allergic to lidocaine or adhesives, do not use this patch. If you develop a rash around the adhesive backing, pull the patch off and notify your doctor. This modality has proven to be extremely effective for the management of pain.

Another type of transdermal (skin) drug-delivery system is a clonidine *transdermal patch*. This is placed over the area of your maximal pain. This drug is a drug that controls an individual's blood pressure. If you are suffering from postherpetic neuralgia, however, your nerve endings may release certain chemicals that increase your pain. Scientists have demonstrated that the use of a clonidine transdermal patch can decrease components of your burning pain. This type of patch is changed on a weekly basis. One advantage of these patches is that they provide you with a constant blood level. If you take pills, you have peaks and troughs in your bloodstream after taking the pill and after the pill is excreted from your body. In contrast, the patch provides a constant flow of the drug. If you are elderly, remember that the clonidine patch is a blood pressure patch. It can decrease your blood pressure. If you get out of a chair or out of bed too quickly, you may become dizzy (a result of orthostatic hypotension). Orthostatic hypotension could cause you to become dizzy and fall. If you have been prescribed this patch, be aware of this side effect.

Oral Medications

You may need to take pills by mouth. If you are elderly, you must be aware that changes exist in your body with respect to target organ sensitivity to drugs. This means that the receptors that sit on the cells of some of your organs may not be as responsive to certain drugs as they would be if you were much younger. As you age, the absorption of drugs through your gastrointestinal system decreases as your age increases. On the other hand, some drugs are passively absorbed through your gastrointestinal system. This means that there will be no change in your blood level. Your blood level will be the same as that of a younger individual who takes the same drug.

Drugs such as tricyclic antidepressants are passively absorbed through your gut. Tricyclic antidepressants are frequently used for the management of pain associated with postherpetic neuralgia. (R.B. Smith, et al. *Anesthesia and Pain Control in the Geriatric Patient.* New York: McGraw Hill, 1995) As a matter of fact, tricyclic antidepressants are used to treat a variety of chronic pain syndromes. The exact mechanism by which these drugs decrease your pain is unknown. The pain-relieving effect of amitriptyline (Elavil) has been shown in rats to decrease pain caused by certain nerves. The correct dose of amitriptyline needed by elderly patients suffering from postherpetic neuralgia is currently unknown. Higher doses definitely produce a greater decrease in your pain. However, the problem with using higher doses is that you may develop a significant decrease in your blood pressure. This is similar to that caused by clonidine. If you become dizzy and fall, you could fracture your hip or one of your other bones. Your doctor will steadily increase your dose of this drug every three weeks. If you become sedated with this drug, another tricyclic antidepressant will be substituted.

Some doctors advocate the use of sedatives for relaxation and to help you sleep in addition to your other medications. If you are elderly, it may be wise for you to refrain from using drugs such as Valium. Valium can have long-acting effects. If you are elderly, Valium is not readily metabolized or excreted. If you take enough of this drug, you may become excessively sedated and even stop breathing. If you have significant sleep deprivation and are becoming agitated as a result of sleep deprivation, a shorter-acting and less-potent drug may be of some benefit to you. A drug called temazepam may have some advantage as a sedative for you. (R.B. Smith, et al. *Anesthesia and Pain Control in the Geriatric Patient.* New York: McGraw Hill, 1995)

You may benefit from the administration of a nonsteroidal anti-inflammatory drug because you may have a portion of your pain caused by your prostaglandins. An example of this drug is ibuprofen. The new COX-2 inhibitors may be somewhat safer for you because their incidence of side effects is less than the older NSAIDs. Because the virus does cause inflammation in your nerves and surrounding tissues, you can benefit from the use of nonsteroidal anti-inflammatory drugs.

If you have ulcers, however, avoid nonsteroidal anti-inflammatory drugs. You should use the smallest dose of the anti-inflammatory drug. For example, one of the new COX-2 inhibitors, Vioxx, comes in a 12.5 mg dose, a 25 mg dose, and a 50 mg dose. You should use the 12.5 mg dose. Remember, however, that these drugs can affect not only your gastrointestinal system, but can also adversely affect your kidneys and your liver. It is best to try to avoid narcotics unless they are absolutely indicated. Some narcotics, such as Demerol and Talwin, are associated with psychiatric side effects. It is best to avoid these two drugs in the geriatric population. If narcotics are to be used, mild narcotics should be initiated, as previously stated. Propoxyphene (Darvon) has been successfully used in a geriatric population. Morphine is commonly used for severe pain. (R.B. Smith, et al. *Anesthesia and Pain Control in the Geriatric Patient.* New York: McGraw Hill, 1995)

Be aware if you are over 65 that geriatric patients have decreased renal function and can be at risk for the breakdown produce of morphine. The same holds true with other narcotic medications. However, morphine does have a breakdown product that is pharmacologically active, meaning that it can cause sedation just as the intact morphine can. Be aware that the breakdown products of Demerol can cause seizures. Muscle relaxants are sometimes used for the management of postherpetic neuralgia pain. They are also used in elderly individuals. Baclofen, which does stimulate some receptors in your spinal cord, can decrease the pain associated with postherpetic neuralgia. It can also relieve any muscle spasms that occur as a result of this painful entity. Amantadine is a drug that can also provide some relief for the management of postherpetic neuralgia. It is an anti-Parkinson's medication. However, it also has NMDA receptor antagonist activity. These receptors can cause you severe pain when they are activated. If you suffer from postherpetic neuralgia, you may not feel like eating.

Baclofen, Amantadine, and Elavil can decrease your burning pain associated with postherpetic neuralgia while anticonvulsant medications can lessen your sharp, shooting pain. Another topical drug that is sometimes used is capsaicin cream. It can be purchased over the counter and can also be purchased by prescription at a higher concentration. This substance is found in hot peppers. It depletes and prevents the re-accumulation of *substance P* in your nerves. However, this medication does cause burning. The burning sensation caused by the capsaicin prevents some individuals from using this drug. However, it can provide excellent benefits. It takes several days to deplete the substance P in your nerve endings.

Physical Therapy

Shingles may benefit from physical therapy. Heat, cold, and massage are frequently used for the management of your pain. Sometimes a *transcutaneous electrical nerve stimulator* (TENS) can be helpful. The TENS unit, however, is not frequently prescribed because on occasion it could worsen the pain associated with shingles. Water therapy can be helpful because the warm water can be soothing and may also desensitize the nerves that are causing the severe pain. If your activities of daily living are limited because of your pain, consult an occupational therapist to learn how to preserve your daily-living activities.

Anesthetic Injections and Nerve Blocks

Sometimes your doctor may want to put numbing medicine mixed with a steroid around your nerve. If you are experiencing pain in your chest wall, for example, your doctor may place an injection into the nerve that provides sensation to your chest. This nerve is called the *intercostal nerve.*

Nerve blocks for the treatment of postherpetic neuralgia were mentioned earlier in this chapter. The type of block that is used to relieve your pain depends on the type of pain that you have. The pain associated with postherpetic neuralgia can be somatic, sympathetic, or central.

(R.B. Smith, et al. *Anesthesia and Pain Control in the Geriatric Patient*. New York: McGraw Hill, 1995) The somatic pain follows a certain nerve that is affected. Sympathetic pain can decrease the blood flow to your tissues and causes you to have a burning pain. Central pain is a result of rewiring of your central nervous system. For this type of pain, you need a different type of block.

Your pain-medicine doctor will evaluate you to determine whether and what type of block can provide you with relief. A somatic block is an injection of your nerve with a local anesthetic. If you have significant relief but your pain returns, your doctor could do a permanent nerve block using a cold-producing modality. This is called cryo analgesia. A stellate ganglion or a lumbar sympathetic block can be used to manage the pain of your chest, lower extremities, upper extremities, or even your face. If you experience central pain, you will have burning as well as pain sometimes from light touch.

Sometimes an epidural injection using local anesthetics can provide relief. Further research is being done to evaluate the effects of the administration of epidural ketamine for the treatment of your pain. For your acute lesions, just an injection under the skin with a local anesthetic can provide pain relief. The different type of nerves that can be injected with a local anesthetic include your trigeminal nerve, your brachial plexus, the nerves under your ribs (called intercostal nerves), as well as your sciatic nerve.

It has been shown that sympathetic nerve blocks, if done early, can relieve pain associated with shingles and can also decrease the incidence of developing postherpetic neuralgia. To be effective, they should be performed within the first two months after the onset of your symptoms. Stellate ganglion blocks are used for pain in your head, neck, and arms. Thoracic epidural blocks are used for pain in your midback and chest wall, whereas lumbar sympathetic blocks are used for the management of postherpetic neuralgia pain in your lower extremities. The purpose of nerve blocks is to interrupt your pain impulses and to facilitate therapy and to help you increase your daily-living activities. Nerve blocks should be used if your pain is becoming too severe and cannot be controlled by nonnarcotic medications.

If you have sympathetic pain that does not respond to the previously mentioned modalities, more permanent blocks of your sympathetic nervous system can be done using a modality called radiofrequency thermocoagulation. This device provides some heat around your sympathetic nerves. This device does not burn your nerves, but the heat essentially knocks your nerves out of commission. The procedure is done on an out-patient basis with only minimal discomfort. Radio-frequency thermocoagulation can provide you with a long-term interruption of your pain fibers and pain impulses. Occasionally a dorsal column stimulator can be placed in your epidural space.

Electrical Stimulation

Remember from the other chapters that the epidural space is the space that surrounds the fluid that surrounds your spinal cord. The dorsal column stimulator is essentially an epidural catheter that has electrodes on it. The number of electrodes that are used depends on the pattern of your pain. The dorsal column stimulator is placed within your body on a trial basis. The catheter is placed on an out-patient basis with x-ray. The end of the catheter attaches to a battery pack. How the dorsal column stimulator actually works is debated. It is believed that the electrical interference with ascending pathways may be the mechanism for decreasing your pain impulse transmission.

The use of this device has been demonstrated to be effective for the management of postherpetic neuralgic pain that is refractory to all other modalities. (R.B. Smith, et al. *Anesthesia and Pain Control in the Geriatric Patient.* New York: McGraw Hill, 1995) The goal of the stimulation is to decrease your pain by at least 50 percent. If you do obtain adequate pain relief, the stimulator is implanted surgically for permanent use. For pain that persists in your arms or legs and is refractory to other treatments, a nerve stimulator can be placed in your extremity to provide you with pain relief. Chemical substances that disrupt nerves have been used since 1930 for the treatment of postherpetic neuralgia.

Neurolitic Blocks

Phenol is an alcohol-like drug used frequently to disrupt your nerve impulses. (R.B. Smith, et al. *Anesthesia and Pain Control in the Geriatric Patient.* New York: McGraw Hill, 1995) It also has some local anesthetic properties. The first reported use of a neurolitic solution was in 1863 by Luton. Neurolitic blocks for chronic pain management were further developed by neurosurgeons. In 1925, Dr. Doppler used phenol for disruption of nerves. In 1955, phenol was administered in the spinal fluid of patients to disrupt their chronic pain. Alcohol has also been used to disrupt nerves.

However, the use of the alcohol can cause post-block pain called a neuritis. Whenever neurolitic chemicals are used, the procedure must be done under x-ray guidance to know where the solution is going. Sometimes the phenol must be re-administered to provide you with a good long-term block of your nerves.

Narcotic Pump

If all the previous modalities fail to provide you with relief, a narcotic pump can be placed within your body. (R.B. Smith, et al. *Anesthesia and Pain Control in the Geriatric Patient*. New York: McGraw Hill, 1995) The pump consists of a reservoir about the size of a hockey puck. It is connected to a tube that runs into the fluid that surrounds your spinal cord. Essentially this pump gives you a drop of a narcotic drug every minute or so and is another way of controlling your pain. The drug-delivery system is refilled approximately every 45 days. Before placing this pump, your doctor will do a trial of morphine and compare it to a salt solution to see whether you actually obtain pain relief from this device.

If your pain persists, you may require surgery. There is no single standard surgical procedure that is effective for the treatment of your postherpetic neuralgia. A procedure called a dorsal root entry zone (DREZ) lesion has been shown to be effective for the management of postherpetic neuralgia in some patients. Sometimes a neurosurgeon can interrupt your pain pathways by doing a procedure in your spinal cord.

Nutrition

Nutrition needs to be addressed with regards to shingles pain. If you are in severe pain, you may not feel like eating. Poor eating habits in combination with a lack of mobilization can cause you to become depressed and weaken your muscles. If you have another chronic pain syndrome such as arthritis, this immobilization and lack of proper nutrients can worsen this pain.

For Men

- Prevent a shingles recurrence by decreasing stress and eating a proper diet.
- Several alternative therapies can be used to relieve your pain, such as aromatherapy, heat or cold therapy, and acupuncture.

- Sedatives will often help you sleep, but do not help the pain.
- Analgesics such as ibuprofen or Tylenol 3 can help relieve some of your pain.
- Apply a topical anesthetic over the area of your shingles pain to get some relief.
- Your doctor may want to place an epidural injection of anesthetic into your spine if your pain is severe.
- Prescription medications such as pain patches, tricyclic antidepressants, anticonvulsants, and narcotics can be use to help relieve your pain.

For Women

- Prevent a shingles recurrence by decreasing stress and eating a proper diet.
- Several alternative therapies can be used to relieve your pain, such as aromatherapy, heat or cold therapy, and acupuncture.
- Sedatives will often help you sleep, but do not help the pain.
- Analgesics such as ibuprofen or Tylenol 3 can help relieve some of your pain.
- Apply a topical anesthetic over the area of your shingles pain to get some relief.
- Your doctor may want to place an epidural injection of anesthetic into your spine if your pain is severe.
- Prescription medications such as pain patches, tricyclic antidepressants, anticonvulsants, and narcotics can be use to help relieve your pain.

Chapter 28

Understanding Sports-Related Pain

The current trend today in the United States is physical activity. Physical exercise can help you maintain or lose your weight, maintain strength, and can be protective for your heart. However, you can develop aches and pains in your body associated with moderate physical exercise. As more individuals become more aware of the benefits of physical exercise, the incidence of exercise-related injuries is increasing. Furthermore, gender-specific differences exist as to the types of injuries that occur.

This chapter will teach you about the different types of sports-related injuries, including tennis elbow, muscle, tendon, and joint injuries. You will also learn about sports-related pain coming from the knee, ankle, Achilles tendon, and joints. Tips on avoiding injury, the injury differences between both genders, and how to treat sports-related pain will also be discussed.

Muscle, Tendon, and Joint Injuries

As you know, pain is your body's signal of telling you that something is wrong in an area of your body. Pain essentially is your body's protective mechanism to prevent further injury to your tissues. Most pain is relatively mild and goes away relatively quickly. If your pain is severe and persists for more than seven days, however, your body is trying to tell you that something is wrong. Most significant pain should not last for more than one to three days unless you have sustained a significant injury. Your pain can be caused by muscle injury or an injury to one of your ligaments or tendons.

You can also have an inflammation of one of your *peripheral nerves*, which are nerves outside of your brain and spinal cord. You can even have a small fracture of one of your bones. If you have pain that persists for seven days or longer, you should call your primary-care doctor. Your doctor will determine whether you need to come into the office for an examination. If you have an injury to a tissue in your body, this tissue is usually a muscle, tendon, or ligament. Tendons and ligaments can tear apart or tear away from their attachments. The same holds true for muscles.

Your bones can also be injured with physical activity. You can have small fractures in one of your bones that occur with repetitive motions such as running. Usually small fractures in bones heal quickly. The most common bone injuries are stress fractures of your small bones, such as those in your feet. These stress fractures usually take approximately eight weeks to heal. The cover of your bone called a *periosteum* is a wrapper around your bone that contains many small nerves. If you sustain a bruise to your periosteum, you can have significant pain for several days to several weeks.

You can develop an abnormal bone growth about the bone in your heel. This abnormal bone growth, which can be painful, is called a spur. Usually a podiatrist or an orthopedic surgeon may have to remove your bone spur if it causes you significant pain. Muscles, ligaments, and tendons are composed of fibers that run parallel to each other. These fibers are like the strings of a guitar. They are wrapped in an outer layer. If these fibers are stretched beyond their normal length, they can tear. Usually these fibers grow back together. However, sometimes scars can prevent the ends of the fibers from reattaching. As a result, scars in these areas can become painful.

Myofascial pain can occur when your muscle fibers are stretched beyond their normal elastic limits. (M. Read and P. Wade. *What to Do When it Hurts: Self-Diagnosis and Rehabilitation of Common Aches and Pains*. n.p.: People's Medical Society, 1997) When this happens, it is called a strain. Where the muscle is torn it can develop a scar. The scar can be very tender to the touch. Occasionally you may need an injection to the scar with a local anesthetic and steroid. The tender areas in your muscles are called trigger points, and these cause a myofascial pain syndrome. Usually ice or heat over the painful muscle can significantly relieve your pain. Massage therapy can also provide you with significant muscle pain relief as well. You also have cartilage in your joints.

Cartilage is a substance that exists between your bones and can be compressed. This compressive ability makes the cartilage act as a shock absorber in some of your joints. Cartilage allows your bones of your joints, such as your knee joints, to slide over each other. If you do not have the cartilage, one bone will slide over another bone. You would have increased friction applied to your bones in your joint, which could cause you significant pain.

You can also stretch and injure a tendon, which is called a sprain. An acute sprain is a stretch of a ligament after your injury. If you don't heal within six weeks, you are showing signs of chronic pain. If you still have pain after six months, you have chronic pain.

A tendon is composed of a group of fibers that attaches your muscles to your bones. A tendon is composed of tough fibers. A tendon injury can take a long time to heal. Muscle injuries, on the other hand, can heal faster than tendon injuries. The reason for this difference is that muscles have a greater blood flow than tendons. The flow of blood to injured tissue is necessary to bring nutrients that can heal tissue. A tendon injury can be potentially serious because if it does not heal properly you can be prone to re-injury. In other words, if your tendon does not heal properly, there can be a weak area in the nonhealed part of your tendon. If you exercise again, you may re-injure this tendon. If your tendon is partially injured or torn, you can develop inflammation in your tendon. This inflammatory process is called tendonitis. Improper healing can cause you to have scar tissue and make you prone to re-injury.

Some tendons in your body are bathed in a fluid that is surrounded by a sheath. If your tendon becomes inflamed from overuse, it may swell. When it swells, it rubs against your outer tendon sheath, which can cause you to have significant pain. This type of pain is called *tenosynovitis*. (M. Read and P. Wade. *What to Do When it Hurts: Self-Diagnosis and Rehabilitation of Common Aches and Pains*. n.p.: People's Medical Society, 1997)

You need to realize that all tendons have this fluid sheath that surrounds them. Another type of tissue in your body is a tough fibrous tissue composed of fibers, as previously mentioned.

The purpose of ligaments is to hold bones together. For example, vertebrae, the bones that are stacked on top of each other in your back, are held together by ligaments. If too much stress is placed on your ligaments, the ligament may tear. As with the other tissues mentioned previously, a tear in your ligament can cause inflammation. Your ligaments can heal properly or improperly. Again like the other tissues that were mentioned previously, improper healing can make you prone to re-injury. Ligaments are an example of another tissue that does not have a great blood supply. As a result of a minimal blood supply, this tissue is slow to heal.

You have probably heard the term "bursitis." (Carl Germano and William Cabot. *Nature's Pain Killers*. n.p.: Kensington Books, 1999) Some people have bursitis of their shoulder, whereas others have a bursitis around their hip. A bursa is a sac that is filled with fluid. This fluid-filled sac is placed between either a tendon and a bone or between a ligament and a bone. A bursa allows a tendon to glide about the bone of your shoulder or hip, for example. When your tendon glides smoothly over your bone, the tendon does not become inflamed or injured. However, sometimes your bursa can become inflamed, leading to what is called bursitis. If the inflammation in your bursa progresses, then fluid can accumulate within your bursa. This expansion of the bursal sac will cause you to have pain. If this happens, you develop bursitis.

You need to be aware that scarring can form within your bursa. If a scar does form, you can have chronic irritation of your bursa. As a result, this can cause you to have chronic pain.

You know what a muscle is. You may have never heard of a fascia. The fascia is a tissue that covers your muscles and separates one muscle from another. The fascia is present throughout your body. This fascia enables one muscle to slide smoothly over another muscle. Sometimes an area where your fascia and muscle come together can be separated, causing pain at this junction. This can also be an origin of what is called myofascial pain. So in a sports injury, you can have pain related to an actual tear in your muscle or pain related to an injury at the junction of your fascia and your muscle.

Tennis Elbow

You usually are not aware of your elbow until you develop pain in your elbow joint. Your elbow joint is formed by one bone from your upper arm and two bones from your forearm. You can have irritation of your elbow joint or you can have a tennis player's or golfer's tendonitis. An injury to your elbow is usually in the tendons of the muscles that attach to the bones around your elbow. In tennis elbow, the pain runs to your outer elbow. You may also have pain around your inner elbow. This usually occurs when you play golf. Tennis elbow was named because it affected tennis players. However, anyone can develop a tennis elbow. Tennis elbow means that you have an inflamed tendon around your elbow. You can have pain on the outside of your elbow. You can develop tennis elbow if you are a weightlifter, play tennis or racquetball, or wait tables.

The problem with tennis elbow is that you can sustain a re-injury. If you have pain on the outside of your elbow, you should stop the activity that caused your pain. You should use ice over the elbow. Nonsteroidal anti-inflammatory drugs may help you control your pain. You probably have tennis elbow if the pain in your elbow is so bad that you cannot even lift a coffee cup. You usually have tenderness over a dime-sized area on the outer aspect of your elbow. X-rays of your elbow are not necessary. A Velcro wrist splint can be helpful in controlling your pain as well. If your pain persists after four weeks, sometimes a short arm cast needs to be used. At 6 to 10 weeks, you should be feeling much better. (M. Read and P. Wade. *What to Do When it Hurts: Self-Diagnosis and Rehabilitation of Common Aches and Pains*. n.p.: People's Medical Society, 1997) (Carl Germano and William Cabot. *Nature's Pain Killers*. N.p.: Kensington Books, 1999) If not, you will be referred to an orthopedic surgeon. You should gradually resume your activities. Physical therapy does play a role, but it is a minor role in the treatment of this painful entity.

You may also develop pain on your inner elbow. This inner elbow pain is called golfer's elbow. If you are scrubbing a floor vigorously, you can develop pain in your inner elbow. The pain usually starts several days after you were doing an activity. The treatment for golfer's elbow is the same as that for tennis elbow. You may also develop pain in your elbow joint. This type of pain may be due to osteoarthritis. Nonsteroidal anti-inflammatory medications will help this pain. (Carl Germano and William Cabot. *Nature's Pain Killers*. N.p.: Kensington Books, 1999)

Rarely will you need a steroid injection into the joint. You can also develop a bursitis in your elbow. You can develop a sudden red, swollen area over your elbow. Your range of motion around normal. You do not need x-rays. If your pain is aggravating and persisting, your doctor may want to use a needle and syringe to remove the fluid from your bursa (a process called "aspiration") and send the fluid to a laboratory to test for crystals, bacteria, and so on. If your tests determine that you have gout, you will be treated appropriately. Injection of a steroid into your bursa can provide you with pain relief. If your pain persists, you will be referred to an orthopedic surgeon. Usually ice and nonsteroidal anti-inflammatory drugs will control this pain.

Knee Pain

Your knee, which is the largest joint in your body, may be injured if you are active in sports. Many different types of injuries can affect your knees.

Jogging or running have gained popularity in the past 10 to 15 years. However, this activity has led to an increase in knee injuries. The knee is made up of your thigh bone and your shin bones. There is also a bone in front of your knee called the kneecap (patella). Your bones around your knee are held together by ligaments. There is a ligament at either side of your knee. These ligaments provide your knee with stability. Your knee also contains cartilage, which coats your bones. Your cartilage allows your bones to slide over each other with ease. If your cartilage wears out, it can cause you to have arthritis. Between your thigh bone and your shin bone is another cartilage called a meniscus. These cartilages are attached to your shin bone (tibia). You also have muscles that control your range of motion. These are called the quadriceps and hamstrings. When your quadricep muscles contract, they make your knee straighten. When your hamstring muscles contract, these muscles make your knee and lower leg pull backward at the knee joint. To cushion your knee, you have several bursa in your knee. You can have several areas of pain within your knee.

Have you ever had pain under your kneecaps after you run? Have you ever had problems where you can't squat or kneel any more? What is the grinding noise that I hear when I bend my knee? These symptoms are compatible with a disease called *chrondromalacia patellae*. This disease involves a painful kneecap. You will have pain when you bend your knee and will feel areas around your knee that feel like Rice Krispies crushing. You may have swelling around your knee. If you have no swelling, you will have a normal range of motion. If your knee is arthritic, you will have the symptoms of chrondromalacia patellae. An x-ray eventually will show signs of osteoarthritis in the joint where your patella meets your femur. Injection of a local anesthetic around this area can be diagnostic of your disease. Arthroscopy, which involves inserting a scope into your knee, can identify the pathology going on with your knee. If you have pain in your knee, you should apply ice and elevate your knee. You should avoid squatting as well as kneeling. Swimming is preferred to jogging or any impact exercises. You may want to use a Velcro strap over your knee. You should take a non-steroidal anti-inflammatory medication following your injury. If your pain persists after three months, you may benefit from an oral steroid.

After three to four months, you will need to continue daily straight-leg-raising exercises as well as doing range-of-motion exercises. Physical therapy is one of the main treatments for this disorder. Swelling around your knee can last for several months. You should attempt to improve your quadriceps and hamstring tone. If you do exercises to strengthen your quadriceps and hamstring muscles, you can slow down the progression of the chrondromalacia to an osteoarthritis. Occasionally, surgical procedures are done. (Carl Germano and William Cabot. *Nature's Pain Killers*. n.p.: Kensington Books, 1999) However, injection therapy or surgery is not a substitute for increasing your muscle strength. Sometimes you can develop swelling just below your kneecap. You will feel as if you have a "fever" inside your knee. As your knee becomes swollen, you will find that you are unable to bend or straighten it.

Osteoarthritis or chrondromalacia patellae or an infection in your knee joint may cause you to have swelling. When this happens, usually an x-ray of your knee is recommended by your doctor. Your doctor may need to aspirate the swelling in your knee. Your doctor will send the knee fluid to the lab to determine whether you have blood cells, glucose, or even bacteria in your knee. You should use ice around your knee and elevate your knee. You should not do squatting and kneeling exercises nor should you run. You may need crutches for the time to avoid weight bearing. You should do straight-leg-raise exercises without weights. If your pain persists for two to four weeks, you may need to get fluid taken off your knee again. You should take a nonsteroidal anti-inflammatory medicine.

If you have not improved after two months, an MRI of your knee may need to be done. You may also need to have an arthroscopic procedure done by your orthopedic surgeon to determine what type of therapy you actually need. Physical therapy is an extremely important modality for swelling of your knee. You can have steroids injected into your knee as well. If you have rheumatoid arthritis, your surgeon can operate on your knee to improve your function and to decrease your pain. When playing sports or running, you may tear a cartilage in your knee.

The cartilage in your knee acts as shock absorbers. These shock absorbers cushion the movement between your thigh bone and your shin bone. You can have a slight tear of your cartilage or a more severe tear. With a slight tear, you may have mild to moderate pain and experience a clicking sound when you move your knee. When you have a severe cartilage tear, your knee may give way. It can also get stuck in a bent position. With a severe tear, your knee will be painful and you will notice swelling around your knee. A plain x-ray of your knee can be helpful in the diagnosis of the cause of your knee pain.

A loose body in your knee may be noted in an imaging study. An MRI image may or may not be useful. An arthroscopy can be helpful in diagnosing the cause of your pain. There is a chance that you may need surgical treatment of your torn cartilage. You should stop sports following your injury. You should not squat or kneel. You should apply ice to your knee when it swells and elevate your knee. You may need crutches so that you can avoid weight bearing. A pull-on knee brace can provide you with relief. If you still have pain after two weeks, your doctor may want to aspirate the swelling about your knee. If you still have pain at four weeks, you will probably be referred to an orthopedic surgeon. You need to be aware that a knee injury can predispose you to premature arthritis. Physical therapy does not play an important role in the treatment of a cartilage tear. Sometimes a steroid injection into your knee will prove helpful.

Ankle Pain

You have probably suffered an ankle sprain before. An ankle sprain is a partial tear of the ligaments in your ankle joint. Your ligaments can be pulled away from the location where they attach to your bones. A sprain can be classified as acute, recurrent, or chronic. If it is an acute sprain, you may have recently stepped off a high curb and come down wrong on your foot. You may have tried to turn a corner while running and your ankle suddenly gave out or playing basketball and jumped up and landed on the side of your foot. All of these instances are examples of an acute sprain.

Did you ever injure your ankle years ago and were recently playing basketball and re-injured your ankle? This is an example of a recurrent sprain. Did you ever injure your ankle years ago but continued to have weakness and pain in your ankle? This is an example of a chronic sprain. Usually following an acute sprain your ankle will be swollen and may be discolored on the side of the injury. Have you had a previous ankle injury and every time you play basketball your ankle gives out? This could be the result of a chronic sprain. Your ligament may not have healed properly if you continue to have chronic pain. When this happens, you should be examined by your doctor. If you have had an ankle injury, you will have tenderness and swelling over the injured side. If you try to move your ankles sideways, you will have an aggravation of your pain.

In an acute injury, your range of motion around your ankle will be limited. With chronic pain, your range of motion will be greater. Your doctor will examine you for lack of stability of your ankle. If you have a minor ankle sprain, you will have tenderness over one of your ankle bones. These ankle bones are projections that stick out to the right and left of your ankle—that is, perpendicular to your ankle. You will usually have tenderness around one of these ankle bones or both. Your acute pain can be so intense that you may have the pain while the doctor tries to examine you. You must, therefore, tell your doctor if the examination is painful. As your symptoms resolve, you may have pain with movement of your ankle. Your pain will improve gradually.

You may develop pain on the outer side of your ankle, which can be a result of a tendon injury. This tendon is called the *peroneus.* Sometimes the bone that forms your fifth toe could have a small fracture. When your pain has resolved, your range of motion should return to normal. (M. Read and P. Wade. *What to Do When it Hurts: Self-Diagnosis and Rehabilitation of Common Aches and Pains.* n.p.: People's Medical Society, 1997) (Carl Germano and William Cabot. *Nature's Pain Killers.* n.p.: Kensington Books, 1999) After your pain subsides, you may continue to have instability of your ankle. If you rock your ankle back and forth with your hand, you may notice a knocking within your ankle. This could signify a separation of your tibia and fibula, which are the two lower bones in your leg. The lower parts of these bones form your ankle joint. If you notice this problem, consult a doctor. A chronic instability of your ankle could lead to a decreased range of motion around your ankle as well as pain with motion. As a result, you may develop arthritis of your ankle.

Following an ankle injury, you may have pain around your inner ankle or around your outer ankle. Pain just behind your inner ankle bone usually results from a tendon injury. This type of injury usually develops slowly. It can get progressively worse. If you sustain trauma to your ankle, you may injure this tendon. When this happens, your ankle may swell. This type of injury is usually caused by running or jumping sports. A lack of a proper warm-up or a lack of conditioning can contribute to this injury. This injury can be seen in soccer players or kickers in football who kick with the inner aspects of their foot. If you have an injury, stop exercising until your pain improves. Apply ice to the painful area. Also elevate your foot and ankle on a pillow. Remember that you may re-injure yourself if your injury is not properly treated.

If your pain persists for a prolonged period, your doctor may have you do physical therapy and may possibly prescribe an orthotic for you (to be placed in your shoe). Remember that you should see your doctor if your acute injury does not resolve in four to seven days. Your primary-care doctor may even refer you to an orthopedic surgeon. Steroid injections may provide you with relief if other modalities fail. You may need x-rays of your ankle to exclude a tear of your ligament from your bone. Upon examination of the x-ray, your doctor may notice small flecks of bone. If your pain persists beyond your normal healing time, a magnetic resonance imaging (MRI) scan may be necessary. The overall goal of treatment is to allow your injury to heal. As previously stated, immediately after the injury you should apply ice and rest the ankle. You should also limit weight bearing. You can immobilize your ankle with an Ace wrap. You may need to temporarily use a crutch. Usually after a week or two you can begin to do some stretching exercises. You may need to wear a Velcro ankle brace or high-top tennis shoes at this time. You should not engage in stop-and-go sports such as basketball, running, or impact aerobics. You must realize that injury healing is measured in months rather than weeks.

You need to be patient following an orthopedic injury. If you still hurt after six weeks, your doctor will probably give you an injection with a steroid as well as numbing medicine. (Carl Germano and William Cabot. *Nature's Pain Killers*. n.p.: Kensington Books, 1999) The injection can be repeated again in two to four weeks if your pain has not significantly improved. After four weeks, you will need to increase your stretching exercises. Three to four days after your initial injury, you may notice that heat provides you with pain relief. Not only can a tendon around your outer ankle be injured, the ligament around your ankle can be injured as well.

Ligaments attach bone to bone and thus stabilize your ankle. You may experience a snap if your ligaments are injured. It takes several hours for swelling and pain to occur. Pain with this injury is similar to that when you injure your peroneal tendon. Treatment for this injury is the same as the pain associated with your peroneal tendon. You must stop activity, elevate your leg, and wrap your ankle in ice. If the pain persists, you must see a doctor. Do not attempt to bear weight on the ankle until you have a decrease in your pain. You may need physical therapy as well as injection therapy. If your pain has not improved over time and if your ligaments are totally ruptured, for example, if your arm, leg, hand, or foot does not move when you consciously try to move, you may need orthopedic surgery. If a total tear of your ligament is suspected, see an orthopedic surgeon quickly. The longer you wait, the less chance that surgery will be successful.

If you have severe pain and swelling after your acute injury, your doctor may want to cast your ankle. The cast may need to be placed for two to three months. In most instances, your pain will resolve with conservative management. If your ankle continues to swell and is discolored and if you have severe pain, you need to see a doctor. You can also sprain your inner ankle. This happens if you have an injury where your ankle collapses inward, such as from playing football or basketball. The treatment for this injury is the same as the treatment for the outer ankle injury.

Whenever you have an ankle sprain, remember that improper immobilization with improper healing can cause you to have a weak ankle, which will subject you to recurrent injury. If you need medications, usually a nonsteroidal anti-inflammatory medication will help you control your pain. If your pain is severe, your doctor may prescribe a more potent medication to you.

Achilles Tendon Pain

An injury to your foot and ankle is not uncommon because your feet and ankles are under a lot of stress. They support the weight of your body. You need to know that your foot has 26 joints in each foot. Furthermore, in your foot and ankles you have 15 different tendons. You also have 10 different ligaments and several bursa. With all of these anatomic structures, it is easy for you to realize that your foot and ankle can be a common source of pain if you are physically active. Your foot and ankle act independently of each other. Examine your foot and ankle. The ankle bones are at the very ends of your lower leg bones. These two bones are connected to each other and to your foot by ligaments. Within your ankle is a joint that enables you to walk on uneven surfaces (and engage in many different types of sports). You have a strong ligament that attaches the muscle of your calf to your heel. This tendon is called your Achilles tendon. Your foot has tendons and muscles that help pull your toes downward or upward.

Another relatively common orthopedic injury is an injury around your ankle, which is an Achilles tendon injury. Do you ever get sharp pains at the back of your leg when you jump? Do you have to stop running because the back of your ankle begins to hurt? Were you ever playing basketball and developed a sudden pain right behind your ankle? If you have injured your Achilles tendon, you will experience tenderness above your heel. If you try to press your foot down to the floor, you will have an aggravation of your pain. If you bring your ankle back toward your knee, you will feel pain as well. Usually your range of motion around your ankle will be normal. The tendon attaches your calf muscle to your ankle. An x-ray will not help with the diagnosis of an Achilles tendonitis. An MRI scan will help with the diagnosis.

Immediately after your injury, stop bearing weight and apply ice and elevate your foot and ankle. A nonsteroidal anti-inflammatory medication such as ibuprofen may be of help. (M. Read and P. Wade. *What to Do When it Hurts: Self-Diagnosis and Rehabilitation of Common Aches and Pains*. n.p.: People's Medical Society, 1997) (Carl Germano and William Cabot. *Nature's Pain Killers*. N.p.: Kensington Books, 1999) You may need an ankle brace. If your pain persists more than six weeks, you may need high-top tennis shoes. Increase your activities gradually if your pain persists. If pain persists more than two weeks, see an orthopedic surgeon. An injection with a steroid may provide with some relief. However, realize that physical therapy plays an important role in this type of injury. If pain persists, you may need surgery.

You have a bursa around your Achilles tendon. This bursa can become inflamed. If this occurs, you will have pain in the back of your heel. X-rays are not helpful in the diagnosis of a bursitis in this area. Usually the diagnosis is made if you have pain immediately above your heel. An injection of local anesthetic in this area can confirm the diagnosis. Your doctor may apply a steroid. Injection may be repeated. You should have physical therapy. Occasionally your doctor may want to immobilize your ankle.

Joint Pain

If you are doing repetitive exercises, you may injure one of the joints in your body. A joint is an area that exists between two bones. Your knee is an example of a joint. Your joint is surrounded by a tissue called a joint capsule. Within your joint is a fluid that is called synovial fluid. This is a viscous liquid that lubricates your joint. Your joint capsule contains many pain fibers. When this capsule becomes inflamed, you may have a painful joint. When your joint is injured, fluid increases in your joint, which can cause you pain. This increase in the fluid in your joint can decrease the range of motion of your joint.

Your doctor may need to aspirate fluid from your joint to decrease your pain. You have cartilage in your joint to separate two bones. If a piece of the cartilage tears, you may have what is termed a loose body in your joint. This loose body can cause significant pain.

Avoiding Injury

To prevent any of the injuries described in this chapter, warm up before doing any exercise. If you have sustained an injury, remember that if your sports injury did not heal properly you may be prone to re-injury. Persistent injury can predispose you to osteoarthritis.

Exercise may cause you to have shoulder pain. You may also sustain a rotator cuff tendon tear. This tendon attaches a muscle to the bone in your upper arm called the humerus. A tear in this tendon can cause weakness and pain in your shoulder. You may sustain this injury if you fall or do violent pulls on a starter cable. Excessive pushing and pulling can cause tears as well. These tears usually respond to stretch exercises as well as nonsteroidal anti-inflammatory medications. On occasion, you may need an injection with a steroid. If you do not respond to conservative care within four weeks, see an orthopedic surgeon. If you have a moderate to large rotator cuff tendon tear, you are a probable candidate for surgery.

With respect to sports injuries, you must try to avoid injury. Avoid the urge to run too much too soon. Take time off if you feel pain. Change your training routines. Get proper rest between high-intensity workouts. Stretch before and after exercise regimens.

The figure that follows shows the femur, hip bone, patella (knee cap), tibia, fibula, and foot. These are common areas for sports-related injuries and pain as described in the sections on knee pain, ankle pain, Achilles tendon pain, and foot pain.

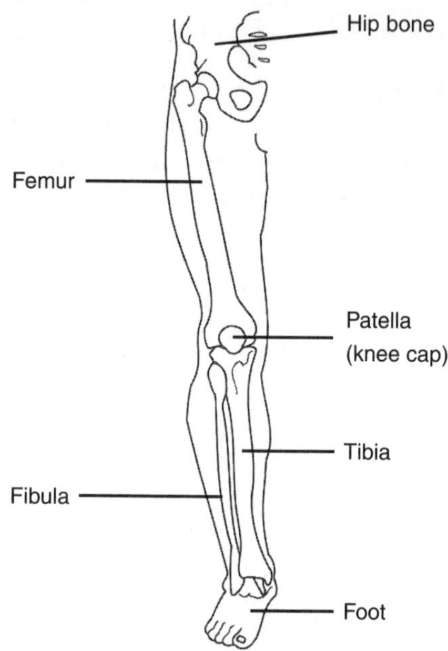

Common areas for sports-related injuries and pain.

Gender Injury Differences

Studies are currently being done looking at women's health in sports and exercise. Studies are currently being done to determine whether there are gender-specific differences in movement patterns that could affect injury risks. Women suffer certain sports injuries more than men. Women are at greater risk of injury to the anterior cruciate ligament in the knee, the kneecap, and knee joint, as well as cartilage in the knee, than are men playing the same sports. In contrast, ankle injuries show no gender-specific differences. (M. Read and P. Wade. *What to Do When it Hurts: Self-Diagnosis and Rehabilitation of Common Aches and Pains*. n.p.: People's Medical Society, 1997) (Carl Germano and William Cabot. *Nature's Pain Killers*. n.p.: Kensington Books, 1999)

What is definitely known is that there are gender-specific differences with respect to sports injuries. (1998 Injury Statics report from the U.S. Consumer Product Safety Commission) Studies are also currently being done looking at the effect of exercise on pre- and post-menopausal women. By comparing these two groups, the effects of hormones on sports injuries may be more easily studied. These studies (or others) may lead us to a greater understanding of the effect hormones play on injury.

The question that remains to be answered is why women have a higher injury rate than men. (1998 Injury Statistics report from the U.S. Consumer Product Safety Commission) Progesterone hormone therapy is being studied. Progesterone stimulates the injury healing process in connective tissue in women. It is imperative for the female athlete to keep her progesterone levels at the maximum level to keep ligaments and tendons strong. You should also know that women with menstrual disturbances are at a greater risk of a sports injury. Menstrual disturbances are more prevalent in female athletes than in the general female population. Stress fractures are more frequent in female athletes with such disturbances. Lower estrogen levels may be associated with such conditions. Lower estrogen levels may have a negative effect on bone strength as well as the retention of calcium within the women's bones. (M. Read and P. Wade. *What to Do When it Hurts: Self-Diagnosis and Rehabilitation of Common Aches and Pains*. n.p.: People's Medical Society, 1997) (Carl Germano and William Cabot. *Nature's Pain Killers*. n.p.: Kensington Books, 1999)

With respect to anterior cruciate ligament injuries in women, women who are mid-cycle in their menstrual cycle are more prone to anterior cruciate ligament injuries. Hormonal differences between men and women influence a tendency toward ligament laxity in women. This ligament laxity may predispose women to sports injuries. Ligament laxity also increases during pregnancy.

High-energy intakes during the Iron Man triathlons help male athletes to accomplish faster times but have the opposite effect on females. In other words, increasing carbohydrate ingestion during the running portion of the contest may help improve performance in male athletes but not in female athletes. The reason for this finding is unknown. On the other hand, men show greater fatigue during exercise and slower recovery time than women.

Studies have shown that women don't slow down as much as men do when they are running a marathon. This is because males may have lower fat-burning properties than females. Fat burning does provide an athlete with energy. As you can see, there are differences among studies comparing men and women athletes. The reason for this controversy appears to be hormonal. (Carl Germano and William Cabot. *Nature's Pain Killers*. n.p.: Kensington Books, 1999) For this reason, hormonal studies with respect to athletic performance continue to be studied.

Treatment for Sports-Related Pain

Physical therapy may help in the management of your pain and possibly prevent its reoccurrence. When you suffer the initial pain, ice, massage, and padding are indicated. Ice needs to be applied for at least 10 minutes to exert its effect. Injection therapy may also provide you with relief.

For Men

- Proper warm-up techniques before exercise activities and cool-down techniques after exercise activities can help prevent some sports-related injuries.
- Physical therapy and stretching exercises can help relieve muscle pain from a sports-related injury.
- Rest, ice, compression, and elevation for strains and sprains will help decrease your pain.
- Over-the-counter pain medications such as ibuprofen and Tylenol can help reduce the pain and inflammation caused by your injury.
- Your doctor may want to prescribe muscle relaxants to help your muscles recoup from the injury.

For Women

- Proper warm-up techniques before exercise activities and cool-down techniques after exercise activities can help prevent some sports-related injuries.
- Physical therapy and stretching exercises can help relieve muscle pain from a sports-related injury.
- Rest, ice, compression, and elevation for strains and sprains will help decrease your pain.
- Over-the-counter pain medications such as ibuprofen and Tylenol can help reduce the pain and inflammation caused by your injury.
- Your doctor may want to prescribe muscle relaxants to help your muscles recoup from the injury.

Chapter 29

Understanding Reproductive System Cancer-Related Pain

As you know, cancer can affect your reproductive organs. Cancer can cause you to experience pain in some instances. If you are a female, you can develop cancer of your breasts, cervix, uterus, or ovary. If you are male, you can develop cancer of your testicles or prostate gland. Cancer-related pain can be excruciating in some cases. Various treatment methods and therapies are available to help relieve your pain if it is related to cancer.

Various pain medicine societies as well as the World Health Organization have studied cancer pain management. It is possible that in the United States cancer pain is frequently inadequately managed. The inadequate management of cancer patients' pain is usually due to a lack of training or a doctor's inability to properly assess and treat cancer pain. If you do not respond to pharmacologic therapy, your doctor may think that you have a psychological problem. Inadequate cancer pain management is decreasing because of proper education of doctors who are treating cancer pain. Your cancer pain can be both acute as well as chronic. Relief of your pain associated with your cancer is an ethical necessity.

In this chapter, you will learn about the different forms of reproductive system cancers, including breast cancer, cervical cancer, uterine cancer, ovarian cancer, and prostate cancer. You will learn about the wide variety of treatments that are available to help control and manage the pain you may have that is associated with your cancer. The effects and side effects of these treatments are covered as well. While the focus of cancers in this chapter is related to the reproductive system, the treatments discussed can be used to treat other types of cancer. Be sure to discuss all of your options with your doctor.

Breast Cancer

Breast cancer is the most common malignancy in women in the United States. Approximately 182,000 women develop breast cancer and more than 46,000 die with it. (L.M. Tierney, et al. *Current Medical Diagnosis and Treatment*. New York: McGraw Hill, 2001) It occurs in one in eight women. Approximately two thirds of cases occur after menopause. Fifteen percent of cases occur before the age of 40. The actual cause of breast cancer is not known. There are different types of breast cancer. Some breast cancers can affect the ducts of the breasts, whereas other types affect lobules of the breasts. Cancer of the ducts usually occurs on one side of the body, whereas lobular cancer is bilateral. The majority of women detect their own breast cancer, therefore, you must be taught how to do a self-examination of your breasts. You should have a breast examination by your doctor at the time of your regular physical examination if you are over age 40. Mammography is recommended every 1 to 2 years if you are older than 40 years of age.

If you have a history of breast cancer, you should have a mammogram yearly. If you are over 40 and have a family history of breast cancer, you should also have a mammogram every year. The survival rate is lower if your cancer is detected by a mammogram as opposed to palpation. Breast cancer is usually painless and presents with a palpable mass in a postmenopausal woman. If it had associated pain, the diagnosis would be more early diagnosed. You should perform routine self examinations as your cancer can be diagnosed early as opposed to waiting for your doctor or mammogram to make the diagnosis.

Accurate diagnosis of breast cancer requires a needle aspiration, a percutaneous needle biopsy, or an incisional (surgical) biopsy. A biopsy should be done on every suspicious breast mass. You must have a chest x-ray to see if your breast cancer may have spread to your lungs, ribs, or spine. A bone scan may also be required to see if your breast cancer has spread to your bones.

If you have breast cancer, your doctor will want to get a CT scan of your abdomen to see if your liver has been affected by the cancer. Your doctor will also obtain a liver function test from you because your cancer can spread to your liver. Risks for breast cancer include increasing age, a family history of breast cancer, previous cancer in one breast, early menstruation (meaning before age 12), late menopause (meaning after age 52), a history of having no children, obesity, a high fat diet, alcohol use, and a family history of cancer of the ovary, uterus, or colon. Cancer will be staged by your pathologist. Staging determines the severity of your cancer. A 0 stage cancer is confined to an area of your organ. A stage greater than III usually means that the cancer has spread beyond your reproductive organ. Your survival rate depends on the stage of the cancer. The stages are based on the severity of the cancer. If you have cancer in your breast that has not spread to your bones or other organs, your 5-year survival rate is greater than 95 percent. However, if your cancer has spread to other areas of your body, your 5-year survival rate is only 10 percent. If your cancer is only in your tissue, you may only need removal of that part of the tissue from your breast.

Cancer treatment is complex and new methods are being developed to treat advanced metastatic cancer. (L.M. Tierney, et al. *Current Medical Diagnosis and Treatment*. New York: McGraw Hill, 2001) However, you are encouraged to do your own breast exams. This may help you to discover the cancer much earlier than if you wait to have an exam at your yearly check-up or during a mammogram at age 40.

If your cancer has spread to other areas of your body, you will most likely require a mastectomy (removal of your breast, radiation therapy, chemotherapy, as well as hormone therapy). Your oncologist will discuss with you the best options for your treatment.

Did you know that breast cancer can also occur in males? (L.M. Tierney, et al. *Current Medical Diagnosis and Treatment*. New York: McGraw Hill, 2001) Males can have an enlargement of their breast tissue. Estrogens stimulate breast development. Androgens such as testosterone inhibit breast development. Male breast cancer is usually on one side and presents as a firm mass that appears to be fixed to the male's underlying tissue. There may even be a nipple discharge. There may also be retraction of the skin around the male breast.

Cervical Cancer

If you are a female, you can also develop cancer of your cervix. Cervical cancer accounts for approximately 2 to 3 percent of all cancers involving women in the United States. More than 15,000 cases of cervical cancer are diagnosed each year, and approximately 5,000 women die from this disease. (L.M. Tierney, et al. *Current Medical Diagnosis and Treatment*. New York: McGraw Hill, 2001) Risk factors for developing carcinoma of the cervix include suppression of the immune system, a history of genital herpes or genital warts, multiple sexual partners, partners with penile warts or cancer, low economic status, intercourse before age 17, and cigarette smoking. Usually cancer of the cervix is painless. Many cases of cervical cancer are detected by a Pap smear. If you have abnormal vaginal bleeding, vaginal discharge, or bleeding after intercourse, you may have advanced cervical cancer. Cancer from your cervix can spread and can cause you lower back pain, leg pain, weight loss, or swelling in your legs. If you have an abnormal Pap smear, you will have a biopsy of your cervix. If the biopsy is unable to determine whether suspicious-looking tissue is cancerous, you will have a bigger portion of your cervix removed, which is called a cervical conization. Your doctor will obtain liver function tests from you, a creatinine level, and a squamous cell carcinoma antigen level. A chest x-ray will be obtained to see whether the cancer has spread to your ribs or lungs. An MRI of your pelvis and abdomen will be obtained to see whether the cancer has spread to other organs. Your gynecologist may place a scope in your bladder and one in your signoid colon to see whether the cancer has advanced to your gastrointestinal tract or urinary tract.

As with most cancers, a pathologist will assign a numeric stage to your cancer. (L.M. Tierney, et al. *Current Medical Diagnosis and Treatment*. New York: McGraw Hill, 2001) If your cancer is only confined to your cervix, you have a 5-year survival rate of 100 percent. If your cancer has spread throughout your pelvis and involved your bladder or rectum, your 5-year survival rate is 20 percent. If your cancer is in an advanced stage and has spread outside of the cervix to other areas of your body, your oncologist will probably prescribe radiation therapy and possibly chemotherapy. If your cancer has spread to your upper vagina, your gynecological oncologist may elect to do an abdominal hysterectomy as well as removal of your lymph nodes. On the other hand, this doctor may elect to do radiation therapy. Many times the therapy chosen depends on your overall health status. After your treatment, your gynecological oncologist will perform a comprehensive pelvic examination as well as a Pap smear every three months for the first two years following your initial treatment; after that, the examination and Pap smear should be every six months from years three to five. If you develop a recurrent cancer of your cervix, you will then probably experience vaginal bleeding or discharge. You can develop pain in your back and legs as well. Again you may experience weight loss. If this happens, you may be treated with radiation therapy or with an extensive removal of the organs in your pelvis.

Uterine Cancer

Approximately 34,000 cases of cancer of the uterus occur each year in the United States. (L.M. Tierney, et al. *Current Medical Diagnosis and Treatment*. New York: McGraw Hill, 2001) The incidence of this tumor decreases yearly. The death rate has decreased each year since 1950. Usually this cancer will occur if you are a postmenopausal woman. Women who undergo menopause after age 52 are more prone to develop uterine cancer. Obesity contributes to an increase in this type of cancer. If you are taking estrogen replacement and are over age 52, you have an increased risk of developing uterine cancer. If you are taking hormones that contain progestins, your incidence of developing this cancer are decreased.

As with the other cancers mentioned in this chapter, there are stages. Stage 0, which is the cancer in your uterus, has a 100 percent success rate. If your cancer involves your bladder or your rectum, your survival rate decreases to 20 percent. If you have stage 0 uterine cancer, a simple procedure that removes the area of the cancer can be done. If you have the fourth stage, which involves your bladder, pelvis, or rectum, you will have radiation therapy. If you have stage 2A, you will have a radical hysterectomy with removal of your lymph nodes followed by radiation therapy. The clinical presentation of this cancer is abnormal uterine bleeding. If you are in menopause and begin bleeding, you should be evaluated by your gynecologist or primary-care doctor immediately. If your cancer becomes advanced, you can have pelvic pain as well as back and leg pain. You will also sustain weight loss. Almost 5 percent of women with uterine cancer have no symptoms. (L.M. Tierney, et al. *Current Medical Diagnosis and Treatment*. New York: McGraw Hill, 2001) You should have a careful and comprehensive pelvic and abdominal evaluation. If you have abnormal bleeding, you should have a biopsy taken from your uterus or a D&C. Most of the uterine cancers detected by your doctor are at an early stage. This means that your prognosis for a five-year survival is good.

Standard therapy for uterine cancer is an abdominal hysterectomy with removal of both your ovaries. As with other cancers mentioned in this chapter, you should have a pelvic exam and Pap smear every three months for the first two years after treatment. Other tests should be done only if you have a recurrence of symptoms. If you do have recurrence of the cancer, a major surgical procedure will need to be done.

Ovarian Cancer

Ovarian cancer develops in 1 in every 70 women. Approximately 1 percent of women die from this cancer. Approximately 24,000 cases of ovarian cancer are diagnosed in the United States each year. More than 13,000 women will die with ovarian cancer each year. (L.M. Tierney, et al. *Current Medical Diagnosis and Treatment*. New York: McGraw Hill, 2001) The incidence of cancer of the ovary is increased in women who have never been pregnant and is more prevalent in women who have had late onset of menopause or have been on a high-fat diet. If you are female and have a history of colon cancer or breast cancer, you are at a higher risk. If you are using oral contraceptives, have had more than one baby, and are breast-feeding, you will have a decreased risk of developing cancer of the ovaries. If someone in your family has a history of ovarian cancer, you are at an increased risk. If your cancer is confined to your ovary, you have a stage 1A cancer. You have a five-year survival rate of approximately 90 percent. If you have a stage 4 ovarian tumor, the cancer has spread to your liver or lung or so forth. Your five-year survival rate is 5 percent.

Unfortunately, most women who have cancer of their ovaries will have an advanced disease at the time of their diagnosis. The reason for this is that the symptoms of ovarian cancer are vague. You may have vague pelvic or abdominal pain. You may only have altered bowel habits. As your cancer develops, you can have obstruction of your intestines and can have swelling and fluid in your abdomen. Sometimes the tumor can be noted on a routine physical pelvic examination. You can have abnormal uterine bleeding. If you are a postmenopausal female and if your doctor can palpate your ovary on a routine pelvic exam, this suggests that you may have cancer of your ovary. Usually, normal ovaries cannot be palpated. If you have an enlarged ovary, an ultrasound of your pelvis may be helpful in diagnosing cancer of your ovary. Your pelvis, abdomen, and chest will be carefully examined as well. Liver-function tests will be done as well as a CT scan of your abdomen. Occasionally a further gastrointestinal workup is indicated. If you have cancer of your ovaries, you will have your ovaries removed as well as a hysterectomy. You will also have surgical sampling of your lymph glands to see whether your cancer has spread to your lymph glands. Chemotherapy may be prescribed to you after surgery. Your prognosis is good if you are relatively young, if you have an early stage of the cancer, and if you have a rapid rate of your ovarian tumor response to the therapy mentioned. As we have seen with all of these tumors, the higher the number of the stage, the worse the tumor. If you have an extremely malignant tumor, your prognosis of survival over five years may be poor. This is the reason that you must get your gynecological examination on a regular basis. The reason for this is that if your tumor is diagnosed early, you have an excellent prognosis.

Prostate Cancer

Men can also have cancers affecting their reproductive organs, including their testes and prostate gland. The testes secrete testosterone and estradiol, which are two hormones. Testicular cancer represents approximately 2 percent of all cancers in men. (L.M. Tierney, et al. *Current Medical Diagnosis and Treatment*. New York: McGraw Hill, 2001) It is the second most common cancer in men between the ages of 20 and 34 years of age. These tumors usually manifest as an enlargement of the testicle. You may have pain and tenderness in your testicle. A male with a testicular tumor can have breast enlargement. Approximately 10 percent of these tumors will have distance spread of the cancer at the time of the diagnosis. These tumors are staged through measurement of certain chemical markers in the bloodstream as well as imaging studies or surgery. Some of these cancers are quite sensitive to radiation therapy. Other tumors that are confined to the testes are cured through removal of the testicle followed by radiation therapy. If your tumor has spread throughout your body, the disease is treated with both radiation therapy and chemotherapy. If your cancer is localized to your testicle, your 5-year survival rate approximates 100 percent. If your cancer has spread throughout your body, your survival rate drops to 20 percent.

Most men over 55 years of age will have an enlargement of their prostate gland. Almost two thirds of these men will have symptoms of prostatism. They will have decreased force of their urine stream and retention of their urine in their bladder after they urinate. They wake up frequently at night to urinate. Over time, they may not be able to hold their urine. Prostatism is a benign entity. However, prostatism can be a symptom of cancer. Cancer symptoms may be without significant symptoms initially but as the cancer advances can become severe.

Prostate cancer, on the other hand, is the second most common tumor in men. Approximately 200,000 new cases are diagnosed each year. Prostate cancer is more common among African Americans and men who have a family history of prostate cancer. The problem with prostate cancer is that it is usually painless and has no other symptoms that are seen with prostatism. Prostate cancer can be detected by routine digital examination or elevation of your prostate specific antigen (PSA). (L.M. Tierney, et al. *Current Medical Diagnosis and Treatment*. New York: McGraw Hill, 2001) Sometimes if you have surgery to remove an enlarged prostate gland, cancer tissue can be found in your prostate gland. When the cancer leaves your prostate and goes to your bone, you can have severe back pain or other bone pain. In many instances, an MRI will be done to see whether your tumor has spread to other organs. Other chemical body markers can be measured as well if cancer is suspected to be present in another organ. A bone scan may be necessary to detect a cancer that has gone to your bones. If you have prostate cancer, your surgeon may do a prostatectomy (removal of your prostate gland), radiation therapy, hormone therapy, or chemotherapy.

If your tumor is confined to your prostate, a prostatectomy, radiation therapy and/or hormone therapy is appropriate. If your prostate cancer has spread beyond your prostate, radiation therapy is usually the treatment of choice. If your prostate cancer has disseminated throughout your body, you will be treated with hormone therapy. Your prostate cancer is usually testosterone sensitive. Your doctor will prescribe hormone therapy that will lower your testosterone in your bloodstream. This can be done through castration. Your doctor can give you large doses of estrogen, which will eventually lower your testosterone blood level. Chemotherapy is usually not effective for the management of prostate cancer. Following treatment, your PSA will be monitored regularly to determine the effects of your therapy. If your PSA continues to rise, this indicates probable residual cancer. Prostate cancer can be detected early; if it is detected early, your prognosis for survival is excellent. This means that you need to follow up with your primary-care doctor regularly and have a regular rectal examination so that your doctor can feel your prostate to see if it is enlarged or if it has possible cancer masses in it. You will also need to have your PSA done on a regular basis.

Treatment for Cancer-Related Pain

If you do develop cancer and have pain related to this cancer, there is no reason why your pain cannot be controlled. However, to receive the maximum benefit from pain management, it is recommended that a team approach be utilized. Remember that you are a member of this team. If you are not experiencing adequate pain relief from the methods that are given to you, you must notify your doctor. In other words, you should not suffer in silence.

Psychiatric Treatment

If you have been diagnosed with cancer, you face a wide range of psychological and physical problems throughout your cancer. You may have a fear of a painful death or disfigurement. These types of fears exist in all cancer patients. However, the degree of your psychological distress caused by these psychological factors varies from person to person. One of the most feared consequences of cancer is pain. To treat your pain appropriately, a multidisciplinary approach may be necessary, including your oncologist, your psychologist or psychiatrist, and your pain-management doctor. When you have been diagnosed with cancer, you will usually have an initial episode of shock and disbelief and possibly a denial that you actually have cancer. Then you will develop anxiety as well as depression. Your emotional distress usually resolves over several weeks to two to three months. Psychological referral is not usually necessary in most cancer patients. Sometimes, however, relaxing medications such as valium are necessary to restore normal sleep patterns.

You can develop psychiatric symptoms associated with your cancer. Almost 90 percent of psychiatric disorders noted in cancer patients are a reaction to the disease itself or treatments used to cure the cancer. An extremely painful disease is the most feared effect associated with cancer. Approximately 15 percent of cancer patients whose cancer has not spread develop significant pain. If the disease is advanced, 60 to 90 percent of patients report significant pain. Unfortunately, 25 percent of all cancer patients die while still experiencing considerable pain.

Depression occurs in approximately 25 percent of all cancer patients. (J.D. Loeser. *Bonica's Management of Pain*. n.p.: Lippincott Williams and Wilkins, 2001) Your depression can increase depending on your level of disability as well as your pain. You may experience a loss of appetite, an inability to sleep, fatigue, and weight loss. Your depression will be treated with appropriate antidepressant medications. Sometimes stimulants such as amphetamines are used for the treatment of depression in some cancer patients. Furthermore, if you do require a significant dose of narcotics, the amphetamine drugs can keep you alert. They may also improve your depression. Opioids can cause sedation in some instances. Sedation can decrease your activity.

It is not uncommon for you to develop anxiety after you have been diagnosed with cancer. You may develop anxiety while waiting to hear of your diagnosis or recurrence, before procedures that need to be done or even surgery. This anxiety can disrupt your ability to function.

Medications used to treat your cancer, such as some chemotherapy drugs, as well as your pain that is not properly controlled or infection can cause you to have anxiety. You can also develop panic attacks. Your doctor may prescribe a short-acting anti-anxiety drug such as alprazolam or a long-acting anti-anxiety drug such as valium. As your cancer becomes advanced, you may become delirious and disoriented. Your delirium can be reversed. However, your delirium usually is not reversible in the last 48 hours of life. If your cancer is advanced and you develop multiple organ failure, your delirium will become worse. You can become agitated as well as restless. If you are being treated with high doses of narcotics, you may develop delirium as well. Chemotherapy drugs can also cause you to have delirium. Steroids have also been associated with causes of delirium.

A drug that can help control your delirium is a valiumlike drug called lorazepam. Sometimes cancer pain can be so severe that you could consider suicide. The majority of suicides observed among patients suffering with cancer had severe pain that could not be controlled. Cancer pain patients in general can have an increased risk of suicide. If their pain remains severe, they may want to escape their pain. A method that will be continued to be debated by lawmakers, doctors, and the general public now as well as in the future is doctor-assisted suicide. Doctor-assisted suicide has become a topic of public debate. This issue is left to religious leaders as well as legislatures.

Antiseizure and Anticonvulsant Medications

Your pain is easily caused by tissue damage from your cancer. As your tumor grows it can compress nerves in your body, which can cause you pain. In some instances, however, you may not have pain as the cancer destroys your tissue. Remember that you have pain fibers in your skin, your muscles, your connective tissue, and your organs. Your cancer pain can cause you sharp, aching, and throbbing pain as well. Pain from your organs is more diffuse as well as gnawing and cramping. Most of your pain can respond to narcotic drugs.

If your pain is in your *central nervous system* or if it affects some of your nerves outside of your brain and spinal cord, you can have what is called *neuropathic pain.* (J.D. Loeser. *Bonica's Management of Pain.* n.p.: Lippincott Williams and Wilkins, 2001) Neuropathic pain causes you to experience symptoms which are sharp and electrical shocklike. This type of pain can be controlled by antiseizure medications such as Neurontin. You can have pain that is severe and excessive for the extent of tissue damage that has occurred. This type of pain is called idiopathic and usually has a psychological pathology associated with it.

Anticonvulsant medications such as Neurontin and Klonopin can relieve severe lancinating pain when your tumor affects one of your nerves. In case you are wondering why a seizure medication would be prescribed, it's because these medications are also pain medications. (J.D. Loeser. *Bonica's Management of Pain.* n.p.: Lippincott Williams and Wilkins, 2001) In the United States, about 5 percent of all anticonvulsant medications are prescribed for pain management. Nerve injury caused by cancer, chemotherapy, or radiation therapy is controlled with anticonvulsant medications.

Nonsteroidal Anti-inflammatory Medications

When using nonsteroidal anti-inflammatory medications, the COX-2 inhibitors are probably the safest drugs in this category for you to use. (J.D. Loeser. *Bonica's Management of Pain.* n.p.: Lippincott Williams and Wilkins, 2001) These drugs will not affect your body's ability to form blood clots and usually will not cause you to have bleeding stomach ulcers. The principles of using pain-relieving drugs are essential tools for any clinician who is treating cancer pain. The most common reason for your pain being unrelieved is the failure of your doctor to routinely assess your pain and to assess your pain relief. This is also true if you have been admitted to a hospital. Your pain is recognized by your report to your doctors.

Narcotics and Their Effects

At one time it was thought that narcotics worked only within the brain and spinal cord to relieve pain. However, recent research has demonstrated that morphine can be present in some cells that migrate to the inflamed tissue. In other words, if cancer cells have migrated to other tissues outside of the area, injection of narcotics into these areas can cause you a significant decrease in pain. If you have these injections into the inflamed tissue, you may have decreased adverse effects such as sedation, nausea, vomiting, and respiratory depression.

Furthermore, you should not suffer any mental clouding. Morphine can be used in the management of your cancer pain. Morphine is the standard of comparison for the rest of the narcotic analgesics. A sustained-release preparation is available called MS Contin; it releases the drug over 8 to 12 hours. There is also a drug that you can take once a day that will give a sustained release over 24 hours called Kadian. Dilaudid is stronger than morphine, but it has a shorter duration of action than morphine. Methadone is another drug that can be prescribed for cancer pain; it is very effective when given in a pill form. Another stronger drug than morphine is Levo-Dromoran. It is stronger than morphine and can last up to 16 hours per dose.

Fentanyl is a potent drug which is more potent than the drugs mentioned. It is given by a transdermal fentanyl patch. There is also an oral fentanyl lozenge that is available for treatment of your breakthrough pain when you are taking around-the-clock opioids. Breakthrough pain can always occur even when you are taking your narcotic. Breakthrough pain means additional pain which can occur when your activities increase. For example, if you go bowling you can have additional pain which must be treated. (*Principles of Analgesic Use in the Treatment of Acute Pain and Cancer Pain*. Illinois: American Pain Society, 1999) (American Pain Society, Quality of Care Committee. "Quality Improvement Guidelines for the Treatment of Acute Pain and Cancer Pain," *JAMA* 274 [1995]: 1874-1880) (E. Bruera, et al. "Opioid Rotation in Patients with Cancer Pain: A Retrospective Comparison of Dose Ratios Between Methadone, Hydromorphone and Morphine," *Cancer* 78 [1996]: 852-857)

Demerol is another drug that is available. It is not recommended because the breakdown products of this drug can cause seizures and also because of its relatively short duration of pain-relieving action, one and a half to two hours, as compared to other opioid preparations. Other types of drugs such as Nubane and Stadol, which act on your kappa receptors, are not readily prescribed for the management of cancer pain. Another drug called Ultram is a weak narcotic-binding receptor drug that decreases the amount of pain that will reach your brain. It also inhibits the reuptake of norepinephrine and serotonin, which are two chemicals that exist in your central nervous system that can also modulate your pain. Sometimes if you take the tramadol you can develop dizziness as well as nausea and vomiting. If you take more than eight tablets per day, you run the risk of seizures. (*Principles of Analgesic Use in the Treatment of Acute Pain and Cancer Pain.* Illinois: American Pain Society, 1999) (American Pain Society, Quality of Care Committee. "Quality Improvement Guidelines for the Treatment of Acute Pain and Cancer Pain," *JAMA* 274 [1995]: 1874-1880) (E. Bruera, et al. "Opioid Rotation in Patients with Cancer Pain: A Retrospective Comparison of Dose Ratios Between Methadone, Hydromorphone and Morphine," *Cancer* 78 [1996]: 852-857)

You must remember that if you are taking a narcotic, you may become drowsy, constipated, and develop nausea or vomiting or itching. On occasion, your breathing rate may significantly decrease. If your side effects are severe, they can be decreased by a decrease in your dose of the narcotic that you are taking. If you are receiving significant pain relief from a certain drug but do become drowsy, your doctor can also prescribe caffeine or an amphetamine. If you are experiencing constipation, you should take a stool softener such as Colace. If you develop nausea and vomiting associated with your narcotic medication, you may need a scopolamine skin patch. Another way of controlling your nausea and vomiting is with a rectal suppository of a medication that will stop your nausea and vomiting.

Remember that tolerance means that it takes a larger dose of narcotic to maintain its original effect. You and your doctor should watch for tolerance and treat it appropriately. You can confuse tolerance with worsening of your cancer. In most instances, your cancer has not progressed but you have become tolerant to your narcotic drug.

Be aware the tumor progression itself may increase your pain intensity. Be sure to discuss your pain progression with your doctor. This is important so that you and your doctor can determine the cause of your increased pain.

Epidural Injections

Clonidine has been approved by the FDA for epidural use. The epidural space is the spinal fluid that surrounds your spinal cord. Clonidine administered into your epidural space can control some pains that are caused by your cancer.

If you are not receiving adequate relief of your pain with these methods, be aware that narcotic medications can be placed into your epidural space or actually even placed into the fluid that surrounds your spinal cord. Narcotics bind to your narcotic receptors in your spinal cord. As a result, an extremely small amount of drug can be given when compared to either an oral route or an intravenous route. The most common drugs used either administered epidurally or intrathecally (into your spinal fluid) are morphine and fentanyl. Morphine remains in your spinal fluid for an extended period of time. As a result you have a longer duration of pain relief as the morphine slowly spreads up your spinal fluid to your brain stem. Fentanyl, on the other hand, is rapidly taken up into your bloodstream. The duration of your pain relief will not be as long as that of the morphine.

The common way of administering narcotics into your spinal fluid is by continuous infusion technique. When using this technique, the drug is placed into a pump. The pump gives you a continuous flow of the narcotic medication. This system provides you excellent pain relief with minimal sedation. The administration of narcotics into your spinal fluid or into your epidural space has an excellent safety record. The most common complication of these systems is infection in your skin.

Oral, Rectal, IV, and Patch Treatments

Your oral route of all the narcotics mentioned is usually the preferred route for chronic narcotic treatment. The reason is because it is usually convenient for you to take a pill and you can always take an extra pill for the control of your cancer pain. If you cannot swallow, many narcotics are available in a liquid form. These narcotic drugs can be given to you by injection into your muscle called an intramuscular injection. The problem with this mode of administering a narcotic is that the injection itself can be painful. The absorption from your muscle fluctuates from person to person. There can be a one-hour lag before the medicine begins to work. The medicine may not last as long as the same drug given by a pill. The narcotic drug may work more rapidly if it is given into your shoulder muscle as opposed to your gluteal muscle. Intramuscular injections of narcotics are rarely used. If you receive too many of these injections, you can develop abscesses or actual injury of your muscle tissue.

Sublingual (under the tongue) morphine when it is in a high concentration (Roxanol 20 mg/ml) can provide you with pain relief if you cannot swallow pills. Actiq is a fentanyl preparation on a stick which resembles a lollipop. Actiq works quickly to provide you with pain relief.

If a narcotic is given to you through your vein, called an intravenous injection, you will have the most rapid onset of effect. However, the length of action of the drug will be less than oral or intramuscular injections. The advantage of the intravenous dose is that if after you have received a dose and if your pain persists, you can be given another dose until your pain is tolerable. Sometimes you can receive an intravenous infusion of a narcotic medication. This infusion will be given on a continuous regimen. You can also have a patient-control analgesia (PCA) machine that enables you to press a button to give yourself an intravenous bolus of a narcotic drug. Sometimes you can receive intravenous boluses of fentanyl until you have pain relief. This total dose, to provide you with pain relief, can be extrapolated by your doctor who can prescribe you a fentanyl patch with an equivalent dose of pain-relieving medication. However, if you are using the fentanyl patch, you can still have episodes of pain. When this happens, you will be prescribed a short-acting narcotic medicine. One of the best rapid ways of controlling your breakthrough pain is oral transmucosal fentanyl. An example is Actiq. This is a lozenge that is sweetened and has a raspberry taste. This medication is rapidly absorbed if the lozenge is placed between your cheek and gum. If you use this lozenge, you can receive relief in 5 to 10 minutes. The transmucosal fentanyl preparation should not be given unless you are taking 60 mg or more of oral morphine per day or if you are using a fentanyl transdermal patch of 50 mcg/hr or more. Approximately 76 percent of cancer patients can have adequate pain relief using the oral transmucosal fentanyl lozenges.

Another way of providing you with narcotic medications is rectally. Rectal suppositories are available for hydromorphone, oxymorphone, and morphine. (*Principles of Analgesic Use in the Treatment of Acute Pain and Cancer Pain*. Illinois: American Pain Society, 1999) (American Pain Society, Quality of Care Committee. "Quality Improvement Guidelines for the Treatment of Acute Pain and Cancer Pain," *JAMA* 274 [1995]: 1874-1880) (E. Bruera, et al. "Opioid Rotation in Patients with Cancer Pain: A Retrospective Comparison of Dose Ratios Between Methadone, Hydromorphone and Morphine," *Cancer* 78 [1996]: 852-857)

The rectal administration of morphine, for example, can produce an onset of action within 10 minutes. This route can be used if you cannot swallow. Narcotic medications can also be given immediately under your skin, which is called a subcutaneous route. The onset of action of a drug given in this manner is slower than some of the other routes of administration mentioned. If you are placed on strong medications, your doctor should see you frequently. The narcotic medications will only benefit you if your doctor monitors your pain relief and adjusts your dose frequently to not only decrease your pain but to allow you to be as active as possible. Occasionally you are unable to tolerate one drug and may need another drug that won't cause you significant side effects.

If your doctor changes you to a new narcotic medication or uses a different route of administration, your doctor should use what is called an equianalgesic dose. The reason for this is that two narcotic drugs are usually not of the same potency. There is a published table that your doctor will use to calculate the analgesic dose of a new medication that is equivalent to the old medication. If this is not done and if your medications are changed, you run the risk of overdosing or underdosing. If your doctor changes you from an oral to an intravenous administration or transmucosal administration, again equianalgesic dosing must be calculated by your doctor. Sometimes if you have been prescribed a narcotic medication for a long time, your body can become tolerant to it. This means that you are not receiving the same pain relief that you received previously from your narcotic drug. When this happens, your doctor will probably want to switch you to another drug. The other drug can be given until you develop tolerance to it. When this tolerance occurs, you can go back to the original drug prescribed to you and your body will then respond well to the initial drug that you were given.

Treatment for Bone Pain

You must be aware that if you have cancer that you have an increased risk of developing post-herpetic neuralgia pain. Not only can your cancer compress some of the nerves throughout your body, it can also go to your bone and destroy it, which can cause you pain as well. You can develop pain in any of your bones. You can note pain in your back, neck, as well as your head or even your mid-back. If you have had a mastectomy, you may develop phantom breast pain. When a cancer has spread to your bones, bone pain is the most common cause of chronic pain associated with cancer. Cancers of the breast and prostate gland can frequently go to the bone. Almost 60 percent of cancer that spreads to the bone can go to the mid-back. Your lower back can be involved 20 percent of the time and your neck 10 percent of the time.

More than one level of the bones in your back is involved in 85 percent of patients. When the cancer goes to your bones, it can make your bone prone to fractures. In the majority of instances of bone pain associated with cancer, nonsteroidal anti-inflammatory medications can provide relief. In many instances, the nonsteroidal anti-inflammatory drugs need to be combined with a narcotic medication. In many instances, the use of nonsteroidal anti-inflammatory medications for the treatment of bone pain is overlooked. There have been many reported instances where the administration of a nonsteroidal anti-inflammatory drug decreased the need for increasing narcotics in the management of cancer associated with bone pain. In managing your cancer pain, your doctor should strive to prolong your survival, optimize your comfort, and optimize your function.

Communicating Your Pain to Your Doctor

If you have difficulty communicating with your health-care provider, you are at risk of undertreatment. (*Principles of Analgesic Use in the Treatment of Acute Pain and Cancer Pain*. Illinois: American Pain Society, 1999) (American Pain Society, Quality of Care Committee. "Quality Improvement Guidelines for the Treatment of Acute Pain and Cancer Pain," *JAMA* 274 [1995]: 1874-1880) (E. Bruera, et al. "Opioid Rotation in Patients with Cancer Pain: A Retrospective Comparison of Dose Ratios Between Methadone, Hydromorphone and Morphine," *Cancer* 78 [1996]: 852-857)

Pain scales are one way of determining how severe your pain is. A numeric scale of 0 being no pain and 10 the worst pain ever imaginable is an easy way of communicating your pain to your doctor. You and your doctor need to cooperate with each other and use the scale that is easy for you to use and easy for your doctor to interpret.

If you have been prescribed a nonsteroidal anti-inflammatory drug and continue to have pain associated with your cancer, your doctor will add opioid medications to manage your cancer-related pain. If oral opioids are causing you a problem or sedation, and if your cancer is confined to a certain area, your doctor can inject a narcotic medication into your affected tissue.

The Pain Stepladder

The World Health Organization has recommended a pain "stepladder" for the management of your cancer pain. This consists of using nonnarcotic analgesics such as nonsteroidal anti-inflammatory drugs or Tramadol. The next step up the ladder is narcotic medications. It is recommended that your doctor begin with a mild narcotic and progress to a stronger narcotic. If you still have not experienced pain relief, it is recommended that your doctor combine the narcotic drugs with other drugs such as anticonvulsant drugs and antidepressant drugs for the management of your pain.

The purpose of the World Health Organization analgesic ladder is to individualize your treatment. If this ladder approach is used for the management of your cancer pain, studies have shown that you can have adequate pain relief 90 percent of the time. Increase in the intensity of your pain is the prime consideration in using this ladder.

Keeping a Pain-Intensity Diary

Your doctor's decision-making pharmacologically will be based on your pain-intensity diary. Your pain intensity will also provide your doctor with feedback about how you are responding to therapy. You need to keep a diary as to whether your pain is localized to one area or if it is more diffuse throughout your body. You also need to keep a diary as to whether your pain is constant or whether you have pain and then it goes away only to recur again. Surgery, chemotherapy, and radiation therapy can account for 25 percent of your chronic cancer pain. If you have had new or increasing pain symptoms following any of these methods, you need to keep a diary and notify your doctor. If your activities of daily living are limited as a result of your pain or as a result of your narcotic treatment or anticonvulsant medication treatment, you need to notify your doctor. In addition to decreasing your pain, your doctor will attempt to maximize your daily activity. Your pain-medicine doctor will obtain a detailed history from you. You will also have a physical examination which will concentrate heavily on a neurological evaluation. If you have any changes in your skin or develop severe skin pain, notify your doctor.

For Men

- Keep a detailed pain-intensity diary to help your doctor determine when you are experiencing most of your pain. This will help your doctor determine the most effective approach to treating your pain.
- Medications prescribed by your doctor such as antidepressants and anti-anxiety can help relieve some of your psychological issues associated with coping with your cancer.
- Antinausea and antivomiting medications prescribed by your doctor will help relieve some of the side effects caused by some of your other cancer treatment medications.
- Narcotic medications may be prescribed by your doctor to help control your cancer-related pain. Do not be worried about dependence, because high doses may be needed to control your pain adequately.

For Women

- Keep a detailed pain-intensity diary to help your doctor determine when you are experiencing most of your pain. This will help your doctor determine the most effective approach to treating your pain.
- Medications prescribed by your doctor such as antidepressants and anti-anxiety can help relieve some of your psychological issues associated with coping with your cancer.
- Antinausea and antivomiting medications prescribed by your doctor will help relieve some of the side effects caused by some of your other cancer treatment medications.
- Narcotic medications may be prescribed by your doctor to help control your cancer-related pain. Do not be worried about dependence, because high doses may be needed to control your pain adequately.

Chapter 30

New Pain-Management Research and Therapies

Currently, clinical drug trials are being conducted for the control of pain. You need to be aware of these trials. Overall, in this new century, medical advances occur every day. However, with respect to pain medicine, many factors remain unknown. The biological causes of pain are being studied, as well as the histological causes (the study of the structure of your tissues which includes tumor classification). Furthermore, different therapies that can help you with your acute and chronic pain syndromes are being studied. Placebo trials are explained for you in Chapter 31, in the section "The Benefits of Self-Education."

You need to be aware that the "magic bullet" for the treatment of your pain syndrome has not been developed. However, the ideal medication to help you with your pain syndrome is expected to be developed within the next decade. However, remember when this drug is discovered, it will take time for this drug to be studied in the human population. As you can see, potentially exciting modalities exist on the horizon for the management of pain. It is thought that some of these endeavors may hold promise for new treatment modalities for the treatment of pain. The purpose of pain research is to offer you a better quality of life.

In this chapter, you will learn about new research in pain management including chiropractic therapy, acupuncture therapy, thermal therapy, and spinal column stimulator therapy. New drugs for managing your pain including nasal anesthetics, new opioids, new drugs to treat neuropathies, epidural anesthetic research, injections, and the pain pump will be discussed.

Chiropractic Therapy Research

Chiropractic therapy is also being studied in a scientific manner. Scientific research on the effects of chiropractic care with lower back pain has focused on how well it can help relieve pain.

Scientific studies comparing chiropractic care with conventional medical care were found to be comparably effective. This study included individuals with acute, subacute, and chronic painful conditions.

Chiropractic therapy has been compared with physical therapy for the management of back pain. Individuals who received chiropractic manipulative therapy (hands on therapy) or physical therapy were better off than those who received no therapy. There were no differences between those who received chiropractic manipulative therapy and those who received physical therapy.

Chiropractic therapy has been compared for the management of acute lower back pain with primary-care practitioners as well as orthopedic surgeons. Not only was pain control studied but also how long it took to return to functional status. There were over 1,500 individuals in the study and each individual had back pain of less than 10 weeks duration. (B. Goldberg. *Alternative Medicine, The Definitive Guide*. Berkeley: Celestial Arts, 2001) The results of the study revealed that the time to recovery was essentially the same no matter which provider provided the medical care.

Chiropractic care was also compared to hospital out-patient clinics in 11 centers for the treatment of lower back pain. Individuals were randomized to receive either chiropractic care or hospital out-patient management. It is interesting to note that chiropractic care was found to be more effective than conventional medical treatment in hospital out-patient clinics.

Chiropractic care was studied comparing spinal manipulation with placebo manipulation in a back pain educational program. The sham manipulation was done to be used as a placebo. Participants in the study did not know if they were receiving chiropractic therapy or a sham therapy. The results of the study revealed that there was greater improvement found in the chiropractic-treated group than in the other groups. Chiropractic therapy has also been compared to massage therapy, use of a corset (contracting the muscle followed by relaxation), and transelectrical muscle stimulation (which can build muscle mass). (B. Goldberg. *Alternative Medicine, The Definitive Guide*. Berkeley: Celestial Arts, 2001) Chiropractic therapy had the most improvement compared to the other therapies with respect to pain and range of motion. Chiropractic is not a new pain-therapy modality. However, scientific studies looking at chiropractic therapy for the management of pain is new.

Acupuncture Therapy

Accupuncture is a traditional Chinese system of healing by the insertion of acupuncture needles into defined points below the skin. Traditional Chinese acupuncture is being investigated for the treatment of pain associated with osteoarthritis (refer to Chapter 16). Individuals performing this study hypothesize that traditional Chinese acupuncture is effective for the control of pain of osteoarthritis. (B. Goldberg. *Alternative Medicine, The Definitive Guide*. Berkeley: Celestial Arts, 2001) This study is being compared to a sham non-acupuncture needle treatment. These individuals are looking at improvement in not only pain but also in function and range of motion around the affected knee joints. Differences in age and gender are also being investigated.

Nasal Anesthetics

Powerful anesthetic drugs that can be administered through nasal passages are also being studied. It is not known at present whether these drugs will be used for the treatment of severe pain. These new drugs—administered nasally to allow your surgeon to operate—have been shown to be safe and effective in preliminary studies. Continued research is being done on these new anesthetic agents.

New Opioids

Scientists continue to search for new pain medications that are non-addictive. According to the National Institute of Health website, www.NIH.gov, researchers at the University of Arizona are currently trying to develop a new analgesic that could help you with respect to your pain but eliminate dependency on a drug. The purpose of their study is to create an alternative drug to morphine.

Morphine can have side effects such as nausea, vomiting, respiratory depression, and even addiction. According to the National Institute of Health website, www.NIH.gov, this new drug that may replace narcotic medications is called Biphalin. The drug has been tested on animals. It is hoped that this new drug can decrease the psychological and physical effects of addiction. This new drug is being researched to bind on a different receptor than the mu receptor. Morphine as well as the other narcotic medications, with the exception of two, binds to the mu receptor.

The other two medications, such as Stadol, bind to the kappa receptors. The new drug currently being researched at the University of Arizona will bind to your delta receptor. If this drug is proven to be beneficial, it will potentially help individuals who are suffering from severe pain.

New Drugs to Treat Neuropathies

A new study is currently being done examining the effects of a drug called EAA-O90. This drug is being used in individuals with diabetic neuropathy (refer to Chapter 17). It is a selective drug that binds to what are called NMDA receptors. Stimulation of NMDA receptors can cause you to have significant pain. The purpose of this study is to assess the safety and efficacy of this new drug. It will be compared with a placebo pill. This study is currently being sponsored by Wyeth-Ayerst Research.

Another study is presently being done investigating the effects of a drug for the treatment of postherpetic neuralgia. Essentially this study will assess the efficacy and safety of a high concentration capsaicin skin patch at three different dose levels. These researchers are trying to establish an optimal dose for the treatment of postherpetic neuralgia. Capsaicin is a substance derived from red peppers. This substance can cause you to have burning pain. However, it is effective for the treatment of postherpetic neuralgia. The drug works by depleting your nerve endings of a chemical called substance P. Depleting substance P from your nerve endings will deplete this pain transmitter and cause you to have pain relief.

This clinical trial, like any new drug study, has to go through three phases before it can be marketed. In phase I, these researchers are testing this new drug treatment in a small group of people. The study is done on approximately 50 people for the first time to see if the drug is safe, to determine a safe dose, and identify any side effects. In the phase II, the drug is given to approximately 200 people to see if it is effective and to evaluate its safety. In phase III, the drug is given to more than 1,000 individuals to ensure that it is effective for the treatment of pain to monitor any side effects and to compare it to other treatments to see if it is more effective. The FDA strictly defines these drug-study phases according to federal law.

Another drug, called NGX-4010, is being investigated for the treatment of painful HIV-associated neuropathy. The purpose of this drug is to assess the efficacy, safety, and the tolerability of this drug at different doses for the treatment of HIV neuropathy. The drug is being investigated for not only the infection of nerves with the HIV virus but also the effects of this drug on pain caused by antiretroviral drug use. Neuropathy associated with the HIV virus can be extremely painful and disabling. Hopefully, this new drug that is being studied for use in this patient population will ease the suffering of these individuals.

New Epidural Drug Research

A current study is also being conducted looking for the reason why a block with a local anesthetic can reduce pain for a longer period of time longer than a local anesthetic. For more than 20 years, we have known that epidural steroid injections can provide significant relief. It is now known that epidural opioids can also provide some relief. The epidural space is the area over the outermost of the three membranes which cover your spinal cord. Medicines can be applied in this space to provide you with pain relief.

Research is also being done on epidural ketamine. Ketamine is a medication that can cause your brain to disassociate like LSD. A study has used epidural ketamine, and it has been shown to provide pain relief in individuals who have disc herniations or who have had back surgery, and this relief can last several months. The epidural space is the space that surrounds the fluid that surrounds your spinal cord. If you have had a back injury, you can have inflammation in your epidural space. Sometimes this inflammation can cause small scarring and you can develop what is caused epidural fibrosis. Epidural steroid injections can help with this type of pain syndrome. Your epidural space extends from your tailbone to the base of your skull.

A deposition of a drug into your epidural space is better than into your spinal fluid space because it eliminates the chance of you developing a spinal headache. The epidural steroid or the nonsteroidal anti-inflammatory drug will eventually reach your spinal cord. However, extremely small needles are available for spinal injection that should not cause you to have a headache. Other drugs besides the ones that we have already mentioned can also be placed into your epidural space.

Clonidine is an antihypertensive medication. This means that it can decrease your blood pressure. However, this medication can also be an effective analgesic administered into your epidural space. Sometimes Clonidine can be mixed with a narcotic medication such as morphine to provide you with significant pain relief. Clonidine can be helpful for the management of your pain associated with reflex sympathetic dystrophy. There is a chance that it can also help control pain associated with post-herpetic neuralgia in some patients as well.

Midazolam is a drug that will relax you during surgery. However, it has been shown to be effective for the management of some postoperative pain when administered epidurally as well. Further study is being done on this drug. You should be aware, however, that there was failure in animal pain models using epidural midazolam. The research on new drugs being used in the epidural space for the management of both your acute and chronic pain syndromes is exciting. However, to date there have been no gender-specific studies using any of these drugs including the Indomethacin.

Injections

As research in pain management continues into invasive pain medicine, more and more patients will eventually have injections of local anesthetics and steroids by specialists trained in pain medicine. Different sections throughout this book have mentioned various injections of local anesthetics. Epidural injections for chronic pain are being examined further to see if other drugs besides steroids can relieve your pain. There has been a recent publication that advocates the use of a nonsteroidal anti-inflammatory in place of a steroid for epidural steroid injection therapy in patients who have pain following back surgery. The results of this study were promising. Studies are being done using nonsteroidal anti-inflammatory medicines such as indomethacin for facet joint injection therapy.

We have known for a long time that the injection of a local anesthetic into a nerve or into the epidural space or spinal space following surgery can decrease pain for a duration. However, we now know that the duration of pain relief exceeds the duration of the local anesthetic. In 1990 a study was reported that was done on individuals who had neuralgia and had an injection of their nerves. The blocks did provide pain relief in patients in this study that lasted much longer than the duration of the numbing medicine.

Some individuals in the study had pain relief that lasted weeks to months. (J.D. Loeser. *Bonica's Management of Pain*. n.p.: Lippincott Williams and Wilkins, 2001)

Thermal Pain Management

You might benefit from two relatively new procedures that can be done for your back pain (performed by your pain-medicine doctor or your surgeon). Your disc has an outer layer called an annulus and an inner layer called a nucleus. If you have back pain caused by your discs in your lower back, you may be a candidate for either one of these procedures. If you have a bulging disc and back pain that did not respond to conservative therapy including medications, physical therapy, or epidural injections, you may be a candidate for an intra-discal electrothermal annuloplasty.

Your discs contain pain fibers in some areas of your disc that are capable of generating pain. These pain fibers are located in great numbers on the back lateral part of your discs. Pain originates from these pain fibers and is transmitted to your spinal cord. Sometimes you may have some tears in the outer ring of your discs. As a result, you can have leakage of material within your discs. The leakage of this substance can be acidic and irritate the nerves that are on the outside of your discs.

If you can imagine an old asphalt parking lot, it will have fissures in it. This same phenomena happens to your discs. When it leaks acidic material out of the disc space, it can cause you to have pain. This procedure is not indicated if you have back pain and pain running down your legs that is related to stenosis or if you have a large disc herniation with compression of your nerve. Using an x-ray, a needle is placed into your disc. After satisfactory placement of the needle is noted on your x-ray, a catheter is placed through the needle. The heating portion of the catheter is placed in the back part of your disc. The purpose of the procedure is to produce a high-enough temperature to produce thermal injury within the disc but at the same time avoid injury to your surrounding tissues. In other words, the pain-causing tissues in your disc need to be heated. You can have pain following the procedure that last three to seven days. This is normal. Your doctor will reassure you that following the procedure this pain is normal. Pain relief will begin gradually and will occur up to six weeks. After 8 to 12 weeks, you should begin a physical therapy back-stabilization program. If you do heavy lifting, you should not return back to work for 60 to 90 days. Otherwise, you should be able to return back to work in approximately 14 days.

You can also have placement of a thermal needle in the center of your disc. This procedure is called percutaneous intradiscal nucleoplasty. This procedure is a straightforward technique. If you have a disc protrusion as well as back pain and pain down one of your legs, you may be a candidate for this procedure. You must have failed conservative therapy as just mentioned. The thermal needle is placed into the nucleus of your disc. Following the procedure, you may feel some minor discomfort. More and more studies are being published demonstrating the efficacy and safety of the two thermal procedures just mentioned.

Gender specificity of these thermal procedures as well as the epidural medications including steroids and other steroid injections have not been defined at the present time.

Spinal Column Stimulator

Spinal cord stimulators have been around for the control of pain since the late 1960s. Improvements, however, have been made recently in spinal cord stimulators. The leads (soft catheters or wires that contain the electrodes which provide you with pain relief) have been designed so that the device can help you with your back pain. Previously the device was used for pain in your legs or arms. New technology has made multilead (more than one catheter placement) placement possible so that you can have multisite stimulation. By using dual stimulation, relief of your back pain is now possible.

The spinal cord stimulator modulates how many pain impulses can actually reach the brain. Your pain fibers terminate in an area in the back of your spinal cord called the dorsal horn. By causing vibration of the large fibers going into your spinal cord, the pain fibers are essentially turned off. Dorsal column stimulators stimulate large A-beta fibers. At first, the spinal cord stimulator was called a dorsal column stimulator because it was believed that the electrical activity in this area would block pain responses. However, now it is known that the electrical stimulation can occur anywhere in the spinal cord and the term dorsal column stimulator has been changed to spinal cord stimulation.

A computer program can turn your leads on and off or you can have the ability to control the dorsal column stimulator electrical activity by carrying a handheld device. If you have tingling, burning, shooting, and lightninglike pain, the dorsal column stimulator could provide you with relief. The device administers a small current of electricity toward the back of your spine. This is where the pain impulses come into your central nervous system.

Because the stimulators work in other areas besides the back of your spinal cord, the exact mechanism of how this device works is unknown. The device is also used now for vascular disease in extremities. In Europe this is the leading indication for a spinal cord stimulator. It can also be used if you have anginal (heart) pain that is refractory to other treatments. Before using this device, all other pain modalities must have been tried and failed. You should have had a psychological consultation before receiving a dorsal column stimulator.

If you have had damage to your nerves from surgery or reflex sympathetic dystrophy, the spinal cord stimulator could provide you with significant pain relief. It is not designed to completely relieve your pain. The goal of the dorsal column stimulator is to significantly decrease your pain and to decrease the amount of medications that you take to control your pain.

Before receiving a permanent dorsal column stimulator, a trial stimulator will be done. The device, which is essentially an epidural catheter with electrodes, will be paced into your epidural space under x-ray guidance. You use this catheter for three to five days. It is hooked to a battery pack that you can wear on your belt. You do have some control over the stimulator. If this device works for you, it will be removed and you will be scheduled for surgical implantation of the stimulator.

If you have reflex sympathetic dystrophy, have had back surgery that did not provide you relief, or have postherpetic neuralgia and phantom limb pain, the dorsal column stimulator could provide you with significant relief. If you have pain in your arms or legs related to a disc in your spine compressing on these nerves or if you have scar around your nerves from previous surgery, the dorsal column stimulator could provide you with some pain relief.

The "Pain Pump"

If you have cancer pain over your body, osteoporosis, head and neck pain, or pain related to multiple sclerosis, you would probably receive better pain relief with an implanted narcotic pump. Different types of narcotics can be used in the pump system. Narcotic medications do not have to be used exclusive in the pump.

Baclofen has been used for muscle spasms. However, there are some anecdotal reports that Baclofen can provide significant pain relief in place of narcotic medications. It was once thought that Baclofen was used for muscle spasms. Sometimes the Baclofen is mixed with the narcotic medications or can be used entirely by itself. Baclofen has been reported to be effective for the management of pain following back surgery. The reason for this finding is totally unknown. The drug does work on a receptor in your spinal cord called a Gabba B receptor. Investigators think that stimulation of this receptor could provide you with relief of your back pain when narcotic medications fail to do so. The narcotic drug-delivery system, like the spinal cord stimulator, has batteries. The batteries need to be replaced surgically periodically.

There is a spinal cord stimulator that attaches to an external battery. However, few patients elect this option. The advantage to the external battery for the spinal cord stimulator is that it does not have to be surgically replaced. Clonidine is another medication that can be placed into your drug-delivery system. This drug is still investigational for the use in this system. It has, however, been administered in the epidural space successfully, as mentioned previously. Clonidine is currently being studied for use in the pump as well as another drug called tizanidine. Dexmetomidine is also being studied.

No one knows what the long-term effects of these new drugs are when placed into an implanted spinal pump. Animal studies are being done to ensure that patients suffer no injury to the spinal cord from these drugs. The general consensus is unless you are sure that any of these drugs administered into your spinal canal are safe, you should avoid them. Drugs such as calcium channel blockers, tricyclic antidepressants, and two drugs called octreoitide and vapreotide are also being studied. These drugs may be used in the future for the management of your pain to be placed inside your drug-delivery system. These new non-narcotic spinal drugs are important alternatives for opioids for the treatment of chronic pain as well.

Other Drug Research

Current studies are being done to determine whether glucosamine and chondroitin sulfate are effective for the treatment of knee pain associated with osteoarthritis. These substances are sold in the United States as nutritional supplements. However, they have been widely touted by the lay press. A current study is being done to study the efficacy of these agents with respect to your knee pain caused by osteoarthritis.

Another medication that continues to be studied for the treatment of your osteoarthritis is hyaluronic acid. Injection of hyaluronic acid into your knee joint is done to improve the elasticity and viscosity of the fluid within your joint and to, therefore, decrease your pain. The Food and Drug Administration has approved a hyaluronic acid product for injection into your joint in 1997. Hyaluronic acid will improve the mechanical action of your knee joint as well as cause you to have improved lubrication of your joint. To date there are minimal adverse effects associated with this drug. Placebo studies have been done in Europe that demonstrated the beneficial effects of hyaluronic acid therapy. It is also believed that this drug can protect the cartilage in your joint from daily wear and tear.

Toxins from sea animals are being studied. Other types of man-made drugs are being studied as well. The research being done, in combination with the drugs that are currently being developed for placement into your spinal fluid, will eventually provide you with many treatment options which will make a significant difference in the management of your pain.

Further studies on other analgesics continue. It is known that bradykinin is a chemical that transmits pain and is formed when you injure your tissue. A bradykinin receptor antagonist is currently under development. Aprotinin is a drug that is being developed to possibly prevent acute inflammation. New COX-2 enzyme inhibitors are also being studied. Nimesulide is a COX-2-specific drug being developed that has a rapid onset of action. Neostigmine is a drug that is currently being investigated to be placed in your spinal fluid to control pain. Animal studies have demonstrated the efficacy of this drug. Some human studies are being done.

Another modality that is being studied is low-power laser stimulation to manage chronic pain. This modality has been found to be useful to threat pain associated with postherpetic neuralgia. Further studies are being done on other chronic pain syndromes.

Chapter 31

Changing the Perception of Pain Medicine

If you suffer chronic pain or if you are going to have surgery and expect to have acute postsurgical pain (as most of us do), you need to be educated with respect to what causes your pain before you have your surgery. For example, after gallbladder surgery, you can have pain with movement. If you expect pain with movement after surgery, you may avoid some anxiety when you actually experience movement pain. Presurgical postoperative pain education can inform you about what you can expect following surgery.

As always, it is important that you educate yourself about your type of pain. It is equally important to educate yourself about the health-care provider(s) you choose to help you manage your pain. This chapter will give you some ideas on how to find a well-trained pain management health-care provider. You will learn some tips on what questions to ask your health-care provider or their licensing authority before choosing one. It is important that you stay optimistic through the process of choosing a health-care provider to manage the treatment of your pain. In most cases, your pain can be adequately and appropriately diagnosed and treated by a specialist.

Finding a Well-Trained Pain Specialist

You should know that pain medicine as an entity is not a recognized medical specialty by the American Medical Association. An anesthesiologist, physical medicine rehabilitation specialist, neurologist, orthopedic surgeon, or neurosurgeon can all call themselves pain specialists, as can psychiatrists, psychologists, and chiropractors. Alternative medicine specialists, such as an acupuncturists, can call themselves pain-management practitioners, as well.

On the other hand, some practitioners have completed fellowships in pain medicine. These individuals have had comprehensive training at a medical center. These doctors have had training in reading your MRI, CT scan, and so on and training in how to decide whether a patient needs physical therapy, psychological evaluation, medications, or injections therapies to manage pain. The analogy between trained doctors who have done a fellowship versus an individual who has limited training in one field can be given by the example or by the following analogy: If Dr. A only has a hammer, everything appears to be a nail. If Dr. B only has a screwdriver, everything appears to be a screw. A fellowship-trained individual is one who has had special training in his or her specialty, whether it be anesthesiology, physical medicine, rehabilitation, or neurology. These specialty-trained individuals are equipped with the proper tools to treat you as a whole individual. This is not to say that the other individuals are not doing an adequate job for managing your pain. More training positions are being created for the study of pain medicine.

Selecting Your Specialist

Most pain complaints can be handled by one specialist. For example, if you have back pain, a chiropractor can usually manipulate you and satisfy your pain complaints. On the other hand, an anesthesiologist may think that you need a steroid injection into your spine. This method can also decrease your pain. A surgeon may think that your disc is causing problems and operate on you and again decrease your pain. However, some entities such as *reflex sympathetic dystrophy* are more complex and require the expertise of someone who has a more in-depth knowledge of your disease. This individual may be affiliated with a university pain-management program. Most anesthesiology departments at university medical centers throughout the country have comprehensive pain-medicine programs. This ensures you that you may be evaluated by a physical therapist, occupational therapist, or psychologist. These types of programs offer you multiple methods. The problem is that some insurance plans advise you to stay away from multidisciplinary pain centers because they can be expensive.

Before seeking medical care, decide what type of specialist you want to see. Your primary-care doctor can help you make a decision. Your primary-care doctor is trained to do some injections in the office and is trained to prescribe some pills. However, when it comes to prescribing narcotics, most state medical boards regulate the prescription practices of doctors prescribing opiates. The reason for this is that following the dispensing of opiates, there could be problems associated with these drugs. As a result, state medical boards have established guidelines for the prescribing practices of narcotic medications.

If you have been involved in a motor vehicle accident or have sustained a work-related injury, your case may end up before a court. When choosing your pain-management practitioner, you may want someone who not only can treat your pain but also who can be a witness for you in a court of law. No matter what type of individual you choose to manager your pain, remember that individual is ultimately being paid by you. Even if your insurance company is paying the individual, remember that you or your employer are the one who pays the insurance premiums. Because most chronic pain syndromes require long-term care with a health-care provider, you need to ask the health-care provider for a curriculum vitae. Ask other people who have seen that doctor or even other doctors for their opinion if you know of any. Because of current federal laws, your doctor will not be able to give you names of any of their patients.

A curriculum vitae will show you the qualifications of your potential health-care provider. Most individuals are proud of their accomplishments and will readily furnish you with a resumé or a curriculum vitae. If your potential health-care provider does not have this information readily available, you must ascertain the educational background of your health-care provider. You need to know what schools that individual has attended. You may want to know the major areas of study during college and the major areas of study during professional training. Most professional training schools offer elective courses throughout the other course of study. You need to know what areas of study the individual concentrated on. You may be going to a psychiatrist who took elective courses in pain medicine. If your pain is caused by a parasite, someone with extra training in this field may be able to provide you with a better understanding of your pain. This individual may have some extra knowledge that could be of benefit to the management of your pain.

You need to know what type of degree the individual obtained. This assumes that if your potential health-care provider is a member of a state professional society that that individual has completed essential study and examinations to allow him or her to practice. However, in some states where alternative medicine practices are established, such as aromatherapy, acupuncture, and reflexology, there are no state societies or examinations. However, some states do have societies for acupuncture practitioners as well as examinations and education requirements to become a licensed acupuncturist. You may have a plumber who also gives massage therapy outside of the plumbing profession. This individual may do an adequate job. However, a massage practitioner who does massage therapy on a daily basis may be better trained to help you if you have a certain pain injury or a certain area in your body where you have chronic pain. These are examples where training is helpful to you.

Checking a Health-Care Provider's Educational Background

Check with your state to see if there are educational requirements for a massage therapist. Massage therapy can be of extreme benefit to you, but it must be properly done for the treatment of muscle injury and so forth. You need to know what degree your pain practitioner obtained. Chiropractors, medical doctors, and doctors of osteopathy have to meet education requirements and take state examinations in order to be able to practice. You need to also know when your health-care practitioner attained his or her degree. Because pain-management methods are relatively new, individuals who obtained degrees before 1970 may not be adequately trained in pain management. However, individuals are expected to take yearly courses for continuing education in order for them to be updated on the latest methods available for their patients in their respective fields.

Your health-care provider should provide you with any additional courses attended as well as the dates. Some individuals have attended no additional courses. Some individuals have attended no additional courses for several years. However, most state medical boards now require individuals to meet continuing medical education courses to keep their licenses. Other health professions also have this continuing education rule. You need to know if your health-care provider has done a fellowship in pain medicine. This fact is important because remember that anyone can place a shingle outside of his or her office claiming a specialty in pain management.

Most individuals keep a list of the education courses that they have attended in the past 10 years. To be a member of an HMO or certain insurance plans, health-care providers must update their curriculum vitae each year (and submit it to the HMO or insurance company).

Your health-care provider should, therefore, have a curriculum vitae that lists what education courses he or she has taken in the past 10 years. You need to know if your health-care provider has been the subject of any disciplinary actions. Sometimes a health-care provider license will not be renewed for various reasons. A common reason is that the individual forgot to pay his or her dues. This is a much different disciplinary action than a disciplinary action for someone who has injured a patient because of medical negligence.

State medical boards can revoke a doctor's license if the doctor has been accused of improperly prescribing narcotic medications or other medications. For example, if your doctor has been accused of overprescribing narcotic medications to patients and if these patients have either died or have had to be admitted to hospitals, your doctor may not be allowed to practice. Some doctors are allowed to practice but are unable to prescribe narcotics or drugs such as Valium. If you have cancer pain, you will most likely need narcotic medication on occasion. You, therefore, should seek a health-care provider who has a license to prescribe a medication that you could potentially need. You need to know if your health-care provider has ever had his or her license suspended or revoked. A doctor may have practiced in another state, and lost his or her license there. Sometimes that individual will apply for a license in other states. If he or she is able to obtain a license, the doctor will move to that state. You, therefore, need to know if your health-care provider has ever had a suspended or revoked license anywhere. Some practitioners have been suspended from practicing because they were taking drugs. However, most individuals are able to return back to their respective health-care practice after going through a rehabilitation program. You should not hesitate asking what your health-care provider's grades were.

Choosing the Right Type of Health-Care Provider for Your Needs

You may have family or friends who have gone to a particular health-care provider, whether it was a chiropractor or doctor, who has significantly helped their pain. Remember that each individual has different reasons for their pain. For example, if you have read the chapter in this book on back pain, you realize that there are many causes for back pain. Your friend's chiropractor can provide significant relief for him or her if he or she has a misalignment of the spine. However, if you are suffering from osteoporosis and have a significant loss of bone density, chiropractic may not provide you with any relief. If you have significant osteoporosis, you may ultimately need care by a rheumatologist or an endocrinologist.

You may also have had a friend or relative who has had a headache and was treated by a psychologist. A psychologist can provide you with significant pain relief if you are suffering from a muscle tension-type headache. However, if you are suffering from a brain tumor, a psychologist will not help. For this reason, if you are not going to a multidisciplinary pain center, you must do your homework and choose the right individual for your particular need. A neurosurgeon is not needed for the management of your headache if you only have a psychological reason for your headache. Do research before deciding on your pain-care provider. In many instances, you will need a referral from your primary-care doctor to get an appointment with the appropriate specialist. Talk to your primary-care doctor and explain your needs and expectations.

In most phonebooks, you will notice advertisements for pain management. Health-care providers throughout the advertising section of a telephone book will tout their expertise in treating your pain. Chiropractors, podiatrists, anesthesiologists, neurologists, physical medicine and rehabilitation specialists, psychologists, and acupuncturists can all tell you that they will help you with your pain syndrome. The question remains, can they?

It is assumed that you will not buy a new or used vehicle without researching the pros and cons of purchasing that particular vehicle. You do this research because purchasing that vehicle can be expensive. However, you also need to realize that pain management can be expensive. Insurance plans cover only so many procedures and types of procedures. You need to know that not every procedure is covered under a particular insurance plan. Insurance companies usually only cover methods that have been demonstrated by evidence-based medicine to be reliable and therapeutic and not dangerous. You should talk to your customer service representative at your insurance company before choosing a pain-management provider.

If you choose the wrong health-care provider for your particular condition, you can spend enormous sums of money only to find out that you will experience no pain relief. The problem is that most individuals who experience severe pain are looking for some hope that they can escape this pain. If that individual just sees an ad where his or her pain will be totally relieved, he or she becomes excited and rushes to that health-care provider. However, if this happens to you and you have no pain relief, you can become depressed, anxious that your pain will continue, and you will lose faith in the health-care system. However, you need to realize that you are the one who made the decision to go to that health-care provider. If your attorney chose a health-care provider for you and if you are suffering a whiplash injury and if you feel over time that you have had multiple procedures, remember that you made the final choice to go to that health-care provider. The same reasoning occurs if you were injured on the job and you have been referred by your workmen's compensation insurance carrier to a health-care provider and if you have been returned to work without pain relief, remember that you made the final decision to go to that individual. You need to do your homework and choose a provider who has no bias in your particular pain syndrome. Ask your health-care provider if he or she is impartial. If you have been injured, ask your health-care provider how many times he has testified before the court for the defendant (the insurance company) or for the patient.

If you anticipate that you will go to court, you will want someone who has testified 50 percent for an insurance company and 50 percent for their patients. This information usually indicates to a jury or judge that your health-care provider is not biased. It may also indicate to you that you will not be undertreated or overtreated.

Because there are no real state or federal requirements for an individual to be a pain-management provider, you are ultimately responsible for choosing the correct individual. You will also need to know what books, articles, or journals are authoritative in their respective fields. The *Journal of the American Medical Association (JAMA)* or *The New England Journal of Medicine* are well-established and recognized journals in the field of medicine. There are also excellent pain-medicine textbooks. Usually a chapter in each of these books will be more authoritative than chapters in other books. A well-versed and trained pain health-care provider can refer you to these particular chapters, articles, or journals. You can obtain this information sometimes from a website or you can go to your local medical school library to retrieve this information.

Many health-care providers will scan pertinent information from journals or from textbooks onto their computer. This allows that health-care provider quick access to information that you as a patient may need. It is also important to know if your health-care provider did publish articles, book chapters, or reviews on certain pain conditions that you may be experiencing. More specifically, did your health-care provider research and do an article on your particular pain syndrome? It is important for you to know when and where this information is published so that you can obtain copies of these publications. If your health-care provider relates that he or she has written or contributed to publications, you need to know where these publications have been published. Some pain centers have their own publications, which are essentially advertising publications that they give to patients or referring doctors.

Articles published in *JAMA* or *The New England Journal of Medicine* have gone through scrutiny by professionals who are specialists in these particular fields. You can be assured that the information in any of the articles in these journals is correct. On the other hand, if your health-care provider has published a local advertisement in your newspaper, you may want to question the validity of any "breakthrough" discoveries that have been recently made by that particular health-care provider. Has your health-care provider discovered a revolutionary treatment for the management of your pain? If this revolutionary treatment addresses your particular pain syndrome, you may want to rush and make an appointment with that health-care provider. The advertisement can unfortunately give you false hope. Why is that revolutionary treatment not being done at one of the recognized medical centers or at your state university medical center? Why? The answer is that it probably is not a true revolutionary treatment. At major medical centers, any treatment has to go through committees that are composed of various scientists both clinical as well as laboratory based. A procedure that is to be tested has to first be approved by one of these committees. There will be controlled studies comparing the "revolutionary treatment" with a placebo to determine its benefit. In other words, a group of individuals will actually receive the treatment while another group will receive a sham treatment. If the "revolutionary treatment" is actually discovered, you will know about it through the news (either television or newspaper or through a magazine).

Advertisements are not the place to discover new revolutionary treatments. Remember that if this particular treatment was safe and efficacious, the local university pain center would be utilizing this procedure. If you are in doubt about the efficacy of a procedure, do not hesitate calling a university pain center to see whether anyone has heard of the procedure and if they recommend the procedure. You should begin to see that you are going to need to have some involvement in choosing the right caregiver for your particular pain syndrome. You should not be misled by false claims from sometimes unscrupulous practitioners. Unfortunately, health care is a business like any other business. This is the reason why you need to find a health-care practitioner who is knowledgeable as well as ethical.

You also need to know whether your health-care provider has obtained certifications, titles, or designations that in effect he or she purchased and did not truly earn. Unfortunately, health-care providers can attend no courses, take no tests, or obtain designations by being "grandfathered in." An unethical health-care provider will leave unearned credits off of their curriculum vitae. In other words, did your psychologist actually earn a doctorate in psychology or was it given to that individual for life experience? You need to know what professional organizations and societies that your health-care provider is a member of. You need to know what their status is in these organizations. If you are a cancer patient, for example, you may want to go to a health-care provider who is a member of the American Cancer Society.

You also need to know that if your health-care provider has a long and detailed curriculum vitae listing many affiliations, and you need to know if these affiliations are current. For example, if your health-care provider lists a certain membership in a pain-management society, you need to know if that membership is current. This will tell you whether your health-care provider is keeping up with new changes that are constantly occurring in the field of pain management. Hopefully, you are now beginning to see that if you do your homework, you will be able to obtain a pain-management practitioner who is right for your needs.

Pain Medicine as a Medical Specialty

You can see now that it is going to take some effort on your part. Hopefully, in the future, pain medicine will become a recognized specialty by the American Medical Association. It is also hoped that there will be more positions available for training individuals in the field of pain medicine. Currently doctors from each specialty associated with pain medicine, manage problems that fall within that individual specialty. The problem with pain syndromes is that most of them do not fall into categories that usually can be treated by one specialist. Patients who have complex pain problems such as cancer patients sometimes require the skills of several health-care providers to manage their pain. Pain-management techniques are now being taught in some medical schools. It is anticipated that this training will increase at least to where medical students can take an elective in pain medicine.

Hopefully some day pain medicine will become a separate specialty that is recognized as a true specialty by the American Medical Association. It is unreasonable to expect one individual to know and comprehend the entire range of knowledge associated with pain medicine without extra training in pain medicine. This is the reason why a multidisciplinary approach to pain management has evolved. This type of approach utilizes the expertise of various disciplines that are brought together in an effort to provide you with optimum pain-management care. The International Association for the Study of Pain (IASP) has defined a core curriculum that should be common in training programs where individuals are being trained in pain medicine. The core curriculum includes anatomy and physiology of pain conducting systems, pharmacology of the drugs used in pain medicine, basic knowledge of physical therapy, and psychological principles and knowledge in the treatment of AIDS, cancer, and other painful syndromes. Currently there is no true certification process for pain-management practitioners. Individuals can take certification in their respective specialties or professions. Anesthesiologists have their own boards as do neurologists, physical medicine and rehabilitation specialists, chiropractors, and in some states acupuncture practitioners. Some states do have certification exams for massage therapists.

As stated previously, it is hoped that the American Board of Medical Specialties (ABMS) will have a certification program eventually. An important organization in the United States, the American Academy of Pain Medicine has been pursuing this goal for some time. The American Board of Anesthesiology does have a subspecialty qualification in pain medicine. This consists of extra training in pain medicine as well as the completion of an examination. Because pain medicine is not a part of the American Board of Medical Specialties, there is no required training process for practitioners who practice pain management. There are hardly any guidelines for the background necessary for health-care providers to provide pain management. It is anticipated that in the future, health-care providers will need some training to call themselves pain-management caregivers. Psychologists, nurses, and physical and occupational therapists have had no true in-depth study of a pain curriculum. These deficiencies are being addressed with post-graduate training.

A society for pain nurses does sponsor continuing-education programs. The American Pain Society (APS) is a chapter of the International Association for the Study of Pain. Both the ISAP and APS have scientific meetings which combine both clinical and basic science topics. Another society, the American Academy of Pain Management, is an organization devoted to the treatment of pain. Members in this organization include not only doctors but also nurses, chiropractors, physical therapists, and other health-care providers who are interested in the science and treatment of various painful entities. This organization and the other organizations mentioned sponsor lectures in continuing-education courses for pain-management health-care providers. In many states, chiropractors, doctors, osteopaths, and nurses meet to discuss various pain issues that are important to the overall care of a pain patient.

There are also support groups for pain patients. The Internet will advise you of a pain support group in your area. These groups are usually aware of the most recent developments in pain management. Many times they will have speakers who are experts in their particular fields to discuss pain management issues and to answer any questions that you may have. You are encouraged to join one of these organizations if there is one available near you.

Do Your Homework: The Benefits of Self-Education

Now that you have some insight into practitioners of pain management, what about pills or procedures that are available for the management of your pain? Did you receive a flyer in your mailbox touting a new pill called Dr. Bill's back-pain-relieving pill? The ad said that Dr. Bill's pill relieved 80 percent of acute back pain. This sounds fairly impressive, doesn't it? However, if you are going to evaluate any method, especially new methods, you need to know how many patients the method was tested on.

In this case with Dr. Bill's pill, further research reveals that 4 out of 5 individuals (80 percent) had pain relief with this pill. A study that includes only five people is not sufficient to conclude any information. A study should include more than 100 patients. Sometimes a study population of 20 may reveal some interesting results. Remember that the higher the number of individuals that were included in the study, the more reliable the results will be. So let's say that Dr. Bill's pill company studied 100 patients that had back pain and they still reported that 80 percent of these individuals received significant pain relief over two weeks. Would you be inclined to purchase this pill? If so, why? If you do not want to purchase this pill, why not? Even though this new study includes 100 patients, there is one aspect of a scientific study that is missing.

Every scientific study should include a placebo control. This means that there should be a study of 100 individuals who received a sugar pill or equivalent. The results of further study revealed that 80 percent of individuals who took Dr. Bill's pill received pain relief over 2 weeks, whereas 80 percent of individuals who took the sugar pill received pain relief over 2 weeks. The results of this study should tell you that there is no medical difference between Dr. Bill's pill and the sugar pill. This should, furthermore, tell you that the back sprain resolves over two weeks with or without an analgesic. You do not have to have a strong background in statistical analysis to realize that the Dr. Bill's pill is a substance of probably no medical significance.

You must do your homework when evaluating any method for pain-relieving medicines and devices sold over the counter that range from scientific nonsense to fraud. Some companies will include testimonials from patients in their advertisements. There is no way of knowing whether these individuals actually exist. Testimonials can be a marketing tool not only for health-care products but for almost any type of product. Most of the time, you can take the testimonials that appear in advertisements with a grain of salt. If you are evaluating a medicine or a product, look for studies on the Internet or in your library that include the method being studied as compared to a placebo control. If Dr. Bill's pill provided 100 percent relief in 1,000 patients and the placebo provided 0 percent relief in 1,000 individuals, all who have had an acute back sprain, you can feel reasonably assured that Dr. Bill's pill may be of some benefit to you if you have had a recent back sprain.

Dr. Bill's pill essentially appeals to those individuals with no science background. Unfortunately, individuals who cannot afford a pain method suffer the most when they purchase a method that provides them with little or no pain relief.

Over a century ago in the United States, patent medicines were touted for the cures of every ailment of mankind and were marketed freely. Because of some instances of documented fraud associated with some of these medicines, passage of the 1906 Pure Food and Drugs Act was passed. This law prohibited false claims of a substance. However, there were no enforcement powers to correct misleading claims about a certain substance. The Food and Drug Administration (FDA) was formed in 1927. This agency prevented products from being sold, and the intent was to keep unsafe products off of the market.

Today the FDA requires drugs to be proven safe as well as effective before they can be sold. You need to know if Dr. Bill's pill is a medication or is it a natural dietary supplement. In the 1990s, the Dietary Supplement and Health Education Act of 1994 exempted natural dietary supplements from requirements for testing as required by the FDA. Now the FDA can only take a dietary supplement off the market if it can demonstrate that it's harmful. The FDA is currently doing animal studies on ephedrine. Dietary supplements cannot be promoted as preventing or treating disease. The Federal Trade Commission (FTC) can regulate advertising. However, it is difficult prosecuting testimonials from individuals about a certain product.

If Dr. Bill's pills make blatant, false claims about the pill, the FTC can review these claims as well. You need to know that over any given time, you will probably recover without any sort of intervention. Essentially our bodies have the ability to heal themselves. The problem is that usually before the natural course of the disease has run, there is some intervening method or person who takes credit for your healing. When this happens, we all have a tendency to believe that the healing was the work of a healer. You need to determine whether your healing was the result of a causal relationship between a method and your illness or was it a casual relationship between your body and your illness.

For thousands of years, fraudulent healers have relied on placebos to cure illnesses. In the first part of the twentieth century, doctors usually only had laxatives and aspirin. Some doctors carried placebo pills. In a significant number of individuals, the placebo pills appeared to cure pain and some illnesses. An example of placebo healing involved Franz Mesmer. Franz Mesmer in 1778 would treat patients with magnetic wands as well as magnetic water. The patients would sit in a circle in a vat filled with water that he relayed was magnetized. Magnetized rods were in the vat and held by each patient. Then Franz Mesmer would wave magnetic wands over each patient. Some individuals got relief of their pain as well as relief of their illness with the magnetic baths and the waving of magnetic wands. A scientific study followed Franz Mesmer's claims. (R.L. Park. *Voodoo Science: The Road from Foolishness to Science*. n.p.: Oxford University Press, 2001) The results of the scientific study proved that Mesmer's treatments were due solely to the power of suggestion that he imparted to each one of his patients. It is of interest that magnets have returned to modern alternative medicine as a cure for some pains and as a cure for some diseases. However, there have been some medical school studies using a placebo control indicating that magnets can provide pain relief of some painful conditions. If you are going to purchase magnets, which can be relatively expensive, research the effects of magnets on your particular pain syndrome before buying them.

You can go to many websites to find the information that you need, and a common one is the National Institutes of Health website. This website can give you some insight into conventional or alternative medicine therapies. Remember, if you do not have a computer and you want to research a certain drug or method, you can go to your local library, which most probably will have a computer that you can use for research. Be aware that in 1992 the Office of Alternative Medicine (OAM) at NIH was created. The OAM can report what alternative therapies work and which do not. Be aware that just because a substance is "natural" does not mean it is safe.

For example, ephedra is popular in the United States as a weight-loss aid. The ephedra contains ephedrine, which can increase your heart rate as well as your blood pressure. This increase in heart rate and blood pressure can stress your heart and could cause you to have a heart attack. If your blood pressure becomes too high, you could suffer a stroke from this natural substance. Some people only use "natural" substances as a treatment for their illnesses, whereas others demand the latest in medical technology. It is up to you to decide which type of medicine you think is best for your needs.

If you do your homework, you will find that some alternative therapies can be extremely beneficial to you, whereas some conventional medical remedies can also provide you with significant relief. To know which remedy is the best for you, you need to research each method and ask your pharmacist as well as your primary-care doctor or chiropractor what remedy is the best for you. If you do your homework and research the anatomical area where your pain exists and develop an understanding of what is causing your pain, you will eventually realize that in most instances you do not suffer from a dreaded disease.

If you research the treatments that have been prescribed for you, you can communicate better with your health-care provider as to whether these methods are actually providing you with relief or if they are causing you untoward side effects.

Stay Optimistic

It is important for you to realize that in most instances that your pain can be adequately diagnosed and treated. It is important for you to remain optimistic and it is equally important for you to recognize that you can take control of your pain by developing a pain partnership with your doctor.

When you understand that your chronic pain syndrome can be taken care of by both you and your health-care provider, your body can then release substances such as endorphins to help provide you with pain relief. If you are not optimistic that your pain syndrome can be controlled, stress hormones can be released into your bloodstream that can increase not only your blood pressure and heart rate but also your breathing rate. The problem is that stress can actually impede recovery of any injury that you may have sustained and, therefore, impede your pain relief. Therefore, we recommend that you stay optimistic and control your pain syndrome and not let your pain syndrome control you.

Appendix
Glossary

acquired immune deficiency syndrome (AIDS) A disease of the immune system caused by the HIV virus.

acupuncture A practice that involves inserting fine needles into your body at specific points that have been found to be effective in the treatment of specific health problems.

agonist A chemical substance capable of combining with a receptor on a cell and initiating a reaction or activity.

alcoholic neuropathy Any neuropathy that can be caused by excessive alcohol consumption.

allopathy *See* conventional medicine.

alternative medicine Practices and products that are not currently considered to be part of conventional medicine.

angina Pain in the chest caused by spasm of the arteries of the heart.

ankylosing spondylitis A chronic disease that affects the joints and muscles of the back and may lead to stiffness.

antagonist A chemical that acts within the body to reduce the physiological activity of another chemical substance (as an opiate); especially one that opposes the action on the nervous system of a drug or a substance occurring naturally in the body by combining with and blocking its nervous receptor.

anticonvulsant A medication used to control seizures; sometimes used for pain control.

antidepressant A large class of medications used to treat depression and some peripheral neuropathies.

antispasmodic drug A medication used to decrease spasm of the smooth muscles, including the gastrointestinal tract.

arthritis An inflammatory disease of the joints.

carpal tunnel syndrome Compression of your median nerve in your carpal tunnel is a common compression neuropathy.

causalgia Pain that usually occurs following an injury that included nerve damage.

central nervous system Your brain and spinal cord.

chemical neuropathy Any neuropathy caused by excessive chemical exposure.

chiropractic therapy Therapy that includes manipulating the bones and joints to relieve pain.

complementary medicine Practices and products that are not currently considered to be part of conventional medicine.

complex regional pain syndrome Pain that usually occurs following an injury.

conventional medicine Medicine that is practiced by individuals who have a medical doctor degree (M.D.) or a doctor of osteopathy degree (D.O.); also includes methods practiced by allied health-care professionals such as physical therapists, occupational therapists, psychologists, and registered nurses.

conversion disorder A psychiatric disorder in which emotional distress is expressed through physical symptoms such as pain.

Crohn's disease Inflammation of the gastrointestinal system.

dermatomyositis Inflammation of the muscles.

diabetic neuropathy Any neuropathy that can be caused by diabetes, typically to the hands and feet.

endorphins Naturally occurring molecules made up of amino acids. Endorphins attach to special receptors in the brain and spinal cord to stop pain messages.

fascial pain Neuralgia pain in areas of the face.

fibromyalgia A pain disorder characterized by pain in many locations throughout the body that seem to have no cause.

gout A joint disease caused by the deposition of uric acid crystals in the joints or in the joint space.

growth hormone The hormone responsible for growth.

headache Any pain associated with the head, particularly inside the head.

hemophilia A disorder of your blood's ability to form a clot.

homeopath A specialist that prescribes dilutions of natural substances from plants, minerals, and animals.

human immunodeficiency virus (HIV) A virus that infects certain white blood cells and can eventually lead to AIDS.

hypochondriasis A belief that real or imagined physical symptoms are signs of a serious illness, despite medical reassurance and other evidence to the contrary.

idiopathic There is no defined cause for your pain.

irritable bowel syndrome (IBS) A disorder that interferes with the normal functions of the large intestine (colon). It is characterized by a group of symptoms (crampy abdominal pain, bloating, constipation, and diarrhea).

mainstream medicine *See* conventional medicine.

modulation When a pain impulse reaches your spinal cord and the pain is lessened.

mononeuropathy Only one nerve is affected by a disease state.

muscle relaxant A medication that is used to relax the muscles.

myeloma A cancerous formation of your plasma cells.

myocardial infarction Death of a segment of heart muscle that occurs following interruption of the blood supply to the heart muscle; also known as a heart attack.

myofascial pain A soft tissue disorder that can cause pain and other disabling effects.

narcotic A certain class of drugs that act more in the central nervous system to control pain.

naturopath A specialist that treats disease by using your body's natural ability to heal itself.

neuritis An inflammation of the nerve.

neuroma A cancer of the nerve.

neuropathy Any disease of your peripheral nerves.

neurotransmitters Chemicals stored close to your nerve endings.

nociception The perception of actual physical pain.

norepinepherine One of many neurotransmitters found in the brain.

nutritional neuropathy Any neuropathy caused by nutrient deficiency.

opioid A centrally acting pain medicine.

orthodox medicine *See* conventional medicine.

osteoarthritis Arthritis of the bones and joints.

osteoporosis A disease that causes a reduction and breakdown in the minerals and structural components of bone.

periosteum A wrapper around your bone that contains many small nerves.

peripheral nervous system All the nerves that are not the brain and spinal cord; includes the nerves of the arms, legs, hands, and feet.

placebo-controlled study A placebo-controlled study means that one group in a study receives a sugar pill while the other group receives the study drug. In theory, the group receiving the drug should get better relief than the sugar pill group.

polyarteritis nodosa Inflammation of the walls of the blood vessels.

polyneuropathy When more than one nerve is affected by a disease state.

postherpetic neuralgia Chronic pain syndrome that occurs following the onset of shingles.

prostaglandins Chemical messengers involved in reproduction and inflammatory response.

psychogenic pain disorder Real physical pain caused by a psychological problem.

referred pain Pain that is felt in a place other than where it originates.

reflex sympathetic dystrophy (RSD) *See* complex regional pain syndrome.

Raynaud's disease or phenomenon A burning sensation, typically of the hands, characterized by a tricolor change when going into the cold.

scleroderma A connective tissue disorder characterized by thickening of the skin, hardening of the arteries, and Raynaud's phenomenon.

scoliosis An excessive curvature of the spine.

serotonin-specific reuptake inhibitor A class of medication that selective inhibits the reuptake of serotonin in the central nervous system.

serotonin One of many neurotransmitters found in the brain.

shingles Painful disease caused by the varicella zoster virus.

sprain A stretching or tearing of ligaments.

steroid Steroid medications are chemically similar to some of your body's own hormones and duplicate their actions.

strain A stretching or tearing of muscles.

substance P A neurotransmitter chemical that can cause pain.

sympathetic nervous system The sympathetic nerves control circulation and perspiration and are part of your autonomic nervous system.

synovial tissue Tissue surrounding the joint.

temporal arteritis Inflammation of the large arteries around the temples of the head.

temporomandibular jaw pain (TMJ) Pain in the jaw joint that is formed by your lower jaw and your temporal bone.

thoracic outlet syndrome Pain that results when spinal cord nerves are compressed as they pass between your neck and shoulders.

Transcutaneous Electrical Nerve Stimulator (TENS) unit A method of pain control that uses electrodes applied to your skin to pass an electric current through your muscles.

transdermal Through the skin.

transduction Chemical substances that make your nerves more sensitive to pain.

transmission When pain impulses from injured tissue flow to the junction at your spinal cord and are then transmitted to the back of your spinal cord.

tricyclic antidepressant A type of medication that interferes with certain chemical processes in your brain that cause you to feel pain.

trigeminal neuralgia Pain located in your face caused by the trigeminal nerve.

uremic neuropathy Any neuropathy caused by excessive amounts of urea and other nitrogen waste compounds in the bloodstream.

vasculitis Inflammation of the blood vessels.

vasospastic disease Diseases of the blood vessels; pain is caused when blood vessels constrict and limit flow of blood.

varicella zoster virus The virus responsible for causing chicken pox and shingles.

whiplash A sudden acceleration/deceleration of your neck that results in a lashlike effect.

Index

A

abdominal pains, 251-253
  Crohn's disease, 249-251
  inflammatory bowel diseases, 248-249
  irritable bowel syndrome (IBS), 241-248
  treatment, 253-256
Achilles tendons, sports-related pain, 403-404
acquired immune deficiency syndrome. *See* AIDS
acupuncture, 88, 126-128, 431
adjuvant drugs, 34-42
agonist, opioid drugs, 54
AIDS (acquired immune deficiency syndrome), 337
  causes of pain, 343-345
  gender differences, 347
  high-risk groups, 341-343
  HIV virus, 340-341
  infection risks, 345-347
  research, 348-350
  treatment, 350-351
  understanding, 337-339
alcoholic neuropathies, 221
allopathy, conventional healthcare, 79
Allopurinol, gout, 207
Alpha delta fibers, 13
alternative medicines, 80-88
alternative therapies, 115-128, 382
amino acid, N-acetylcysteine, 85
amitriptyline (Elavil), 33, 96
analgesics, topical, 89-91, 439
  nonprescription creams, 92-94
  prescription creams, 94-96
  skin patch, 96-100
anatomy, drug absorption differences, 6-7
angina, 305
  characterization, 308-311
  diagnosis, 311-314
  injuries to heart muscle, 305-307
  pectoris, 306
  research, 315-316
  treatment, 317-320
  versus cardiac syndrome X, 314-315
ankylosing spondylitis, 204-205
annulus, 132
antagonist, opioid drugs, 54
anti-inflammatory medications
  alternative medicines, 84
  cayenne, 85
  NSAIDs, 67-78
anticonvulsant medications, 36-38, 299, 418-419
antidepressants, 2, 8
antioxidants, 85-86
antiseizure medications, 418-419
antispasmodic drugs, 38-42
anxieties, psychology, 21-23
Aprotinin, 439
aromatherapy therapy, 126
arrhythmia, 306
Arsenic, chemical neuropathy, 223
arthritis
  ankylosing spondylitis, 204-205
  association with Raynaud's disease, 366
  COX-2 inhibitors, 72
  doctor diagnosis, 196-198

gout, 205-207
joint tissue attack, 195-196
osteoarthritis, 198-202
rheumatoid, 202-204
treatment, 208
atypical antidepressants, 35-36
auras, migraine headaches, 183
autoimmune disease, osteoporosis, 228

B

back pains
aging, 157
causes, 145-148
muscle tension, 154-155
osteoarthritis, 153-154
osteoporosis, 154
physical therapy, 111-114
posture, 155-157
research, 158-160
spasms, 154-155
spine, 148-153
spondylolisthesis, 157-158
thermal pain management, 435-436
treatment, 160-162
Baclofen (Lioresal), 39
bamboo spines, 204
benzenesulfonic acid derivatives, 70
Bextra, 68-70, 77
biofeedback, 30-31
bones
cancer treatment, 424-425
osteoporosis, 225-240
spondylolisthesis, 157-158
whiplash, 171
bowel obstruction, 252
bradykinin, 13
brain
responses to pain, 12-15
whiplash injuries, 171-172
breast cancer, 410-411
bursitis, 396
Butorphanol (Stadol nasal spray), 56

C

C fibers, 13
Calcitonin, osteoporosis prevention, 236
cancers
COX-2 inhibitors, 72
reproductive system, 409-427
stomach, 252
cannabinoids, 87
capsaicin, nonprescription topical analgesics, 92-93
carbamazepine (Tegretol), 36
carboxylic acids, 70
cardiac syndrome X *versus* angina pain, 314-315
carisoprodol (Soma), 40
carpal tunnel syndrome, 209, 214-219, 367
causalgia, 322
cayenne, 85
Celebrex, 68-70, 77
central nervous system
differences, 3
irritable bowel syndrome (IBS), 242
opioid drugs, function, 54-56
cervical cancer, 411-413
chemical neuropathies, 223-224
chest pains, angina, 305-320
chlorzoxazone (Paraflex), 40
chondroitin sulfate, knee pain, 439
Cisplatin, chemical neuropathy, 223
clonazepam (Klonopin), 36
Clonidine patch, 100
cluster headaches, 186-187
coccyx, 148
Codeine, migraine headaches, 184
Colchicine, gout, 207
cold packs, physical therapy, 109
cold therapies, 120-122
collateral circulation, 306
complex regional pain syndromes, 321-336
compression fractures, 171, 231-232
compression neuropathies, 213
computerized tomography scan (CT scan), 132

connective tissue diseases, 361
contraceptives, medication absorption, 9
conventional healthcare, 79
conversion disorders, 25
creams, topical analgesics, 90-96
Crohn's disease, 249-251
cryotherapy, 120
CT scan (computerized tomography scan), 132
cyclobenzaprine (Flexeril), 40
cyclooxygenase chemicals, 69
cytokine inhibitors, 86

D

Dantrium (Dantrolene), 39
Darvocet, migraine headaches, 184
Darvon (propoxyphene), 54, 70
degenerative joint disease, 198-202
Demerol (Meperidine), 55
density, bones
  hormones, 232-233
  osteoporosis, 226-227
Depakote (valproic acid), 36
dermatomyositis, association with Raynaud's disease, 366
Desyrel (Trazodone), 35
diabetic neuropathies, 218-221
diagnosis
  arthritis, 196-198
  breast cancer, 410
  chest pains, 311-314
  facial pain, 301-302
  fibromylagia, 258-260
  irritable bowel syndrome (IBS), 243
  myofascial pain, 275-278
  osteoporosis, 229-230
  ovarian cancer, 414
  prostate cancer, 415
  Raynaud's disease, 367-368
  reflex sympathetic dystrophy (RSD), 326-330
  temporal mandibular joint disorder (TMJ), 294-296
  uterine cancer, 413
  whiplash, 174
diathermia, 122
Diflunisal (Dolobid), 76
Dilantin (phenytoin), 36
discography, 150
discs
  back pains, 149-151
  neck injuries, 133-134
  temporal mandibular joint disorder (TMJ), 293-294
  thermal pain management, 435-436
  whiplash, 169-170
Dolobid (Diflunisal), 76
drugs
  absorption differences, 6-7
  abuse, 57, 64-65
  addiction, 57, 65-66
  adjuvant, 33-42
  dependence, 57
  dosage, age effects, 9
  NSAIDs, 67-78
  opioids, 53-66, 431-432
  research, 439
  response differences, 7-9
Duragesic (fentanyl), 55
dysmenorrhea, COX-2 inhibitors, 71

E

Effexor (venlafaxine), 35
Elavil (amitriptyline), 33
elbows, tendonitis, 396-398
electric therapy, 122-123
electrical stimulation, shingles, 389
EMLA cream, prescription topical analgesics, 94-95
emotional disorders, 25-27
endometriosis, 251
endorphins, 16, 124, 261
enolic acids, 70
epidurals
  drug research, 433-434
  reproductive system cancers, 421-422
equianalgesic doses, 424

escitalopram oxlate (Lexapro), 35
estrogens, osteoporosis, 235-236

F

facet joints, 130, 169
facial pains, 289-304
fentanyl (Duragesic), 55
fentanyl lozenge (Actuic), 56
Fentanyl patch, 97-98, 423
fibromyalgia, 257-258
  COX-2-inhibiting NSAIDs, 72
  diagnosis, 258-260
  hormones, 261-263
  muscle pain, 260-261
  research, 263-264
  treatment, 264-271
  versus myofascial pain, 281-283
Flexeril (cyclobenzaprine), 40
fluoxetine (Prozac), 34
fluvoxamine (Luvox), 35
fractures, 227-232

G

GABA (gamma aminobutyric acid), 17
gabapentin (Neurontin), 36
gallbladder, inflamation, 251
gamma aminobutyric acid (GABA), 17
gastritis, NSAIDs, 74
gastrointestinal pains, 251-253
  Crohn's disease, 249-251
  inflammatory bowel diseases, 248-249
  irritable bowel syndrome (IBS), 241-248
  treatment, 253-256
gels, topical analgesics, 90-91
genetics, 17
ginseng, 84
glucosamine, knee pain, 439
gouty arthritis, 205-207

H

head trauma headaches, 188
headaches
  cluster, 186-187
  common types, 179-181
  gender differences, 190-192
  head trauma, 188
  migraines, 182-185
  pain source, 189
  physical therapy, 109-111
  research, 189-190
  temporal arthritis, 188-189
  tension, 185-186
  treatment, 193-194
  whiplash, 171-172
heart, 305-320
heliocobacter pylori, 252
hemophilia, 360
hepatitis, 251
herbal medicines, 84
herbs, nonprescription topical analgesics, 93
herpes zoster, 381
hip fractures, 235
histamines, 86
HIV (human immunodeficiency virus), 337
  causes of pain, 343-345
  gender differences, 347
  high-risk groups, 341-343
  infection risks, 345-347
  osteoporosis, 229
  research, 348-350
  treatment, 350-351
  understanding, 337-339
  virus, 340-341
homeopathic medicines, 82-83
hormones
  affect drug absorption, 7-9
  differences, 2-3
  fibromyalgia, 261-263
  headaches, 191
  osteoporosis, 230-233
  response to pain, 16-17
  temporal mandibular joint disorder (TMJ), 297-298
hot packs, physical therapy, 109
hot therapies, 120-122
human immunodeficiency virus. *See* HIV

hyaluronic acid, osteoarthritis, 439
hydrocodone, 58
hydrocolator packs, 120
hydromorphone, 423
hydroxytryptophan, 86
hyperparathyroidism, osteoporosis, 228
hyperthyroidism, osteoporosis, 228
hypnosis, 31-32
hypochondriasis, 25

I

IBS (irritable bowel syndrome), 241-248
idiopathic osteoporosis, 228
illicit drugs, 64-65
immune system, AIDS
  causes of pain, 343-345
  gender differences, 347
  high-risk groups, 341-343
  HIV, 340-341
  infection risks, 345-347
  research, 348-350
  treatment, 350-351
  understanding, 337-339
indomethacin, 70
inflammatory bowel diseases, 248-249
inhibitors, prostaglandins, 69-70
inhibitory system impairment, temporal mandibular joint disorder (TMJ), 294
injections, 422-423, 434-435
injuries, neck, 132-140
intercostal nerves, 387
interstitial cystitis, 251
intestinal pains, 251-253
  Crohn's disease, 249-251
  inflammatory bowel diseases, 248-249
  irritable bowel syndrome (IBS), 241-248
  treatment, 253-256
intradiscal electrothermal annuloplasty, 435
intramuscular injections, narcotics, 422
intravenous injection, narcotics, 423
iontophoresis, 123
ipriflavone, 86
irritable bowel syndrome (IBS), 241-248
ischemic pains, 260
Isonizid, nerve pain, 212

J-K

joints
  pain, COX-2-inhibiting NSAIDs, 72
  sports-related pain, 405
  tissues, arthritis, 195-196
  whiplash, 169-170

ketamine, prescription topical analgesics, 96
Ketorolac, 76
ketolorac, 70
kidneys
  NSAIDs, 75
  stones, 251-252
  uremic neuropathy, 222
Klonopin (clonazepam), 36
knees
  drug research, 439
  sports-related pain, 398-400

L

labor, NSAIDs, 72
Lamictal (lamotrigine), 36
lamotrigine (Lamictal), 36
Lexapro (escitalopram oxlate), 35
lidocaine, prescription topical analgesics, 96
Lidoderm patch, 98-100
Lioresal (Baclofen), 39
liver, NSAIDs, 75
lupus, osteoporosis, 228
Luvox (fluvoxamine), 35

M

magnetic resonance imaging (MRI), 132
malingering, 25

MAOIs (monoamine oxidase inhibitors), 34
medications
  absorption differences, 6-7
  adjuvant
    anticonvulsant, 36-38
    atypical antidepressant, 35-36
    MAOIs, 34
    muscle relaxants, 38-42
    SSRIs, 34-35
    tricyclic antidepressants, 33-34
  dosage, age effects, 9
  education, 441-455
  herb, 84
  opioid drugs, 53-58
  response differences, 7-9
  whiplash, 175-177
menstruation
  headaches, 192
  medication absorption, 8
  NSAIDS, 73-74
menthol, 93-95
Meperidine (Demerol), 55
metaxalone (Skelaxin), 40
methadone, 55
methocarbamol (Robaxin), 40
methyl salicylate, prescription topical analgesics, 95
migraines, 182
  causes, 182-183
  NSAIDs, 72
  prevention, 183-184
  stress, 184-185
  treatment, 183-184
  women, 185
mixed agonist/antagonist, opioid drugs, 54
modulation, 13
monoamine oxidase inhibitors (MAOIs), 34
mononeuropathies, 209
morphine, 53, 423
  effects, 56
  prescription topical analgesics, 96
  sublingual, 422
MRI (magnetic resonance imaging), 132
multiple myeloma, 360-361
muscles
  back pains, 154-155
  fibromyalgia, 260-261
  myofascial pain, 273-287
  neck injuries, 137-138
  overuse injuries, muscle relaxants, 41-42
  sports-related pain, 396
  relaxants, 38-42
  whiplash, 170
myeloma, 214, 360-361
myocardial infarction (heart attack), 306
myofascial pain, 273
  characterization, 273-275
  diagnosis, 275-278
  latent trigger points, 280-281
  sports-related, 394
  treatment, 283-287
  trigger points, 278-280
  versus fibromyalgia, 281-283

N

N-acetylcysteine, 85
nalbuphine (Nubain), 56
Nalfon, 76
naproxen, 70, 76
naturopathic medicines, 83-84
neck pains
  anatomy, 129-132
  gender differences, 140-142
  injuries, 132-140
  physical therapy, 111
  prevention, 142-143
  treatment, 143-144
  whiplash, 163-178
nerves
  fibers, 13-14
  neck injuries, 135-137
  peripheral neuropathies
    alcoholic, 221
    carpal tunnel syndrome, 214-218
    characterization, 210-214

chemical, 223-224
diabetic neuropathy, 218-221
nutritional, 222-223
treatment, 224
uremic, 222
shingles, blocking injections, 387-389
nervous systems, complex regional pain syndromes, 321-322
diagnosis, 326-330
phases, 330-331
research, 331-334
sympathetic nervous system, 322-325
treatment, 334-336
neurolitic blocks, shingles, 389-390
Neurontin (gabapentin), 36
neuropathies
drug research, 432-433
peripheral
alcoholic, 221
carpal tunnel syndrome, 214-218
characterization, 210-214
chemical, 223-224
diabetic neuropathy, 218-221
nutritional, 222-223
treatment, 224
uremic, 222
neurotransmitters, 13
niacin deficiencies, pellegra neuropathies, 223
nonpain fibers, 14
NSAIDs (nonsteroidal anti-inflammatory drugs), 67, 95-96, 419
Nubain (nalbuphine), 56
nutrition, shingles, 390
nutritional neuropathies, 222-223

O

ointments, topical analgesics, 90
omega-3 fatty acids, 85
opioid drugs, 53
addictions, 58-65
combined with tricyclic antidepressants, 34
function, 54-56
headaches, 192
morphine effects, 56
research, 431-432
treatment, 57-58
oral medications
contraceptives, absorption, 9
narcotics, 422
shingles, 385-387
oral transmucosal fentanyl, 423
orthodox medicines, 79
osteoarthritis, 153-154, 198-202
COX-2-inhibiting NSAIDs, 72
pain differences, 9
osteoporosis, 154, 225
bone density, hormones, 232-233
characterization, 226-231
compression fractures, 231-232
men, 233
prevention, 234-236
research, 236-238
treatment, 238-240
ovarian cancer, 414-415
Oxycontin, 57
oxymorphone, 423

P

Pap smears, cervical cancer, 412
Paraflex (chlorzoxazone), 40
parasites, 252
Pasteur, Louis, vaccines, 339
patches
fentanyl, 423
topical analgesics, 91, 96-100
patient-control analgesia (PCA), 423
Paxil (piroxitine), 35
PCA (patient-control analgesia), 423
pellegra neuropathies, 223
percutaneous intradiscal nucleoplasty, 436
periosteum, 179, 394
peripheral nervous system, 12-14
inflammation, 393
irritable bowel syndrome (IBS), 242
opioid drugs, 54

peripheral neuropathies
  alcoholic, 221
  carpal tunnel syndrome, 214-218
  characterization, 210-214
  chemical, 223-224
  diabetic neuropathy, 218-221
  nutritional, 222-223
  treatment, 224
  uremic, 222
PET scan (Positron Emission Tomography scan), 16
phenytoin (Dilantin), 36
phonophoresis, 122
physical exercises, sports-related pain, 393
  achilles tendon, 403-404
  ankle, 400-403
  gender differences, 406-407
  injuries, 393-396
  joints, 405
  knees, 398-400
  prevention, 405
  tendonitis, 396-398
  treatment, 408
physical therapies, 101-114, 387
piroxitine (Paxil), 35
pneumonia, 252
polyarteritis nodosa, association with Raynaud's disease, 366
polyneuropathies, 209
poplar tree bark, nonprescription topical analgesics, 93-94
Positron Emission Tomography scan (PET scan), 16
post-traumatic headaches, 188
posterior longitudinal ligaments, 129
premenopause, medication absorption, 8
procyanidolic oligomers, 86
progesterone therapies, osteoporosis prevention, 234
prognosis, whiplash, 173-177
propoxyphene (Darvon), 54, 70
prostaglandins, 13, 69-70, 86
prostate cancer, 415-416
Prozac (fluoxetine), 34
psuedoaddictions, 61
psychogenic pain, 25
psychological dependences, 57
psychological testing, irritable bowel syndrome (IBS), 244-245
psychology
  anxiety, 21-23
  gender differences, 20-21
  pain assessment, 51-52
  pain perception, 19-20
  psychologists, 32
  reproductive system cancer, 417-418
  thresholds, 23-27
  tolerances, 23-27
  treatment methods, 27-32
pulposus, 132
pumps, narcotics, 438

Q-R

raloxifene, osteoporosis prevention, 234
Raynaud's disease, 353
  associated diseases, 364-367
  diagnosis, 367-368
  research, 368
  treatment, 368-371
  types, 356-357
receptors, opioid drugs, 54
rectal suppositories, narcotics, 423
referred pain, 14-15, 131
reflex points, 124
reflex sympathetic dystrophy (RSD), 321-322
  diagnosis, 326-330
  phases, 330-331
  research, 331-334
  sympathetic nervous system, 322-325
  treatment, 334-336
reflexology therapy, 124-125
relaxation, 30-31
renal failure, uremic neuropathy, 222
renal stones, 251

repetitive-motions
carpal tunnel syndrome, 214
vibration trauma, 361-362
reproductive system, cancer, 409-427
research, 429
acupuncture therapy, 431
AIDS, 348-350
angina pain, 315-316
back pains, 158-160
chiropractic therapy, 430-431
drugs, 439
epidural drugs, 433-434
fibromyalgia, 263-264
headaches, 189-190
injections, 434-435
narcotic pumps, 438
nasal anesthetics, 431
neuropathy drugs, 432-433
opioids, 431-432
osteoporosis, 236-238
Raynaud's disease, 368
spinal cord stimulators, 436-437
thermal pain management, 435-436
understanding pain, 4-6
responses to pain, 12-17
rheumatoid arthritis, 72, 202-204
risks, NSAIDs, 74-77
Robaxin (methocarbamol), 40
RSD (reflex sympathetic dystrophy), 321-322
diagnosis, 326-330
phases, 330-331
research, 331-334
sympathetic nervous system, 322-325
treatment, 334-336

S

sacroiliac joints, back pains, 151-152
sacrum, 148
scars, 396
sciatica, back pains, 151
scleroderma, association with Raynaud's disease, 364-365
selective serotonin reuptake inhibitors (SSRIs), 34-35
serotonin, 15-16, 261
serotonin-specific reuptake inhibitors (SSRIs), female reactions, 2
sertraline (Zoloft), 35
shingles, 373
associated pain, 377-381
treatment, 381
alternative therapies, 382
assessing pain, 381-382
electrical stimulation, 389
geriatric patients, 383
men, 390-391
narcotic pump, 390
nerve block injections, 387-389
neurolitic blocks, 389-390
nutrition, 390
oral medications, 385-387
physical therapies, 387
topical analgesics, 384-385
women, 391
varicella zoster virus, 373-376
sickle cell disease, 359-360
Skelaxin (metaxalone), 40
skin, topical analgesics
function, 89-91
nonprescription creams, 92-94
patch, 91, 96-100
prescription creams, 94-96
social issues, affect on pain perception, 4
Soma (carisoprodol), 40
somataform disorder, 25
somatization disorder, 25
spasms, back pains, 154-155
spinal cords
neck injuries, 135-137
stimulator improvements, 436-437
spine
anatomy, 129-132
back pain, 148-153
spinous processes, whiplash, 169
spondylolisthesis, back pains, 157-158

sports
- massages, 125
- medicines, chiropractors, 116
- pain, 393
  - *achilles tendon, 403-404*
  - *ankle, 400-403*
  - *gender differences, 406-407*
  - *injuries, 393-396*
  - *joints, 405*
  - *knees, 398-400*
  - *prevention, 405*
  - *tendonitis, 396-398*
  - *treatment, 408*

sprains, whiplash, 170
SSRIs (selective serotonin reuptake inhibitors), 2, 34-35
Stadol nasal spray (Butorphanol), 56
stepladder, cancer pain, 426
steroids
- gout, 207
- osteoporosis, 234
- prescription topical analgesics, 95

stomach-related pains, 251-253
- Crohn's disease, 249-251
- inflammatory bowel diseases, 248-249
- irritable bowel syndrome (IBS), 241-248
- treatment, 253-256

stress
- migraine headaches, 184-185
- temporal mandibular joint disorder (TMJ), 294

studies, 429
- acupuncture therapy, 431
- chiropractic therapy, 430-431
- drugs, 439
- epidural drugs, 433-434
- injections, 434-435
- muscle relaxants, 42
- narcotic pumps, 438
- nasal anesthetics, 431
- neuropathy drugs, 432-433
- opioids, 431-432
- spinal cord stimulators, 436-437
- thermal pain management, 435-436
- understanding pain, 4-6

sublingual morphine, 422
substance P inhibitors, 86, 261
Sumatriptan, migraine headaches, 184
superficial pain, 120
supplements, gaining support, 81-82
sympathetic nervous system, 322-325
synovium, 195
synthetic estrogen, osteoporosis prevention, 234

T

Tegretol (carbamazepine), 36
temporal arthritis headaches, 188-189
temporal mandibular joint disorder (TMJ), 16, 289-290
- abnormal mouth bite, 292-293
- characterization, 290-291
- diagnosis, 294-296
- gender differences, 296-297
- hormones, 297-298
- inhibitory system impairment, 294
- nervous habits, 293
- psychological causes, 291-292
- stress, 294
- worn discs, 293-294

tendonitis (tennis elbow), 396-398
tendons, 395
tennis elbow (tendonitis), 396-398
TENS (transcutaneous electrical nerve stimulator), 123, 387
tension headaches, 185-186
Thallium, chemical neuropathy, 223
thenol group, NSAIDs, 70
therapies
- acupuncture, scientific research, 431
- alternative, 115-122
- chiropractic, scientific research, 430-431
- physical
  - *differing regimens, 106-108*
  - *exercises, 108-114*
  - *expectations, 101-102*

first therapist appointment, 102-105
shingles, 387
team member, 105-106
thermal pain management, 435-436
thiamine deficiencies, nutritional neuropathies, 222-223
thoracic outlet syndrome, association with Raynaud's disease, 367
thresholds, 23-27
tic douloureux (trigeminal neuralgia), 298-299
Tizanidine (Zanaflex), 39
TMJ (temporal mandibular joint disorder), 16, 172, 289-290
abnormal mouth bite, 292-293
characterization, 290-291
diagnosis, 294-296
gender differences, 296-297
hormones, 297-298
inhibitory system impairment, 294
nervous habits, 293
psychological causes, 291-292
stress, 294
worn discs, 293-294
tolerances, 23-24, 57
behavioral medicine specialist, 24-25
emotional disorders, 25-27
Topamax (topiramate), 37
tophi, 207
topical analgesics
function, 89-91
nonprescription creams, 92-94
prescription creams, 94-96
shingles, 384-385
skin patch, 96-100
topiramate (Topamax), 37
traction therapy, 124
Tramadol (Ultram), 56
transcutaneous electrical nerve stimulator (TENS), 123, 387
transdermal patches, 91, 96
Clonidine patch, 100
Fentanyl patch, 97-98
Lidoderm patch, 98-100
shingles, 384
transduction, 13
transmission, 13-15
Trazodone (Desyrel), 35
treatments
AIDS, 350-351
angina pain, 317-320
arthritis, 208
back pains, 160-162
bones, cancer, 424-425
breast cancer, 411
cancer, 412-416
carpal tunnel syndrome, 216-217
chiropractors, 119-120
facial pains, 302-304
fibromyalgia, 264-271
headaches, 193-194
irritable bowel syndrome (IBS), 245-247
migraine headache, 183-184
myofascial pain, 283-287
neck pains, 143-144
NSAIDs, 67
differing responses, 77-78
functions, 67-74
risks, 74-77
opioid drugs, 57-58
osteoporosis, 238-240
peripheral neuropathy, 224
psychology, 27-32
Raynaud's disease, 368-371
reflex sympathetic dystrophy (RSD), 334-336
reproductive system cancers, 417
administering narcotics, 422-424
anticonvulsant medications, 418-419
antiseizure medications, 418-419
bone treatment, 424-425
communicating pain, 425
epidural injections, 421-422
men, 427
narcotic effects, 419-421
nonsteroidal anti-inflammatory medications, 419
pain diary, 426
psychological problems, 417-418

stepladder for pain, 426
women, 427
shingles, 381
alternative therapies, 382
assessing pain, 381-382
electrical stimulation, 389
geriatric patients, 383
men, 390-391
narcotic pump, 390
nerve block injections, 387-389
neurolitic blocks, 389-390
nutrition, 390
oral medications, 385-387
physical therapies, 387
topical analgesics, 384-385
women, 391
sports-related pain, 408
stomach-related pains, 253-256
whiplash, 177-178
trials, 429
acupuncture therapy, 431
alternative medicines, 82
chiropractic therapy, 430-431
drugs, 439
epidural drugs, 433-434
injections, 434-435
narcotic pumps, 438
nasal anesthetics, 431
neuropathy drugs, 432-433
opioids, 431-432
spinal cord stimulators, 436-437
thermal pain management, 435-436
tricyclic antidepressants, 33-34
trigeminal neuralgia (tic douloureux), 298-299
trigger points, myofascial pain, 278-281
triptans, migraine headaches, 184

U

ulcers, 74, 251
Ultram (Tramadol), 56
ultrasound heat, 122
ultraviolet lights, 120
unconventional healthcare. *See* alternative therapies
uremic neuropathies, 222
urinary tract infections, 252
uterine cancer, 413-414

V

vaccines, 339-340
Valium, 39
valproic acid (Depakote), 36
varicella zoster virus, 373-376
vascular diseases
causes, 357
cold temperatures, 358-359
connective tissue disease, 361
hemophilia, 360
multiple myeloma, 360-361
risks, 362-364
sickle cell disease, 359-360
vibration trauma, 361-362
characterization, 353-356
Raynaud's disease, 353-371
vasculitis, association with Raynaud's disease, 365
venlafaxine (Effexor), 35
vibration trauma, 361-362
Vioxx, 68-70, 77
viruses
AIDS, 337-351
shingles, 373
vaccines, 339-340

W

weaknesses, whiplash, 172-173
whiplash, 163-178
whirlpool baths, 120

X-Y-Z

Zanaflex (Tizanidine), 39
Zoloft (sertraline), 35